patient care skills

FOURTH EDITION

Mary Alice Duesterhaus Minor, MS, PT
Program Director
Physical Therapist Assistant Program
Sanford-Brown College
St. Louis, Missouri

Scott Duesterhaus Minor, PhD, PT
Program in Physical Therapy
Washington University School of Medicine
St. Louis, Missouri

Photography by Robert Morrison

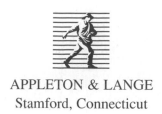

APPLETON & LANGE
Stamford, Connecticut

Copyright © 1999 by Appleton & Lange
A Simon & Schuster Company
Copyright © 1995, 1991, and 1987 by Appleton & Lange
Copyright © 1982 by Reston Publishing Company, Inc.

www.appletonlange.com

99 00 01 02 03 / 10 9 8 7 6 5 4 3 2 1

Prentice Hall International (UK) Limited, *London*
Prentice Hall of Australia Pty. Limited, *Sydney*
Prentice Hall Canada, Inc., *Toronto*
Prentice Hall Hispanoamericana, S.A., *Mexico*
Prentice Hall of India Private Limited, *New Delhi*
Prentice Hall of Japan, Inc., *Tokyo*
Simon & Schuster Asia Pte. Ltd., *Singapore*
Editora Prentice Hall do Brasil Ltda., *Rio de Janeiro*
Prentice Hall, *Upper Saddle River, New Jersey*

Library of Congress Cataloging-in-Publication Data

Minor, Mary Alice D., 1944–
    Patient care skills / Mary A. Duesterhaus Minor, Scott Duesterhaus
Minor ; photography by Robert Morrison. — 4th ed.
        p.   cm.
    Includes bibliographical references and index.
    ISBN 0-8385-8157-9 (pbk. : alk. paper)
    1. Transport of sick and wounded—Handbooks, manuals, etc.
2. Patients—Positioning—Handbooks, manuals, etc.   3. Nursing—
Handbooks, manuals, etc.   I. Minor, Scott Duesterhaus.   II. Title.
    [DNLM: 1. Physical Therapy—methods.   2. Nursing Care—methods.
3. Transportation of Patients—methods.   4. Asepsis—methods.
5. Orthopedic Equipment.   WB 460M666p 1999]
RT87.T72M56   1999
610.73—dc21
DNLM/DLC
for Library of Congress   98-25824

Acquisitions Editor: Lin Marshall
Production Service: Jennsin Services
Designer: JoEllen Ackerman
        Mary Skudlarek
Cover Designer: Mary Skudlarek

0-8385-8157-9

90000

9 780838 581575

PRINTED IN THE UNITED STATES OF AMERICA

*This book is dedicated to
better care for all patients.*

Contents

Preface . . . . *ix*

Acknowledgments . . . . *xi*

Chapter 1   Documentation 1
          Purpose 2
  1.1   Formats of Medical Records 2
  1.2   Methods 3
  1.3   Audit 8
  1.4   Review Questions 8
  1.5   Suggested Activities 9
  1.6   Appendix A 10
  1.7   References 10

Chapter 2   Preparation for Patient Care 11
          Introduction 12
  2.1   Management of the Environment 12
  2.2   Body Mechanics 13
  2.3   Instructions and Verbal Commands 14
  2.4   Patient Preparation 15
  2.5   Transporting 16
  2.6   Wheelchair Wheelies 28
  2.7   Elevators 30
  2.8   Review Questions 31
  2.9   Suggested Activities 31

Chapter 3   Vital Signs 33
          Introduction 34
  3.1   Heart Rate 34
  3.2   Blood Pressure 39
  3.3   Respiration 42
  3.4   Temperature 44
  3.5   Review Questions 47
  3.6   Suggested Activities 47
  3.7   References 48

Chapter 4   Aseptic Techniques **49**
                Introduction. 50
        4.1   Definitions 50
        4.2   Universal Precautions. 52
        4.3   Sterile Field 52
        4.4   Apparel 55
        4.5   Handwashing 56
        4.6   Procedures. 58
        4.7   Wound Dressings 76
        4.8   Cleansing and Sterilizing 84
        4.9   Waste Disposal 89
        4.10   Laundry 91
        4.11   Housekeeping 92
        4.12   Isolation 93
        4.13   Alternative Systems for Isolation Precautions 101
        4.14   Review Questions 113
        4.15   Suggested Activities 113
        4.16   References 114

Chapter 5   Turning and Positioning **115**
                Introduction. 116
        5.1   General Procedures. 117
        5.2   Supine Position 118
        5.3   Turning from Supine to Prone 118
        5.4   Prone Position 122
        5.5   Turning from Prone to Supine 123
        5.6   Turning on the Floor Mat 126
        5.7   Turning from Supine to Sidelying 127
        5.8   Sidelying Position 128
        5.9   Assuming Sitting. 129
        5.10   Review Questions 132
        5.11   Suggested Activities 132
                Case Studies. 132

Chapter 6   Range-of-Motion Exercise. **133**
                Introduction. 134
        6.1   Method. 135
        6.2   Anatomical Planes of Motion. 136
        6.3   Diagonal Patterns of Motion 138
        6.4   Lower Extremity 140
        6.5   Upper Extremity 160
        6.6   Head, Neck, and Trunk 187
        6.7   Review Questions 190
        6.8   Suggested Activities 190
                Case Studies. 191
        6.9   References 191

Chapter 7   Wheelchairs. **193**
                Introduction. 194
        7.1   Wheelchair Brakes. 195
        7.2   Seat Belts 198
        7.3   Caster Wheels 198
        7.4   Drive (Push) Wheels 199
        7.5   Armrests 200

7.6   Front Rigging. 201
7.7   Antitipping Devices 206
7.8   Folding Wheelchairs 207
7.9   Specialized Wheelchairs 208
7.10   Measuring to Determine Wheelchair Size 217
7.11   Standard Wheelchair Measurements. 222
7.12   Review Questions 223
7.13   Suggested Activities 224
       Case Studies. 224

Chapter 8   Transfers 225
       Introduction. 226
8.1   Sliding Transfer—Cart to Treatment Table 228
8.2   Three-Person Carry. 230
8.3   Hydraulic Lift 233
8.4   Two-Person Lift 242
8.5   Dependent Standing Pivot 246
8.6   Sliding Board 248
8.7   Push-Up 250
8.8   Assist to Front Edge of Chair. 252
8.9   Assist to Sitting on Treatment Table 256
8.10   Assisted Standing Pivot 257
8.11   Dependent One-Person Transfer—
       Floor to Wheelchair. 267
8.12   Independent Transfer from Wheelchair
       to Floor and Return. 270
8.13   Review Questions 284
8.14   Suggested Activities 285
       Case Studies. 285

Chapter 9   Ambulation With Assistive Devices 287
       Introduction. 288
9.1   Teaching Tips. 288
9.2   Choosing an Assistive Device 290
9.3   Choosing a Gait Pattern 298
9.4   Guarding 301
9.5   Assumption of Standing and Sitting. 306
9.6   Ascending and Descending Stairs. 308
9.7   Curbs 309
9.8   Moving through Doorways 309
9.9   Tilt Table 310
9.10   Walkers. 313
9.11   Axillary Crutches 344
9.12   Forearm (Lofstrand) Crutches 374
9.13   One Cane 404
9.14   Two Canes 437
9.15   Review Questions 462
9.16   Suggested Activities 463
       Case Studies. 463

Chapter 10   Americans With Disabilities Act 465
       Introduction. 466
10.1   Background 466
10.2   Resources. 467

10.3 General Considerations 468
10.4 Specific Requirements. 468
10.5 Review Questions 493
10.6 Suggested Activities 494
10.7 References 494

Index *495*

Preface

We feel fortunate for the continued acceptance of this text. We hope to meet the responsibility of this faith in our efforts by the addition of new elements in this fourth edition that build on the strengths of the previous three editions.

This manual serves as an introduction to basic procedures of patient care by providing both a written explanation and visual guide for performance. The procedures presented are safe and effective patient care techniques. Each of the procedures presented has alternative methods of performance. Many of the alternatives are presented to provide a spectrum of instruction and practice. The methods included are chosen for their applicability to a variety of patients and situations.

We have benefitted from continued critical commentary and counsel from students and colleagues who have used previous editions of this manual. In response to this feedback, this fourth edition has been enhanced by the addition of:

- *Learner Objectives* (LO)
- *LO* icons linked to text
- *Highlight* boxes
- *Suggested Activities*
- *Case Studies*
- Numbered illustrations

The numbered *Learner Objectives* at the beginning of each chapter serve as a guide to material included within a chapter and as goals to be achieved by studying each chapter. *Learner Objectives* are connected to chapter content by a series of numbered *lightbulb* symbols, indicating which *Learner Objectives* are associated with specific text. *Highlight* boxes provide a brief summary of important concepts in the text and are a guide to finding the full text pertaining to important concepts.

LO-1

HIGHLIGHT BOXES

Brief summaries of important concepts

A large number of procedures and variations are included in this manual, although it is not all inclusive. When choosing from among alternative methods or procedures, the most important consideration is to use the safest and most beneficial method for the patient and therapist. In some cases, this will require modification of previously learned procedures. In all cases, practice will develop safe and efficient performance.

We have found that when teaching these procedures, students can learn both the specifics of the procedures as well as general rules of good body mechanics, patient handling, and safety for patients and therapists. Students may require assistance in problem solving when applying procedures in a variety of patient care situations. To assist student learning and problem solving skills, *Suggested Activities* and *Case Studies* have been included in this edition.

Each chapter and major section is introduced by a general explanation of the basis for performing the procedures to be described and by a presentation of general rules or guidelines that are generic to a series of procedures. Individual rules for specific procedures are associated with each procedure presented. For each procedure presented, numbered step-by-step illustrations are accompanied by brief verbal explanations. By following the sequence of illustrations for a specific procedure, the necessity of extensive text explanations is decreased. This provides students with a visual reference to determine if the steps of the sequence they are performing match the sequence of steps presented. Each chapter concludes with a series of review questions that provide students an opportunity to test newly acquired knowledge. The review questions can also be used as a study guide by reviewing the questions before beginning study of a chapter.

Finally, we wish to comment on the terms "patient" and "therapist." We have used the term "patient" throughout the text to designate the individual receiving care. This term has been used for its general sense of meaning for consistency throughout the text. We have used the term "therapist" throughout the text to designate the individual providing care. This does not mean that only physical therapists can, or will, perform these tasks. We expect that many health care providers, including home health aides, medical assistants, nurses, nurses' aides, nursing home attendants, occupational therapists, occupational therapy assistants, orderlies, and physical therapist assistants, will perform these tasks. Therefore, we hope this manual will be useful to the many people receiving, and practitioners providing, care.

Mary Alice Duesterhaus Minor
Scott Duesterhaus Minor
St. Louis, 1998

Acknowledgments

It is unimaginable to us that any author could create a text and then perform all the additional tasks required to transform the text into a book and place it before the public. With this in mind, we wish to acknowledge those who have contributed significantly to this manual.

We first thank Robert Morrison, photographer, for the photographic illustrations on which this book depends. We are grateful to Bob for the critical eye, suggestions, and attention to detail he brought to his work. It was a pleasure to work with him. We also wish to thank Winifred Anglin, illustrator in Medical Illustration, Washington University School of Medicine, for the graphic illustrations.

We are especially appreciative for the patience and understanding of our daughter Sarah during this project.

To Deborah Bosse, Jeffrey Bosse, Bettina Brown, Suzanne Cornbleet, Kathleen Dixon, Mustafa Koluman, Janice Loudon, Sarah Minor, and Michael Mueller, we offer thanks and appreciation for their participation in photography sessions.

We are grateful to Tamara Versluis for her assistance and suggestions.

We extend our thanks to Arnie Berger of Clasen Home Health Care, St. Louis, for arranging the loan of patient care equipment, and to Clasen Home Health Care for providing the equipment.

We wish to express our appreciation to the Program in Physical Therapy, Washington University School of Medicine, St. Louis, for the use of facilities and equipment for photographic sessions.

We must acknowledge our appreciation to Appleton & Lange personnel who have provided support and assistance. We are grateful to Linda L. Marshall, Editor, and Lisa Guidone, Production Editor, for their guidance and efforts on this fourth edition. We also want to thank the following reviewers: Anne Bello, PTA, MS, Southwestern Community College; Jonathan T. Spry, PT, California State University, Fresno; Susan Flanagan, MHS, PT, Northern Virginia Community College; and Marlene Medin, PT, Linn State Technical College.

Finally, to acknowledge that this is the fourth edition of a successful book, we wish to remember those who contributed to the first three editions. For their work on the first two editions, we thank Jim York, Mary Edna Harrell, Freda Bowden, Marvin Levand, Jennifer McFarland, Gary Bergner, and Julie Leidecker. We thank Cheryl L. Mehalik, Editor-in-Chief, and Sondra Greenfield, Production Editor, for their contributions to the third edition. For their contributions of facilities and equipment we acknowledge Wichita State University, Maryville University, and Washington University.

Documentation

Learner Objectives

The student will be able to:

1 List the purposes of documentation in the health care system.
2 Describe the two formats of medical records
3 Describe the procedures involved in the POMR system.
4 Describe the sections of the SOAP note format.
5 Discuss the requirements of proper goal statements.
6 Discuss the requirements of adequate documentation.
7 List the information provided by a medical records audit.

PURPOSE

There are many aspects of patient care, and a large number of professionals involved in the care of each patient. Coordination of these aspects and professionals requires a high level of communication among all concerned. **Documentation** that is precise and concise is essential in providing the level of communication required, and is thus an essential function of health care professionals.

LO-1

A patient's chart serves as the single repository of pertinent facts concerning the patient's history, illness(es), and treatment. The primary role of adequate documentation by all medical and health care professionals is to enhance communication for medical and legal purposes. Because of its role, any event or action must be documented, and is deemed to have occurred only if documented in the patient's chart.

The most important rationale for appropriate documentation is to provide the highest possible level of patient care at all times. With proper documentation, those involved with providing care for the patient and support for the patient's family will know

> **PURPOSES**
>
> Communication
> Legal record
> Highest level of care
> Research
> Audit
> Reimbursement

1. What has been determined about the patient's condition based upon interviews and tests
2. The specific medical problems identified
3. The goals of treatment
4. Treatment strategies employed
5. The patient's response to treatment
6. The rationale on which goals and treatment are based

Proper documentation provides a valid basis for research. Without proper documentation, initial patient status may not be known, subsequent patient progress may be difficult to monitor, coordination of patient care may be lost, quality assurance reviews cannot be performed adequately, and reimbursement by third-party payers will be compromised.

LO-2

1.1   Formats of Medical Records

There are two major formats of medical records, the **source-oriented method** and the **problem-oriented medical record method** (POMR). Ideally, all departments within a facility should use the same method of record keeping. This simplifies the process of communication between professionals in different departments. Even if all departments within a facility do not use the same method of record keeping, an individual department can implement the POMR.

In the source-oriented method, a chart is divided into sections for each health care provider working with a patient by profession (ie, MD, nursing, PT, etc.). Each professional discipline provides its documentation in a separate section of the patient's chart. The source-oriented system segregates patient information by professional discipline. The ability to identify patient problems and focus treatment resources on the specific needs of a patient is decreased in this format. Documentation of the flow of patient care among professions, and the interaction of professional interventions for the benefit of the patient is lost when using the source-oriented format in medical charts.

> **FORMATS**
>
> Source oriented
> Problem oriented

The **problem-oriented medical record (POMR) system**, introduced by Lawrence Weed,[1] is designed to facilitate care provided to patients by organizing each medical record in a standard format. Since its introduction, the concept of the POMR has been favorably received and put into use in medical schools, hospitals, and rehabilitation settings.[2-4]

The POMR is comprised of a

1. Database
2. Problem list
3. Initial, progress or interim, and discharge notes

The **database**contains subjective and objective information, including medical, family, and social history, and medical examination and test results. The **problem list** is a list of the patient's problems that are identified from the information contained in the database. Problems may be identified from the information contained in the database. Problems may be identified by any professional discipline providing patient care, and may be listed as a(n) abnormal test result, chief complaint, diagnosis, physical finding, physiological finding, or symptom. Notes are a sequential record of decisions, actions, and events describing the course of a patient's treatment by all involved professionals. An **initial note** presents the initial findings and plan of treatment. **Progress (interim) notes present the progression of treatment, the effects of treatment, and changes in the plan of treatment. A** discharge note presents the status of the patient's problems and the current course of treatment at the time of patient discharge.

Proper application of the POMR system provides a medical record for each patient that clearly delineates the

1. Patient's medical history
2. Medical findings of signs, symptoms, and tests
3. Patient's problems, based upon an evaluation of signs, symptoms, and test results
4. Goals of treatment
5. Methods of treatment
6. Patient's response to treatment

When the POMR system is fully implemented, an audit process for peer review and outcome assessment is included. The results of audits indicate areas of strengths and weaknesses in patient care rendered, thus indicating areas for the improvement of patient care.

1.2   METHODS

Procedure

Upon admission or referral, a database is initiated. The database includes identifying information, medical complaints voiced by the patient (symptoms), a brief medical history, and a short review of all physiological systems (signs). The information elicited from this review provides the basis for the initial problem list, determining which health care providers need to be involved in this patient's care, and which systems require more extensive medical review. The problem list is placed in one specific place in a chart, making it readily available to all personnel when needed.

Each problem is assigned a number and title, and is listed with the date the problem was identified when it is entered on the problem list. Subheadings under a general problem may be used to provide more specific delin-

LO-3

PROBLEM LIST

Numbered
Titled
Dated

eation within a major problem. Problems are often clustered under major categories: medical, psychological, and socioeconomic. Any problem may be considered active, resolved, or inactive. A problem is considered resolved when it has been resolved by medical care, or has been resolved of its own accord. A problem is considered inactive when the condition continues to exist, but is not a focus of treatment at this time. When a problem is considered resolved or inactivated, the date on which this occurred is entered on the problem list. In this way, the sequence of medical history for each patient may be maintained in an organized manner.

A **medical team** is comprised of all medical professionals participating in the care of an individual patient. Membership of a medical team will change as a patient's medical, psychological, and socioeconomic needs change. A **case manager** may be any member of the medical team designated to be responsible for the overall organization of care for an individual patient. In many cases, this role is assumed by the patient's primary physician. Any member of the medical team, however, may identify a problem. Depending on procedure in individual facilities, the team member identifying the problem, or the case manager, may enter a newly identified problem on the problem list, or such entries may be made during team conferences. When a problem is resolved or inactivated, the date on which this occurred is entered on the problem list. Again, this entry may be made by an individual team member, case manager, or during a team conference, depending upon facility procedure.

LO-2

NOTE FORMAT

Narrative
SOAP note

Note Format

There are two major formats for writing notes, the **narrative format** and the **SOAP note format**. In the narrative format, statements concerning the patient are written in narrative form. Such notes may or may not have subheadings to organize information. The organization and flow of information within notes written by different personnel vary, making it difficult to identify where or how specific information is contained within the medical record.

The SOAP note format, which may be used in different approaches to medical records, is the usual format used for medical chart notes written by health care providers using the POMR system. SOAP is an acronym that alludes to the section headings.—**Subjective, Objective, Assessment**, and **Plan**—of a SOAP note. In some facilities, the SOAP note format is used without also using the database and problem list sections of the POMR system.

LO-4

SUBJECTIVE

Patient and family
reports

S denotes **subjective data**. Although verifiable, the initial brief identifying data is provided as the first sentence(s) in this section as an introduction to the patient. Relevant data concerning the patient's history that is not verifiable in medical records is considered subjective data. The patient's description of functional problems, pain, and the date of onset are also included as subjective data. Complaints reported by the patient and family are considered to be subjective data, and are classified as symptoms. The patient's goals of treatment are considered to be subjective data, and are included in this section. An example of the Subjective section of a note for a patient with a recently healed fracture is

Subjective

This 43-year-old black female automotive assembly line worker was seen in physical therapy clinic today for the first time. Patient is 8 weeks post fracture L olecranon process and 10 days post cast removal. Patient's chief complaint is inability to use left arm for activities of daily living and for work. Patient's goal is to return to previous job.

O denotes **objective data**. Data that is verifiable from medical records is considered objective data. Evaluation and treatment results documented by health care providers are also included as objective data. Observations by health care personnel and test results are considered objective data and are considered signs. An example of the Objective section of a note for a patient with a recently healed fracture is

	OBJECTIVE
	Verifiable from records
	Observed by you

Objective

Active ROM:	L elbow ext—flex	15–110°
Passive ROM:	L elbow ext—flex	10–115°
Strength:	L elbow ext	3/5
	L elbow flex	3+/5
	L supination	3+/5
	L pronation	3+/5
	L wrist (all)	4/5
	L hand (all)	4/5
	L shoulder (all)	5/5

Pain: L elbow 2/10 in dependent position with no motion
L elbow 4/10 during passive ROM.
L elbow 5/10 during active flexion, supination, pronation.
L elbow 7/10 during active extension.

A denotes **assessment or analysis** by the health care professional of the data included in the Subjective and Objective sections. A list of the patient's problems, identified from the Subjective and Objective information, is included in this section. Information contained in this portion of a note may include professional opinion concerning the patient's problems, and a discussion of reasoning used as the basis of the plan of treatment. Hypotheses concerning patient problems listed in the assessment section are thus documented by available data, and presented for review by all members of the medical team.

ASSESSMENT
Interpretation of the "S' and "O'
Includes goals

Goals of treatment are also included in the assessment section. **Goals** are statements of expected patient capabilities at the end of treatment, when the treatment is successful. These statements of expected outcome are based on the results of the patient evaluation, and are written in terms that describe observable and measurable patient behaviors. Goal statements describe what the patient will be able to do. They should be specific, objective, measurable, and related to function. They do **not** describe what the therapist will do to the patient, or the treatment to be used with the patient.

Long-term goals (LTG) are statements describing functional capabilities the patient will have at the end of treatment. **Short-term goals (STG)** are more discrete activities the patient will have to be able to perform to achieve the functional activities stated as long-term goals. There should be a clear progression of goals, indicating that successful achievement of short-term goals provide the basis for successful attainment of long-term goals.

CLINICAL NOTE:
LTG: Final Outcomes
STG: Building Blocks

The goal statement must be complete to be useful. The nemonic ABCDFT[5] can be used to ensure the inclusion of all components of a goal. The first component of a goal statement indicates the audience, "A." The audience of a goal is the patient. A goal is about how the patient will perform, not what the therapist will do. The second component of a goal is the behavior, "B," a patient will exhibit. Ambulation or dressing are examples of behavior. Behavior is described in observable and measurable terms, which are the conditions, "C." Conditions are distance, use of a type of assistive device, speed of performance, or other achievements that the patient will demonstrate. The degree, "D," is how often the patient is expected to perform the behavior under the described conditions. When no specific degree is stated, the patient is expected to perform the behavior under the stated conditions 100% of the time the behavior is required. Longterm goals are statements of functional behavior. In short-term goals, behaviors may not be functional behaviors. An example, a short term goal may be related to obtaining ROM or strength. In the STG, a functional behavior, "F," or the behavior a patient will ultimately perform when the STGs have all been achieved, should be included to inform others why the described behavior is important. The last component of the goal is the time line, "T." Each goal needs to include an indication of how long it will take the patient to achieve the goal. The time can be stated in terms of number of treatments or days.

An example of the assessment section of a note for a patient with a recently healed fracture is

Assessment

- Problem 1—Decreased ROM L elbow
- Problem 2—Decreased strength L elbow and wrist
- Problem 3—Pain L elbow

Problems 1 through 3 result of recent fracture L olecranon process and casting of L upper extremity.

LTG: The patient will be able to use L arm for washing, dressing, and combing hair.
Patient will be able to perform previous job as automotive assembly line worker.
STG: The patient will have a 5–110 degrees range of motion in L elbow.
The patient will have 4/5 muscle strength in all major muscle groups of the L upper extremity to perform job skills in 2 weeks.
The patient will be free of pain in L elbow while performing job skills in 5 weeks.

P denotes the *Plan* to be followed in providing care for the specific patient. Information provided in the Plan should include

1. The priority given for treatment of each of the patient's problems
2. An estimated timetable for meeting the goals for the patient
3. Enough detail concerning treatment procedures to enable another person to continue treatment
4. The anticipated duration of each treatment and session

The Plan should establish the actions the therapist will take in order to assist the patient in achieving the established goals.

An example of the Plan section of a note for a patient with a recently healed fracture is

Plan

Priorities:	Increase ROM L elbow.
	Increase strength L elbow and wrist.
	Decrease in pain expected as ROM and strength re turn to normal.
Treatment:	Cryotherapy prior to and following each exercise session to decrease swelling and pain.
	Proprioceptive neuromuscular facilitation (PNF) procedures to increase ROM.
	PNF procedures for strengthening exercises in clinic.
	Free weight exercises for strengthening in clinic and as home exercise program.
Schedule:	Clinic visits 45 min 3×/wk for 2 weeks followed by 45 min 2×/wk for 2 weeks.
	Independent ADL using L arm in 2 weeks.
	Return to work in 5 weeks.

Each section of the SOAP note need not be included in every note; however, initial notes generally include all sections. Only the relevant sections are needed for any specific note. Progress notes need to include only those sections necessary for indicating changes in patient status, ie, progress or regression. Discharge notes summarize treatment provided, progress achieved, and the patient profile on discharge. In this way, the initial status, the final status, and thus the effectiveness of therapeutic intervention can be presented in an organized manner.

Requirements

The primary role of adequate documentation is to enhance communication for medical and legal purposes. To perform this role, documentation must be precise, concise, legible, and timely. To be **precise**, measurements and test results must be recorded accurately, and terminology must be used accurately and appropriately. To be **concise**, documentation must be organized effectively, conveying important information in a clear, unfettered fashion. To be **legible**, the method of note entry in a medical record should be one that allows all team members to read the entry of others accurately and without delay. **Timeliness** requires that notes be entered into the medical record immediately after the patient is examined or treated, in order that subsequent patient care decisions are based upon current information.

An important aspect of medical documentation is the presentation of information in a manner that can be read and interpreted quickly and efficiently. Many institutions recommend outline format, rather than fully developed prose descriptions. There are many cases in which charts or tables can be used to report individual and serial test results. The use of such charts or tables enables the communication of large amounts of information quickly and avoids excess use of prose. When prose is used, the rules of proper grammatical usage should be followed. Sentences or phrases that do not contain specific information relevant to the patient's health care should not be used. Confusion and misunderstanding is avoided if abbreviations are customary and standardized within a facility. Do not assume that everyone reading a chart will interpret nonstandardized abbreviations in the same way.

LO-6

REQUIREMENTS
Precise
Concise
Complete
Accurate
Legible
Timely

LO-7

AUDIT
Peer review
Quality assurance

1.3   AUDIT

Periodic and consistent evaluation of patient care activities is necessary to measure and analyze the quality of patient care provided. When appropriate and significant data are reported in a consistent format, **audit** for peer review and quality assurance is facilitated. Records can be audited to determine if actual patient care outcomes are consistent with expected patient care outcomes, and if patient care outcomes are dependent upon the type of treatment employed. There are several potential benefits to be gained in using audits to improve patient care rendered and patient care outcomes. A partial list of information that an audit may yield is whether

1. Individual therapists are including pertinent and required information in medical chart notes
2. Department or individual therapist treatment protocols are appropriate for the patients being treated
3. Changes in department policy or protocols are necessary to improve patient care
4. Continuing education is necessary to improve patient care skills

Only through the availability of properly completed records can useful audits be performed.

1.4 REVIEW QUESTIONS

1. List the general categories of information found in a medical record.

2. Compare and contrast the source oriented-method and the problem-oriented method of medical record keeping.

3. Describe the three components of a POMR.

4. List the information contained in a patient's medical record using the POMR method.

5. What is the procedure for creating and maintaining a POMR?

6. What is the SOAP note format?

7. Define each section of a SOAP note indicating the information contained in each section.

8. What are the requirements of adequate documentation?

9. What information can be obtained from an audit?

1.5 SUGGESTED ACTIVITIES

1. Students indicate in which component of the SOAP note each of the following statements should be by placing the appropriate letter S, O, A, P before the statement.

_____ ROM of the right shoulder flexion is 0–85.

_____ The family reports that the patient frequently falls at night.

_____ The patient will be treated twice a week for 3 weeks.

_____ The patient will ambulate with a straight cane on all surfaces for functional distances without fatigue within 4 weeks.

_____ The patient reported a pain level of 5/10 after treatment.

_____ The patient's pain level decreased following treatment.

_____ The patient was able to ascend and descend 12 stairs step over step using the hand rail 4 times.

_____ The patient's ability to assume standing from sitting is impaired because of weakness of both quadriceps muscles.

2. Students organize the following narrative note into the SOAP note format:

Mr. Ted Jones is a 67-year-old male 2 days post left total knee replacement. Mr. Jones is to be discharged to a skilled nursing care facility in 2 days where he will receive additional therapy. The goal is for Mr. Jones to ambulate independently without an assistive device as a community ambulator. The physician has indicated that when Mr. Jones has 90 degrees of left knee flexion, good strength of knee flexors and extensors, and can ambulate 200 ft × 4, he can be discharged to his home. Mr. Jones reports pain of 4/10 about the incision. The incision is anterior over the left knee in a proximal distal direction. Some clear discharge is noted at the distal end of the incision. The circumference of the left knee at 2 inches above the tibial tuberosity is 3/4 inch larger on the left than the right.

3. Students identify the components of the following goal statement by writing the word or phrase in the appropriate space:

Goal statement: The patient will have full left knee extension ROM for ambulation, dressing, and getting in and out of a chair within 2 weeks of daily treatment.

A:_____

B: _____

C:_____

D: _____

F: _____

T: _____

1.6 APPENDIX A

Answers for Suggested Activities in Chapter 1

1. O, S, P, A, S, A, O, A
2. Mr. Ted Jones is a 67-year-old male 2 days post left total knee replacement.
    S: Mr. Jones reports pain of 4/10 about the incision.
    O: Mr. Jones has an incision on the anterior aspect of the left knee that runs proximal to distal. Some clear discharge is noted at the distal end of the incision.
    The circumference of the left knee at 2 inches above the tibial tuberosity is 3/4 inch larger on the left than the right.
    A: LTG: Mr. Jones will ambulate independently without an assistive device as a community ambulator. STG: Mr. Jones will have 90 degrees of left knee flexion for getting in and out of a chair prior to discharge home. Mr. Jones's strength of the left knee flexors and extensors will be 4/5 prior to discharge home. Mr. Jones will be able to ambulate 200 ft × 4 using a straight cane prior to discharge home.
    P: Mr. Jones is to be discharged to a skilled nursing care facility in 2 days where he will receive additional therapy.
3. A. the patient
    B. left knee extension ROM
    C. full
    D. 100%
    F. for ambulation, dressing, and getting in and out of a chair
    T. within 2 weeks of daily treatment

1.7 References

1. Weed LL. *Medical Record, Medical Education, and Patient Care*. Chicago: Yearbook Medical Publishers; 1970.
2. Dunsdale SM, Mossman PL, Guleckson G, Jr, et al. The problem oriented medical record in rehabilitation. *Arch Phys Med Rehabil*. 1970; 51; 488–492.
3. Editorial. Ten reasons why Weed is right. *N Engl J Med*. 1971; 51; 284.
4. Milhous R. The problem oriented medical record in rehabilitation management and training. *Arch Phys Med Rehabil*. 19782; 53; 182–185.
5. Kettenbach, G. *Writing SOAP Notes*. 2nd ed. Philadelphia, David, 1995.

Chapter

2

Preparation for Patient Care

 Learner Objectives

The student will be able to:

1 State who is responsible for managing the environment.
2 Describe general guidelines for managing the environment.
3 Describe correct body mechanics.
4 Describe therapist position when guarding a patient during gait training.
5 Distinguish between instructions and verbal commands by describing the characteristics of instructions and verbal commands.
6 Describe the purposes of draping and method of draping.
7 Describe proper management of the various tubes, lines, and monitors attached to a patient.
8 Demonstrate transporting patients safely via a cart of wheelchair.

INTRODUCTION

Fundamental to all patient care are such skills as management of the environment, body mechanics, and communication. Safe implementation of a treatment procedure is best achieved when all the components of the procedure are given proper attention. Generally, a few minutes taken at the start of a procedure to plan the steps involved and to prepare for the procedure will increase the likelihood of safe, efficient, and effective implementation. The safety of the patient and the therapist must be of paramount consideration at all times.

LO-1

2.1   MANAGEMENT OF THE ENVIRONMENT

The work area must be organized for the protection of the patient and staff, as well as for efficient use. Managing the environment to achieve these goals is a serious responsibility of all staff members. Some tasks may be delegated to certain personnel; the user, however, always retains final responsibility.

Preparation for the next treatment begins at the end of the previous treatment. Following use, equipment must be returned to the proper storage area in safe functioning condition. unused supplies must also be returned to the proper storage area, and used supplies must be disposed of properly. The person responsible for ordering supplies should be notified in the appropriate manner when consumable supplies are low.

All equipment is required to be inspected to ensure safe functioning. Malfunctions are to be reported in the appropriate manner to the proper person at the time they occur. A simple examination of equipment before each use also helps to ensure patient safety. Patients can, and should, be taught to inspect their own equipment, such as crutch tips, for wear.

House keeping requirements must also be considered in management of the environment. As examples, cleaning of floors, mats, and treatment tables is necessary to provide a clean and safe environment for treatment. Proper cleaning of equipment will prolong its life of safe and effective use. Such cleaning should occur on a regular basis, and be in accordance with facility procedures. The basis of these procedures is outlines by the Centers for Disease Control and Prevention. Specifics of some of these procedures are covered in Chapter 4, "Aseptic Techniques."

By following these simple rules, supplies and equipment will be available and functioning safely when needed. All personnel will know where to find what is needed for the treatment plan to be implemented. The environment will be safe and clean for use.

LO-2

Prior to initiating a transfer or treatment, the bed or treatment table and surrounding areas must be readied. Supplies necessary in a treatment area include linens and pillows. Call bells must be within reach of patients in areas where patients will be left unattended. Treatment tables, mats, or beds should be prepared before the patient arrives in the treatment area. Additional sheets are used as pull sheets for transfers or for draping. Pillows for patient positioning, comfort, and safety must be within easy reach. Trying to support a patient's head while reaching for a misplaced pillow, or leaving a patient in an uncomfortable or unsafe position while equipment is retrieved, is not good patient care.

Specific equipment required for a treatment should be prepared prior to beginning work with the patient. Having equipment and supplies required for treatment available in the area before treatment begins avoids the possibility of having to leave a patient unguarded or interrupting treatment.

Enough room must be allowed for unimpeded movement. Staff and patients must be able to maneuver in the area without bumping into or tripping over equipment. When equipment, such as a diathermy machine, is used in the treatment of a patient, position the equipment and patient to allow easy access to the patient. Improperly positioned equipment may hamper the ability to provide patient assistance quickly.

Equipment and furniture not needed during a transfer or treatment, such as ultrasound device or mobile stool, should be moved away from the area of transfer. Besides getting in the way, many of these pieces of equipment are not stable and become dangerous when a patient tries to use them as support during a transfer.

2.2 BODY MECHANICS

Proper posture is required to limit stress and strain on musculoskeletal structures. when lifting, pushing, or pulling, the stresses and strains upon the musculoskeletal system are increased. Proper posture and body mechanics are based upon alignment and functioning of the musculoskeletal system. **Correct body mechanics** for patient care is guided by the five cardinal rules of lifting. The five cardinal rules with application to lifting or transferring patients are

LO-3

1. Keep the load close—keep the center of gravity of the patient close to the therapist.
2. Maintain balance—use a base of support that is of appropriate size and shape.
3. Use the back muscles isometrically to keep the back in a constant (preferably erect) position—do not extend the back to perform the lift.
4. Lift with the legs—use the larger and stronger muscles of the legs to perform the lift.
5. Don't twist—rotate whole body, not just the spine, as the patient is transferred.

The initial stance for lifting is with the therapist's feet placed in stride and slightly apart. This stance widens the base of support in both the anterior/posterior and lateral directions, negating the effect of small shifts in the center of gravity. In this way, a balanced position can be maintained more easily. Lifting should be initiated from a squatting position. The depth of the squat should be deep enough to permit the therapist to reach the person or object to be lifted, but not so deep that the leg muscles are at a disadvantage in regaining the upright position. This type of squat is achieved by flexing the hips and knees, rather than by trunk flexion. The trunk should be maintained in good alignment so muscles only have to maintain this alignment, and do not have to work to extend the trunk during the lifting motion. Contracting the muscles of the trunk prior to lifting can reduce the potential for injury. Being as close as possible to the person or object to be lifted or carried allows the combined center of gravity to be maintained within the base of support. When the center of gravity is centered within the base of support and near the body's midline, both balance and correct postural alignment are easier to maintain.

Transfers require movements that move the center of gravity away from the center of the base of support. These movements have the potential of causing a loss of balance. Increasing the size of the base of support by setting the feet in stride and slightly apart provides a larger base of support. The therapist's feet should also be unencumbered to move as the situation requires, always allowing the base of support to be reestablished under the moving center of gravity. Crossing of the therapist's legs during movement should be avoided because it decreases the size of the base of support and constrains freedom of foot movement.

When moving large pieces of equipment, such as diathermy machines or parallel bars, or when guarding a patient during ambulation, the therapist should be positioned behind the equipment or patient, facing in the direction of movement. This allows the therapist to

1. Determine a path free from obstruction
2. Use a lifting or pushing motion
3. Use larger muscles and body weight more efficiently during pushing or lifting

LO-4

With the therapist behind the patient, the patient's view and path of movement are not obstructed by the therapist.

When **guarding** a patient during gait training, the therapist should be positioned with feet in stride, at 45-degree angle slightly to the side and behind the patient. If the patient falls forward, backward, or to either side, this position usually allows the combined center of gravity to be maintained within the base of support with only a shift of the therapist's weight, and does not usually require large foot movements. The base of support must be large enough to support such shifts in the center of gravity should the patient start to fall. To permit unencumbered weight shifting or foot movement, the therapist's feet should not be crossed during ambulation or become entangled with the patient's feet or ambulatory equipment.

In all cases, plan movements and prepare the area to be used before starting. Use proper body mechanics and safety precautions. When in doubt about your ability to lift or carry a patient or object safely, always obtain additional assistance.

2.3   INSTRUCTIONS AND VERBAL COMMANDS

Patients must know what they are to do and when they are to do it during transfers and treatment to participate effectively. Verbal commands focus the patient's attention on specifically desired actions. **Instructions** must be simple, informative, and in language that the patient can understand. Terminology used must be appropriate to the patient's level of understanding. Medical terms should be used only when the patient readily understands medical terminology. In some cases, foreign language instructions will be necessary.

The therapist should describe to the patient the general sequence of events that will occur. In addition, the patient should be instructed in the expected responses. This helps the patient to learn the skill for future independent use and increases the safety of the immediate task performance. Therefore, the therapist must determine that the patient understands the instructions. Asking the patient, "Do you understand the instruction?" does not always ensure understanding. Having the patient repeat the instructions in the proper order provides an opportunity for mental rehearsal of the task in addition to indicating an appropriate level of understanding.

LO-5

The therapist should speak clearly and vary the tone of voice as the situation requires. Sharp commands will receive quick responses, while soft commands will elicit slower responses.

Patients must be able to hear commands. When the patient cannot hear, or does not understand the spoken word, gestures and demonstrations can convey the necessary meaning.

A **command** is a cue for activity during a procedure. Commands must be brief, specific, and properly times. Patients often become confused when given a long series of actions to implement when given only one cue. Therefore, each specific action may require a specific command. Commands must be specific to the action desired. For example, counting to "three" does not instruct a patient to do anything specific. When a patient is to look up, count to three and say "look up." "Look up" is a specific command. The specific command "look up" instructs the patient what to do without requiring translation of the word "three" into the action of "looking up." Commands must be timed for each action to occur in the proper sequence and at the appropriate time so that the entire procedure is completed safely and effectively.

2.4   PATIENT PREPARATION

For efficient use of treatment time, patient preparation should be completed prior to transport and treatment. Nursing personnel and transport personnel must be notified of preparation requirements well in advance of the scheduled treatment time. A patient should be properly dressed for transfers and treatment to ensure the patient's right to modesty, for beneficial treatment, and for safety.

When working with patients, including transport and treatment, attention must be paid to appropriate draping or dress. **Draping** is covering the patient with a sheet(s) or towel(s). The purpose of draping are to

1. Protect a patient's modesty
2. Provide warmth
3. Protect wounds, scars, stumps, personal clothing, etc.
4. Expose a specific body segment for treatment

LO-6

When draping, edges of sheets and towels should be secured to avoid inadvertent exposure of the patient. When moving a patient, advance planning is required to maintain appropriate draping during movement.

Hospital gowns are designed for ease in dressing and access during nursing care. They may not provide effective draping during the movements required for transfers and treatment. Properly securing the ties of a hospital gown may provide some coverage. Midlength robes or housecoats, or two hospital gowns, one opening in front and one opening in back, can be used. When necessary, a sheet or towel can be used for additional draping. Long robes or housecoats interfere with movement and their use should be avoided.

Whenever possible, patients should be dressed in slacks or shorts to provide ease of movement without loss of modesty. Shorts are especially important if the lower extremity must be observed. A belt should be used as slacks or shorts will be useless and dangerous if they fall from the waist or restrict leg movement. A halter top or bra is necessary when a female patient's upper trunk must be observed. Shoes that offer support are required if the patient is to stand, ambulate, or practice transfers. When shoes are worn, socks should be worn for comfort and sanitation. When a patients is not ambulatory, slippers may be acceptable as they are easier to take off and put on as necessary. In all cases, decisions concerning dress must be tempered by the patient's needs, the patient's ability to manipulate the clothing, and the requirements of treatment.

Patients will be seen in a variety of settings. In many cases, IV (intravenous) lines, chest tubes, catheters, respirators, cardiac monitors, or combinations of these, will be present. When positioning, transferring, or treating patients, care must be taken not to disrupt the set-up of vital medical equipment. when chest tubes are present, there will be chest tube bottles either hung on the bed rails or taped to the floor. The bottles must not be disturbed or hit while lowering the rails, head of the bed, or the bed itself. The bottles may hit the floor or bed, depending on their placement, before the rail, head of the bed, or bed itself is completely lowered. Breaking these bottles can be a life-threatening situation. When a chest tube bottle is broken, the chest tube should be clamped shut immediately as close to the chest as possible, and emergency help should be requested.

In all cases, tubes and lines will limit the amount of movement available to a patient. Prior to moving the patient, or having the patient move, the therapist must check the amount of movement allowed by the tubes and lines present. Plan in advance for repositioning IV containers, catheter bags, oxygen masks, chest tubes, and the like. Repositioning of containers, tubes, lines, and other equipment, may require additional equipment or personnel. Do not allow tubes or lines to become tangled, pinched, kinked, stretched, or pulled out from their insertion site. Any of these occurrences will interrupt fluid or gas glow. Some of these situations, such as pulling out chest tubes or disconnecting respirator tubes, are life-threatening. IV drop rates and oxygen flow rates must not be changed without a change of the physician's orders. IV containers must remain above the level of the patient's heart. Urinary catheter bags must remain below the level of the bladder. Proper placement of IV containers and catheter bags is necessary to maintain the correct direction of fluid flow.

2.5   TRANSPORTING

Transporting the patient from one area to another is frequently necessary. A cart or wheelchair may be required because of the patient's condition of because of hospital regulations. The patient should be transferred in an appropriate manner, with proper draping during the transfers and transport.

The brakes on the wheelchair or cart must be locked before beginning a transfer. The patient's clothing, draping, and medical equipment (IVs, etc.) must be adjusted to avoid becoming tangled in the wheels or dragging on the floor during transport. Arms and legs must be within the cart or wheelchair to avoid injury during transport. Wheelchairs may have seat belts, and carts may have straps or side rails. Safety belts should be used to secure the patient. Side rails should be used on a cart when available.

A mattress on a cart and a cushion on a wheelchair are used for patient comfort and protection. Additional pillows and padding are positioned for the patient's comfort and protection as necessary.

LO-7

INSPECT PATIENT AND ENVIRONMENT

Prior to moving patient
Look for tubes, monitors, and IV lines

AVOID TUBES OR LINES BECOMING

Tangled
Pinched
Pulled
Kinked
Stretched

LO-8

CLINICAL NOTE

Safety: Always lock wheelchair or cart before moving patient.

We wish to note that in some illustrations throughout the text, the thera-pist's position has been altered from the desired position, or the therapist is absent from the illustration. This has been done to provide a clear view of other detail in the illustration.

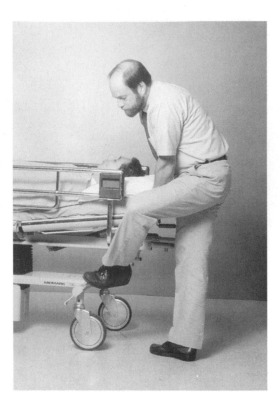

Figure 2.5–1. Locking wheel on cart.

Via Cart

Carts often have four swivel wheels to make it easier to push the cart from either end. Locks are located on each wheel. Generally, there are three positions in which the lock can be used. With the locking lever in the horizontal position, both swivel and rolling movements are permitted. When the locking level is tilted in one direction, swivel movement is locked and rolling motion is permitted. Tilting the locking level in the other direction prohibits both swivel and rolling movements.

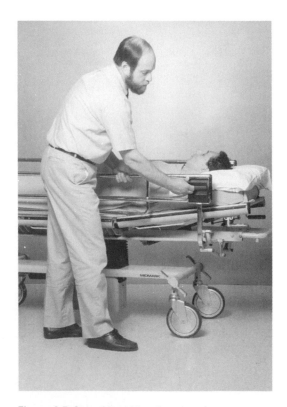

Figure 2.5–2. Locking side rail on cart.

Cart side rails raise or swing up to be used to prevent the patient from falling off the cart. The rails lower or swing down for easier transferring. Cart rails have a locking mechanism to secure them in the up position.

The therapist should push from the head of the cart so that the patient is moving feet first. The pace should be slow and steady. Quick, jerky movements may upset a patient or make the patient nauseated. Control of the cart must be maintained at all times. Corners must be turned cautiously. Additional personnel may be needed to maneuver on and off elevators, in and out of doors, and at blind corners. When necessary, catheter bags and IV containers must be attached to the cart at an appropriate height.

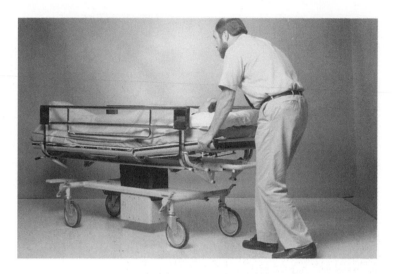

Figure 2.5–3. Pushing from head of cart.

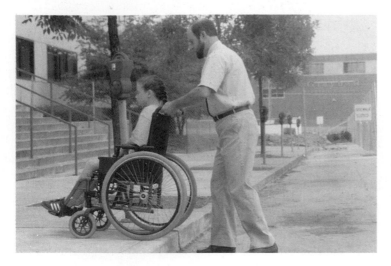

Figure 2.5–4. Starting position to descend curb backward.

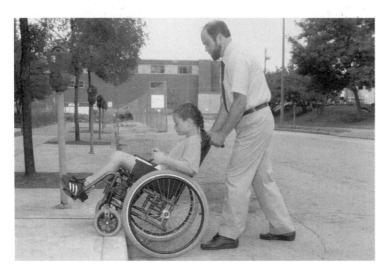

Figure 2.5–5. Rear wheels lowered to street.

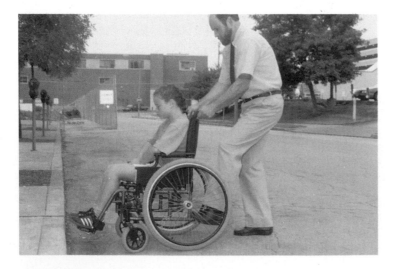

Figure 2.5–6. Lowering front wheels.

Via Wheelchair

Using a wheelchair properly requires the patient to be seated well back on the seat, and that the lower extremities be placed on the footrests or leg rests. Wheelchairs must be pushed at a slow and steady pace without quick and jerky movements. Control of a wheelchair must be maintained at all times. When necessary, catheter bags and IV containers must be attached to the wheelchair at an appropriate height.

Descending Curb—Backward Method

To lower a patient in a wheelchair down a curb, position the wheelchair so the patient is facing away from the curb. This positions the larger rear wheels at the edge of the curb to be descended. The therapist should step off the curb backward, while facing the wheelchair.

Holding onto the handles, the therapist slowly lowers the rear wheels of the wheelchair to the street by rolling them smoothly off the edge of the curb.

Holding the handles securely, the therapist continues to roll the wheelchair backward, maintaining the tilted position of the wheelchair until the front wheels are clear of the curb. The therapist then slowly lowers the front wheels until all four wheels are securely on the lower level.

Decending Curb—Forward Method

An alternative method is to approach the curb forward. The therapist then tilts the wheelchair backward so the front wheels are approximately 8 inches above the ground.

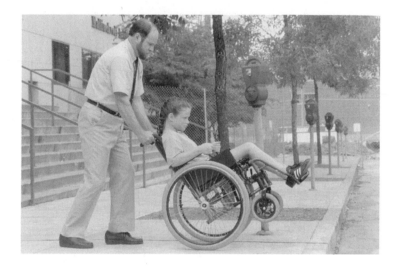

Figure 2.5–7. Tilting wheelchair to descend curb forward.

The wheelchair is then rolled slowly and smoothly off the curb onto the lower level. As the wheelchair rolls over the curb the therapist must assume a crouched position and step forward.

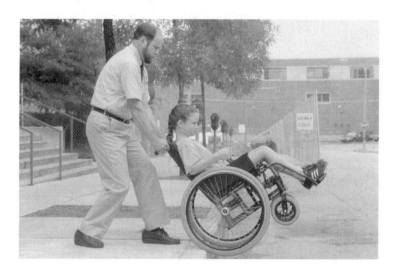

Figure 2.5.–8. Rolling wheelchair off curb.

The therapist then slowly lowers the front wheels until all four wheels are securely on the lower level.

This method places more stress on the therapist while controlling the roll of the wheelchair over the edge of the curb. There is also greater danger of losing control of the wheelchair.

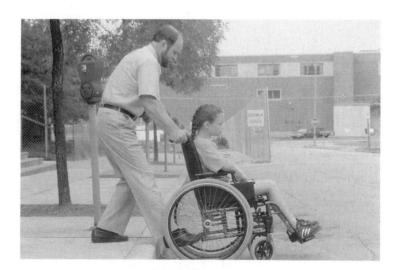

Figure 2.5–9. Lowering front wheels.

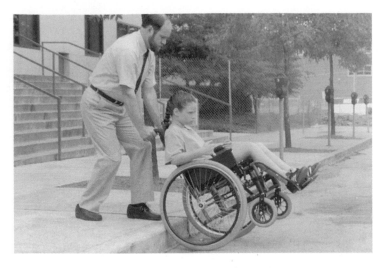

Figure 2.5–10. Tilting wheelchair to ascend curb backward.

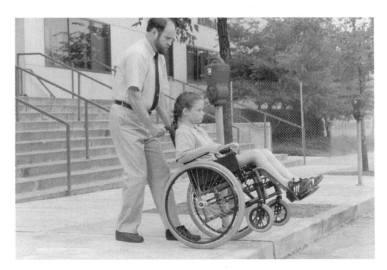

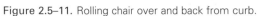

Figure 2.5–11. Rolling chair over and back from curb.

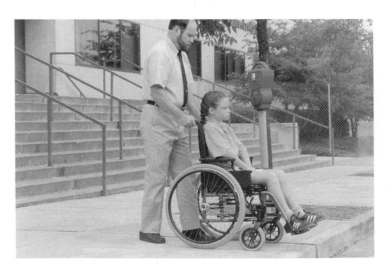

Figure 2.5–12. Completion of ascending curb backward.

Ascending Curb—Backward Method

To raise the wheelchair up a curb, the previous procedures are reversed. The wheelchair is backed up to the curb, with the patient facing away from the curb. The therapist tilts the wheelchair backward onto the rear wheels.

Standing on the curb, the therapist lifts and rolls the wheelchair backward up the curb, maintaining the backward tilt of the wheelchair.

The wheelchair is rolled backward until all four wheels are clearly past the curb and over the higher level. The therapist then slowly lowers the front wheels until all four wheels are securely on the higher level.

Ascending Curb—Forward Method

An alternative method is to approach the curb or step forward. While facing the curb, the wheelchair is tilted backward onto the rear wheels so the front wheels can clear the curb.

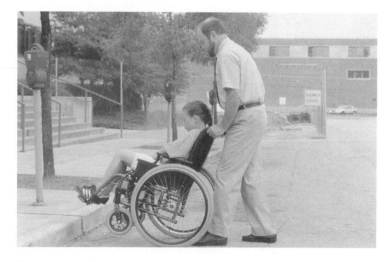

Figure 2.5–13. Tilting wheelchair to ascend curb forward.

The wheelchair is wheeled forward, placing the front wheels on the upper level as soon as they are clearly over the upper level.

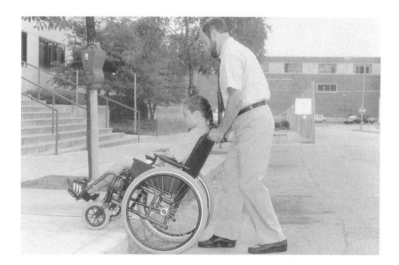

Figure 2.5–14. Rolling wheelchair up curb.

The therapist continues to wheel the wheelchair until the rear wheels contact the curb. The therapist then lifts and rolls the rear wheels up and over the curb.

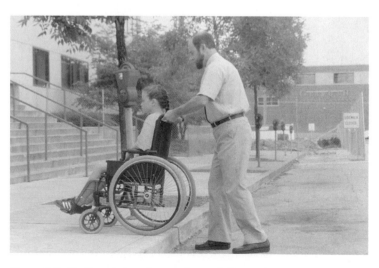

Figure 2.5–15. Completion of ascending curb forward.

Doorways with Automatic Door Closers

The following sections present wheelchair ambulation through doorways. To prevent the therapist from obscuring the desired views in these photographs, the text and photographs depict independent ambulation in a wheelchair. Assisted wheelchair ambulation through doorways is performed in a similar manner, with the therapist providing the force to open the door and propel the wheelchair.

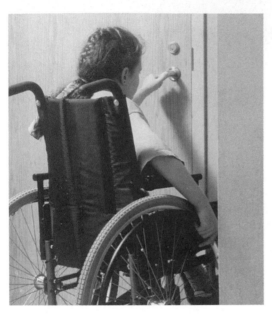

Figure 2.5–16. Grasping door handle.

Door Opens Toward Patient

The patient approaches the latch edge of the door. When possible, the patient positions the wheelchair at the latch edge of the door while facing the hinge edge of the door, and beyond the arc through which the door will open. The patient grasps the door handle.

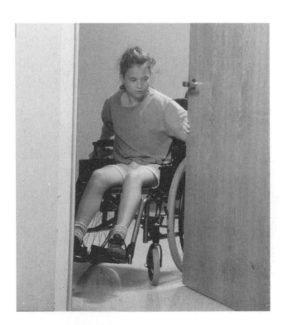

Figure 2.5–17. Pulling door open.

The patient pulls the door open wider than is necessary for her to move through the doorway. The wider opening of the door is necessitated by the fact that the door will start to close automatically as the patient enters the doorway.

The patient must move into the doorway quickly to block the closing door. Care must be taken that the closing door does not strike the patient, or hit the wheelchair hard enough to cause the patient to lose control of the wheelchair. Some wheelchair users do this by pulling on the doorjamb. Others propel their wheelchair in the usual way, or use a combination of doorjamb and normal propulsion. As the patient propels the wheelchair into the doorway, the rubber bumper on the footrest closest to the door, and then the wheelchair wheel, are used to block the door open. Care must be taken to avoid crushing the patient's fingers between the door and the wheel of the wheelchair as the door is blocked.

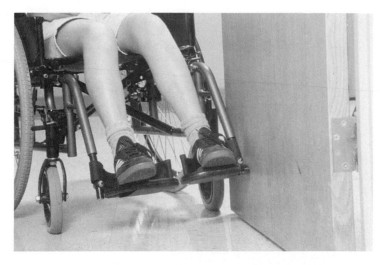

Figure 2.5–18. Using footrest to block door.

As the patient continues to move through the doorway, the wheel of the wheelchair continues to block the door.

When the patient has moved completely through the doorway, the door finishes closing behind the patient.

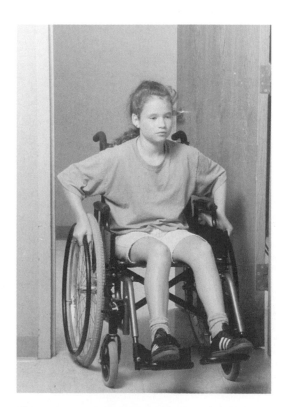

Figure 2.5–19. Completing passage through doorway.

Door Opens Away from Patient

The patient approaches the latch edge of the door and grasps the door handle.

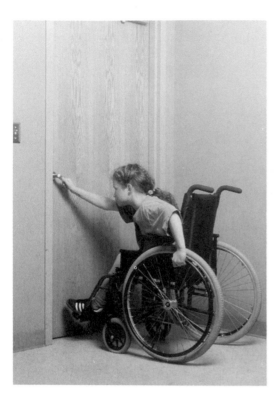

Figure 2.5–20. Grasping door handle.

The patient pushes the door open wider than is necessary for her to move through the doorway. The wider opening of the door is necessitated by the fact that the door will start to close automatically as the patient enters the doorway.

The patient must move into the doorway quickly to block the closing door. Care must be taken that the closing door does not strike the patient, or hit the wheelchair hard enough to cause the patient to lose control of the wheelchair. Some wheelchair users do this by pulling on the doorjamb. Others propel their wheelchair in the usual way, or use a combination of doorjamb and normal propulsion.

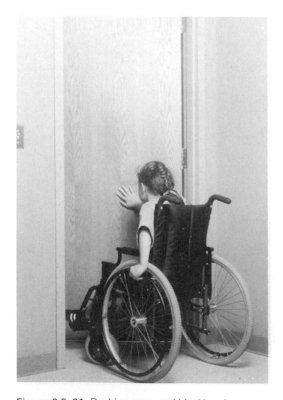

Figure 2.5–21. Pushing open and blocking door.

As the patient continues propelling the wheelchair through the doorway, the rubber bumper on the footrest closest to the door, and then the wheelchair wheel, are used to block the door open. Care must be taken to avoid crushing the patient's fingers between the door and the wheel of the wheelchair as the door is blocked.

When the patient is nearly through the doorway, the door is given one last opening push. the patient quickly propels the wheelchair out of the arc of the closing door, and the door is allowed to close behind the patient's wheelchair. Some patients may turn around the latch side of the doorjamb as they proceed through the doorway. This maneuver allows them to move out of the arc of the closing door quickly. In either case, once through the doorway, and after the door has closed, the patient can turn to proceed in the desired direction.

Doorways Without Automatic Door Closers

When the door does not have a closer, rapid propulsion through the doorway is not necessary. Extra-wide opening of the door is also not necessary. Propulsion of the wheelchair can be slower. Use of the wheelchair bumpers as a doorstop between the door and the patient is not required. The patient must turn to close the door, because the door will not close automatically.

Doorways With Automatic Door Openers.

When doors have an automatic door opener, a push-plate should be placed on the wall along the approach to the door or alongside the door. Some automatic door openers will operate using sensor, and do not use a push-plate.

When the door opens toward the patient, patients should make sure they are clear of the arc of door opening so they are not struck by the opening door. This is not a problem when the door swings away from the patient. When the push-plate is used to activate the door, the door should open, and stay open while the patient moves through the doorway. The patient should not hesitate while moving through the doorway because the automatic door opener will release after a set period of time.

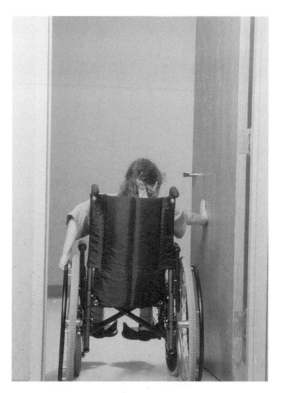

Figure 2.5–22. Continuing to move through doorway.

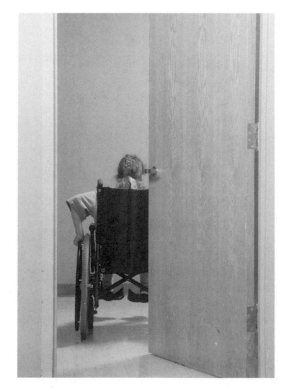

Figure 2.5–23. Completing passage through doorway.

2.6   WHEELCHAIR WHEELIES

A wheelchair wheelie is performed by balancing on the rear wheels of a wheelchair with the caster wheels in the air. A patient must be able to perform wheelies in order to go up and down curbs independently when there are no curb ramps.

It is critical to guard a patient during the learning of a wheelie to prevent injury. The therapist must be behind, and move with, the wheelchair in order to guard the patient during this maneuver. The therapist's hands must always be beneath the wheelchair handles, ready to catch the wheelchair if it tilts backward too far.

A wheelie begins by grasping the anterior portion of the wheel rims.

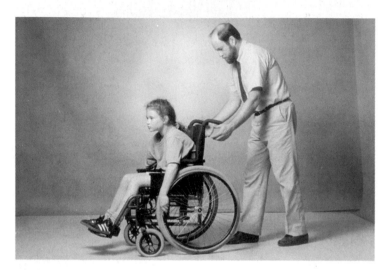

Figure 2.6–1. Grasping anterior portion of wheel rims.

A quick backward movement of the wheels places the hands in position for the forward thrust that achieves the wheelie position.

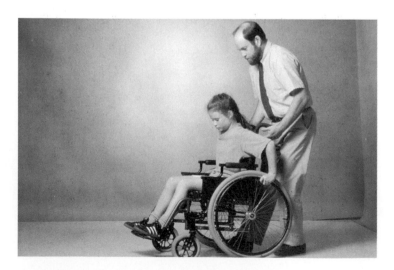

Figure 2.6–2. Pulling backward quickly on wheel rims.

The quick backward motion is immediately followed by a quick forward thrust on both wheel rims, causing the wheelchair to rise onto the rear wheels only.

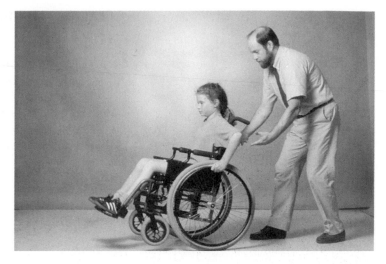

Figure 2.6–3. Thrusting forward on both wheel rims.

The patient controls balance by small movements of the rear wheels.

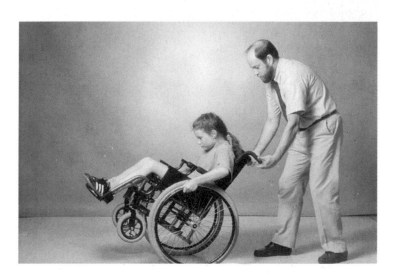

Figure 2.6–4. Balancing on rear wheels.

2.7   ELEVATORS

When using an elevator, the patient should be positioned facing the elevator door. If space is sufficient, the patient may enter the elevator forward and then turn around. When space is limited, the patient should enter the elevator backward. Facing forward allows the patient to monitor the floor display and have easy access to the control panel. Exiting the elevator is usually safer when facing forward. Facing forward is also the position most commonly assumed by elevator users.

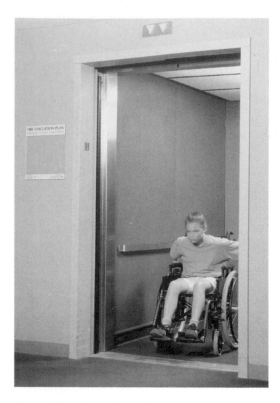

Figure 2.7–1. Facing forward on elevator.

2.8   REVIEW QUESTIONS

1. How is the treatment environment managed to ensure a safe and efficient environment?

2. What are the four rules of proper body mechanics?

3. How are the four rules of proper body mechanics applied when transferring patients, guarding patients, and moving equipment?

4. What is the purpose of verbal commands?

5. What are the purposes of draping a patient?

6. What precautions should be observed while transporting a patient?

2.9 SUGGESTED ACTIVITIES

1. Demonstrate different modes of patient transport to students.

2. Students transport a classmate around the building on a cart.

3. Students transport a classmate around the building in a wheelchair.

4. Students ambulate around the building via a wheelchair with a classmate accompanying to ensure safety.

5. Discuss the experiences in activities 1, 2, and 3, including:

   a. Perceptions of self when being transported compared to ambulating.

   b. Reactions of others in the environment.

   c. Realization of the challenge of being in a wheelchair or on a cart.

6. Students rotate through several stations related to body mechanics. Suggestions for stations include:

   a. Foot placement. Place foot marks on the floor indicating foot placement.
   Make some foot placements correct and some incorrect.
   Students perform tasks such as lifting boxes from a wheelchair to a mat table, from a wheelchair to a treatment table, from a table in front to a table behind, using correct and incorrect foot placement.

   b. COG centered. Have students carry books in a book bag from point A to point B with the book bag on one shoulder, properly positioned on back, held in one hand, and held out in front of them.

   c. Discuss the experiences to determine which were easier and safer.

7. Have students document selected experiences during activities in SOAP note format.

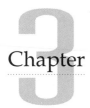

Chapter

3

Vital Signs

Learner Objectives

The student will be able to:

1 Describe the purposes, methods, sites, and norms for vital signs: pulse, blood pressure, respiration, and temperature.
2 Correctly assess pulse, blood pressure, respiration, and temperature.
3 Correctly use terms that describe vital signs outside the normal ranges.
4 Identify vital signs that are below, within, or above normal range.
5 Correctly document vital signs.

INTRODUCTION

All personnel providing health care should be aware of, and able to perform, the simple basic measurements of body function known as vital signs, which are important objective findings. Vital signs are used to monitor a patient's status at any given time during patient care, and to evaluate basic physiologic responses to treatment. Vital signs consist of heart rate (HR), or pulse (P); blood pressure (BP); respiration (R); and temperature (T).

3.1 HEART RATE

LO-1

Purpose

Pulse is a measurement of **heart rate.** Pulse measured after an extended period of rest is defined as basal heart rate. Basal heart rate is one indication of cardiovascular function in the absence of physical stress.

Pulse can also be measured before, during, or following the imposed physiologic or physical stress of treatment or other exercise, as indicated by a patient's medical condition. When measured during rest, the pulse rate is called the resting heart rate, a measurement of heart rate without imposed stresses. When measured during treatment or exercise, pulse is one measurement of the cardiovascular system's capability to provide blood flow during imposed physiologic or physical stress. When measured after treatment or other exercise, pulse is also one measure of the cardiovascular system's recovery rate following the imposition of physiologic or physical stress.

Measurements of pulse are also used to determine the **patency,** or the openness, of the peripheral portion of the cardiovascular system. When used for this purpose, the important measurement is the presence or absence of a pulse at a chosen site. Such measurements of pulse can provide a preliminary indication of arterial occlusion resulting from physical blockage, or peripheral vascular insufficiency secondary to disease states, such as diabetes.

In addition to patency and rate, regularity and quality of pulse can provide information concerning cardiovascular status. Measuring a pulse permits a subjective assessment of the regularity of the heart beat. Regularity refers to the evenness of heart beat. Terms such as strong, weak, full, or thready are used to describe the quality of a pulse. A pulse that varies in rate, regularity, or quality from normal ranges may be indicative of disease or injury.

LO-2

Method

The most common clinical method of measuring pulse is manual palpation. The pads of the index and middle finger are placed over the site where the pulse is to be measured. The pad of the thumb should not be used for palpation when measuring pulse because there is a pulse in the pad of the thumb. If the thumb is used for palpation, one's own pulse may be mistaken for the patient's pulse.

Care must be taken not to press too hard while palpating a pulse. Excessive palpation pressure can obscure the pulse, impede blood flow, or cause arterial spasm. Obscuring the pulse prevents measurement and impeding blood flow or causing arterial spasm can be dangerous to a patient. This is especially true when evaluating the more distal pulses, which are palpated when measuring peripheral vascular patency.

Heart rate is measured in beats per minute (bpm or b/m), but is reported without the use of units. A heart rate of 74 beats per minute is reported as 74.

To obtain a heart rate, a watch or clock that displays time in seconds is used. Once the pulse has been palpated, beats are counted within a specified interval of time.[1,2] The most accurate method is to count beats for a period of 60 seconds. The result can then be reported without additional calculation.

Alternative methods require less time to monitor the pulse, but require additional calculation. Counting beats for a 10-second time period and multiplying the result by six, or using a 15-second time period and multiplying by four, are the most common shortcuts used. Using a shorter sampling period may result in a measurement that is less precise. Many times, a whole number of beats does not occur within a shorter time period. An estimate of the fractional heart beat is not as accurate as an exact count. Irregularities in heart beat are not detected as readily when a shorter sampling period is used. The necessity of additional calculation provides a potential source of error. Sometimes one beat in a time period is missed. In either of these cases, using a shortcut will increase the error, either six-fold or four-fold respectively.

As an example, an error of one beat during measurements taken over a 60-second time period and over a 10-second time period will provide two very different results. For a patient with an actual heart rate of 72 beats per minute, missing one beat during the 60-second count produces an error of 1/72, or 1.4%. Using a 10-second count, the same heart rate should yield 12 beats. If one beat is missed during the 10-second count, only 11 beats will be counted. This is multiplied by six, resulting in a calculation of 66 beats per minute for the same patient, an error of 6/72, or 8.3%. Although shortcut methods are used routinely, and their results recorded without question, care must be taken to provide an accurate and valid measurement.

There are two methods of counting heart rate.[2,3] The key factor in counting heart rate is that the number of heart beats *within* a given time period are to be counted.[2,3] The first,[2] or traditional, method starts the time period of counting at a specific time on a clock or watch, and the first heart beat felt after the time period has started is considered *beat 1*. This is beat 1 because it is the first heart beat *within* the specified time period. The second method[3] starts the time period of counting when a heart beat is felt, and is *beat 0*. This is beat 0 because it does not occur *within* the specified time period, but marks the beginning of the specified time period. Whichever method is used will provide an accurate count if attention is paid to the basis for when the interval begins and the number of counts that fall *within* the specified interval.

CLINICAL NOTE

Heart rate: Beats per minute

LO-5

CLINICAL NOTE

Most accurate method: Count for 60 seconds

Site

The radial artery and the carotid artery are the most commonly used sites for measuring heart rate.

LO-1

The radial pulse is most easily palpated on the volar surface of the wrist, just medial to the styloid process of the radius.

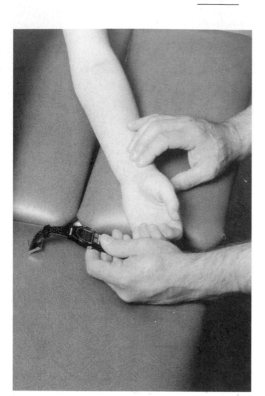

Figure 3.1–1. Palpation of radial pulse.

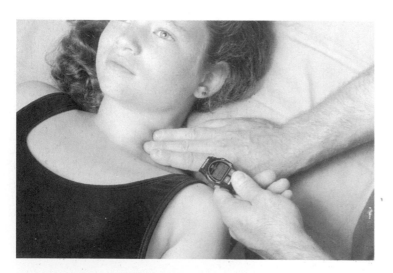

Figure 3.1–2. Palpation of carotid pulse.

The carotid pulse is most easily palpated on the lateral aspect of the neck, just inferior to the angle of the mandible. Care must be taken to palpate the carotid pulse without reaching across the throat. Palpating the carotid pulse on the side of the neck opposite to where the therapist is standing, requires the therapist to place his hand across the patient's throat, providing the potential for compromising the patient's airway.

The most common additional sites for the palpation of pulses for determining vascular patency are the brachial, femoral, popliteal, and pedal pulses.

The brachial pulse can be palpated on the medial aspect of the arm, midway down the shaft of the humerus.

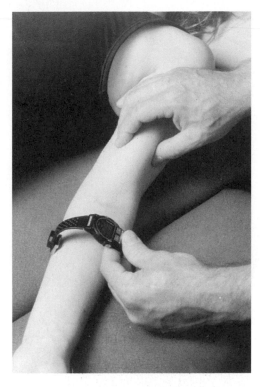

Figure 3.1–3. Palpation of brachial pulse.

The femoral pulse can be palpated in the femoral triangle. Although usually a strong pulse, the femoral pulse lies close to several large muscles, making palpation difficult. Care must be taken to avoid embarrassment for the patient, and pain from palpation that is too firm.

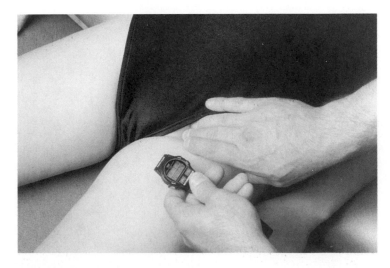

Figure 3.1–4. Palpation of femoral pulse.

Both the popliteal pulse and the pedal pulse are more difficult to palpate than other pulses even in healthy patients. These pulses are most commonly susceptible to degradations of strength in patients with peripheral vascular insufficiency, making palpation even more difficult. Care must be taken when palpating these pulses to avoid pressure that will obliterate the pulse.

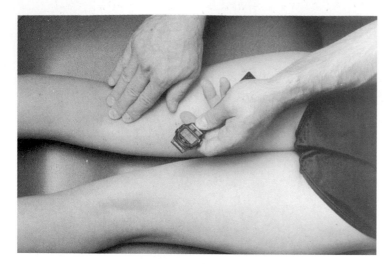

Figure 3.1–5. Palpation of popliteal pulse.

The popliteal pulse is palpated at or just above the knee on the posterior aspect of the leg. Generally the pulse can be palpated just lateral to the medial hamstring muscles.

The dorsal pedal pulse can be palpated on the dorsum of the foot, approximately over the cuboid bones.

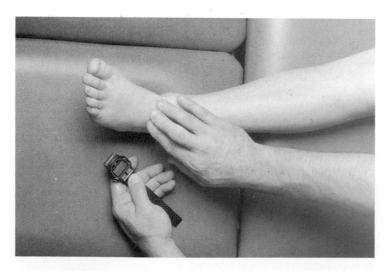

Figure 3.1–6. Palpation of dorsal pedal pulse.

Norms

The following ranges are generally accepted norms for heart rates. Individuals who maintain a high level of physical training may have a resting heart rate between 40 and 60 beats per minute. Individuals who maintain a moderately sedentary lifestyle may have a resting heart rate between 60 and 85 beats per minute. A resting heart rate greater than 85 beats per minute is usually indicative of a state of deconditioning or a medical condition. The normal resting heart rate for infants and young children is between 80 and 100 beats per minute.[4]

Resting heart rate in adults can vary greatly, depending on the state of physical conditioning of each individual. The technical definition of a very slow resting heart rate, or **bradycardia,** is a heart rate less than 60 beats per minute. The technical definition of a very fast resting heart rate, or **tachycardia,** is a heart rate greater than 100 beats per minute.[5] Bradycardia or tachycardia are usually indicative of disease.

Maximal heart rate is the highest heart rate a person without cardiovascular pathology should achieve on maximal exertion. The following guidelines for determining maximal heart rate are based on the absence of cardiovascular pathology in the individual patient. Maximal heart rates are calculated for each individual based on age. A simplified method of determining maximal heart rate, that does not take into consideration individual patient characteristics, is calculated by subtracting the patient's age from 220. For a 43-year-old person, the maximal heart rate is:

$$220 - 43 = 177$$

Target heart rate is the heart rate that an individual without cardiovascular pathology should achieve during exercise for cardiovascular conditioning. To be effective for cardiovascular conditioning for a patient without cardiovascular pathology, the target heart rate must fall between 60% and 80% of the maximal heart rate.[6] Thus, the formula used to determine a target heart rate for cardiovascular exercise for the 43-year-old person discussed above is between:

$$(0.60) \times (220 - \text{AGE}) \text{ and } (0.80) \times (220 - \text{AGE})$$
$$= (0.6)(220 - 43) \text{ and } (0.8)(220 - 43)$$
$$= (0.6)(177) \text{ and } (0.8)(177)$$
$$= 106 \text{ and } 142$$

or between 106 and 142 beats per minute. The target heart rate for a patient with cardiovascular pathology is adjusted by a physician based on clinical findings for the individual patient.

3.2   BLOOD PRESSURE

Purpose

Blood pressure (BP) is a measure of vascular resistance to blood flow. The primary purposes for measuring blood pressure are to determine vascular resistance to blood flow, and to determine the effectiveness of cardiac muscle in pumping blood to overcome the vascular resistance. There are two values reported as a measurement of blood pressure. The first value represents **systolic pressure,** which is a measurement of the pressure exerted by

CLINICAL NOTE

Adults 60–85
Infants 80–100
Bradycardia less
than 60
Tachycardia greater
than 100

LO-3

LO-4

LO-1

blood against arterial walls when the heart is contracting. The second value represents **diastolic pressure,** which is a measure of the pressure exerted by blood against arterial walls when the heart is not contracting.

LO-2

Method

Commonly, measurement of blood pressure is performed by auscultation of an artery using a stethoscope and a **sphygmomanometer.** A sphygmomanometer consists of an air bladder inside a cuff, a device for inflating the bladder, and a device for measuring the pressure in the bladder. Blood pressure measurements are actually measurements of the cuff's air bladder pressure. This pressure corresponds to arterial pressure as arterial blood flow occurs past the occluding cuff.

Blood pressure measurements were originally based on the pressure required to raise a column of mercury in a glass tube. Therefore, blood pressure measurements are stated in millimeters of mercury (mm Hg). To avoid potential exposure to mercury, air pressure gauges or electronic devices are now commonly used for measuring the bladder pressure, but blood pressure measurements continue to be reported in mm Hg. Should a mercury sphygmomanometer be used, care must be taken to avoid breaking the glass tube that contains the mercury, and to prevent the mercury column from separating.

Blood pressure readings are reported as the systolic blood pressure over the diastolic blood pressure, but without the use of units. A patient with a systolic pressure of 120 mm Hg and a diastolic pressure of 80 mm Hg, will be reported as having a blood pressure of 120/80 ("120 over 80").

A blood pressure cuff is placed snugly around the arm, midway between the shoulder and elbow. The inflation bulb must be within easy reach and the pressure gauge must be positioned where it can be read easily. The antecubital arterial pulse is identified visually or by palpation.

A stethoscope is used to auscultate the sounds of arterial blood flow through the antecubital artery in the antecubital fossa. The sounds to be monitored are called Korotkoff sounds.[4] The pressure relief valve on the inflation bulb is closed, and the cuff is inflated to approximately 200 mm Hg, a level well above estimated systolic blood pressure.

When the cuff is inflated above the systolic blood pressure, the artery is totally occluded. Therefore, no sounds of blood flow emanate from the antecubital artery. Air is evacuated from the cuff by opening the pressure relief valve slowly. As the pressure in the cuff falls to the level of systolic blood pressure, blood flows through the antecubital artery during systole (contraction phase), but not during diastole (noncontraction phase). The sounds heard through the stethoscope at this cuff pressure are usually described as tapping sounds. Initially the tapping sound may be difficult to hear as the sounds may be faint or soft, and may not occur evenly. As cuff pressure falls, the tapping sounds becomes more distinct and clear. The tapping nature of the sound is the result of the start of blood flow during systole and the stopping of blood flow during diastole. This occurs because at this level of cuff pressure, arterial flow can only occur during systole. When the first tapping sounds are heard, a pressure reading is noted, and represents the value of systolic blood pressure.

As more air is evacuated from the cuff, pressure falls towards the diastolic level. When the cuff pressure is at the diastolic blood pressure level the distinct and clear tapping becomes muffled, and usually disappears af-

CLINICAL NOTE

$$BP = \frac{\text{Systolic Pressure}}{\text{Diastolic Pressure}}$$

LO-5

CLINICAL NOTE

Systolic reading taken when the first tapping sounds are heard

ter an additional drop of 5 to 10 mm Hg. The muffling of sounds occurs because at this level of cuff pressure blood flows through the antecubital artery during both systole and diastole. When the tapping sounds become muffled a pressure reading is noted. This reading represents the value of diastolic blood pressure.

At this time, the pressure in the cuff can be evacuated rapidly by opening the pressure relief valve completely. The stethoscope and cuff can then be removed from the patient.

Throughout this procedure, care must be taken not to maintain pressure on the antecubital artery for more than 2 or 3 minutes without relief. If cuff occlusion occurs for more than 2 or 3 minutes without relief, the patient may experience symptoms of tingling or numbness, such as when an arm or leg "falls asleep."

CLINICAL NOTE

Diastolic reading taken when sounds become muffled

CLINICAL NOTE

Cuff should not be inflated for more than 2 to 3 minutes at a time

Site

LO-1

The most common site for measuring blood pressure is the left upper arm. This site corresponds closely to the level of the tricuspid valve in the heart, which is considered the "reference level for pressure measurement."[4] Measurements made at the level of the upper arm are within 1 mm Hg of measurements made at the heart in the same body position. Although body position may change blood pressure, such changes are accurately measured when using the upper arm as the reference level.

Norms

LO-3

As a reference point for blood pressure, 120/80 is considered ideal. Blood pressure will change with stress or physical activity, and with age. Approximate ranges of pressure at different ages are presented in Table 3–1.[4]

LO-4

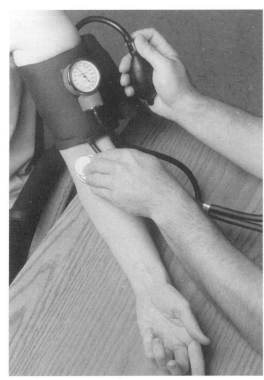

Figure 3.2–1. Blood pressure cuff and stethoscope in place.

TABLE 3–1. Approximate Ranges of Blood Pressure by Age

	Pressure (mm Hg)		
Age	*Systolic*	*Mean*	*Diastolic*
Birth	85 to 100	75	50 to 65
40	125 to 140	110	85 to 100
80	160 to 175	125	100 to 115

LO-4

Table 3–2 presents blood pressure levels which are generally accepted to define normal limits, but are not absolute boundaries. Higher levels are considered to indicate the existence of hypertension, and lower levels are considered to indicate the existence of hypotension. Judgments based on the values presented in Table 3–2 must also include a consideration of age, as presented in Table 3–1, and other medical information gathered on evaluation of each individual patient.

TABLE 3–2. Approximate Hypertension/Hypotension Levels (mm Hg)

	Pressure (mm Hg)	
Type	*Hypertension Pressure*	*Hypotension Pressure*
Systolic	140	90
Diastolic	90	60

Changes from resting blood pressure can result as patients change position or increase activity. A drop greater than 10 mm Hg, or a reading greater than 250 mm Hg, for systolic pressure indicates a need to stop activity and assess the patient's cardiac status. The same is true for an increase greater than 20 mm Hg for diastolic pressure. Failure of systolic pressure to rise in proportion with increased intensity of activity is also of concern.

3.3   RESPIRATION

LO-1

Purpose

Respiratory rate is the measurement of breathing rate. Each **respiratory cycle** includes one inspiration and the subsequent expiration. Respiratory rate can be measured and the quality of respiration can be observed.

LO-2

Method

The methods of measurement and observation are visual, auditory, and at times, palpation. In many cases, auditory measurement and observation can be performed without using a stethoscope. Unobtrusive visual and auditory observations can be made just prior to, or just following, taking a pulse. In cases where shallow or quiet breathing patterns make visual and auditory observation difficult, a stethoscope may improve auditory observation, and palpation can also be used.

A therapist's hand placed lightly on the patient's thorax will allow the therapist to feel the rise and fall of the chest during the inspiratory and expiratory phases of respiration.

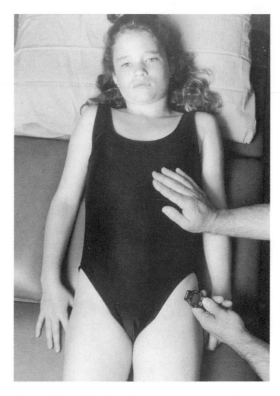

Figure 3.3–1. Palpation of respiratory rate on chest wall.

An alternative method of palpation is for the therapist to place the back of a hand close to, but not touching or occluding, the patient's mouth and nose. Changes in the direction of air flow during respiration can be felt as slight pressure and temperature changes on the dorsal surface of the hand.

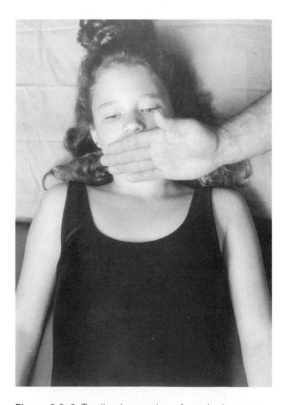

Figure 3.3–2. Tactile observation of respiration over nose and mouth.

LO-5

Respiratory rate is measured as the number of breathing cycles per minute. To obtain a respiratory rate, a watch or clock that displays time in seconds is used. Once respiration can be visualized or palpated, cycles are counted for a set period of time. Each complete respiratory cycle consists of two major phases, inspiration and expiration. Only complete respiratory cycles, those consisting of both inspiratory and expiratory phases, are counted. Measurements may be over a 60-second time period, or shorter time periods may be used. The same problems of accuracy noted previously for determining heart rate when using shortcut methods also apply to measurements of respiratory rate. Respiration is measured as cycles per minute but is reported without the use of units. A respiration rate of 12 respirations per minute is reported as 12.

Duration of inspiratory and expiratory phases can also be measured. Depth of inspiration, regularity of inspiration, and use of accessory muscles of respiration can be observed as indicators of the quality of respiration.

Norms

LO-3

LO-4

The normal respiratory rate for adults is approximately 12 breaths per minute.[4] Breathing rates at rest of less than 10 breaths per minute, or greater than 20 breaths per minute, are considered abnormal.[4] A normal breathing pattern should be even and relatively quiet, with a slight pause between the end of expiration and the initiation of inspiration. Only a very low-level hiss of air movement through the nose or mouth should be evident. Small variations may be noted, depending upon an individual's level of physical training and state of anxiety. Children normally have a respiratory rate of approximately 20 breaths per minute. The ratio of inspiration time to expiration time within one complete respiratory cycle (I/E ratio) is normally 1 to 2.[7]

Following periods of exercise, or during respiratory distress, respiration may increase to 40 or 50 breaths per minute for short periods of time. At these times, breathing will be more shallow, and accessory muscles of respiration around the neck and shoulder region will more likely be involved in the breathing pattern. When a patient is in respiratory distress, increased sounds of respiration, termed stridor, may be evident. In patients with obstructive lung disease, an I/E ratio as high as 1 to 4 may be observed.[7]

3.4 TEMPERATURE

LO-1

Purpose

Body **temperature** is one indication of the metabolic state of an individual. Temperature measurements provide information concerning basal metabolic state, possible presence or absence of infection, and metabolic response to exercise.

Method

Originally **thermometers** were made of a graduated glass tube with a bulb to hold a small quantity of mercury. Changes in temperature cause the mercury to expand or contract, indicating different temperatures. A minimum of 3 minutes is necessary for a stabile reading on a mercury thermometer. After extracting the thermometer from the measurement site, the measurement at the highest level of mercury should be read and recorded as the temperature.

LO-2

Electronic thermometers with disposable probes or probe covers have supplanted glass thermometers in many instances, and may take less time. Electronic thermometers can be used in measuring axillary or oral temperature. A tympanic thermometer is required when measuring temperature at the ear. Electronic thermometers produce a digital reading of the temperature and often make a sound when the maximum temperature is reached. The digital display of temperature will hold the value of the highest temperature until the instrument is reset.

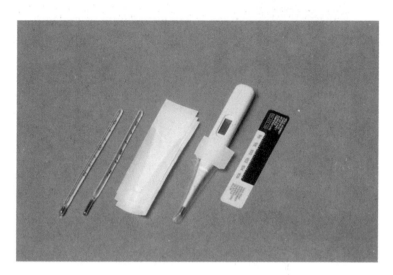

Figure 3.4–1. Examples of thermometers and accessories.

Measurements can be made on the forehead using heat sensitive strips that indicate a temperature range rather than a specific degree. When used on the extremities, such strips can also be used as indicators of the adequacy of peripheral circulation.

Prior to each use, inspection of the thermometer should be performed to determine that (1) the mercury in the thermometer has not separated, (2) the mercury in the thermometer has been shaken down to a point below the expected temperature, and (3) the glass that comprises the thermometer is not cracked, split, or chipped, and does not present any danger of cuts or mercury leakage to the patient. Reusable thermometers must be cleansed and sterilized between uses. When probes are used, a new probe cover must be used with each patient.

In all cases, the patient should remain quiet during the time a temperature measurement is being taken. Close supervision of young children and incompetent patients is necessary for safety and to obtain an accurate measurement.

LO-5

Measurements of body temperature can be recorded in degrees Fahrenheit or degrees Celsius.

Site

LO-1

Oral, rectal, and axillary temperature measurements are most commonly used. Traditionally, oral and rectal temperatures are considered the most accurate measurements of core temperature. Axillary and tympanic temperature measurements are used primarily for children, and when the patient has a medical complication that prevents easy and safe access to the mouth or rectum.

Oral temperature is taken by placing the thermometer or probe under the tongue. The tip of the thermometer or probe should be placed as far back as is comfortable for the patient. Probe covers must be changed for each patient.

Rectal temperature is taken by inserting the thermometer into the rectum carefully. The thermometer may be lubricated to provide comfort and safety for the patient during insertion and extraction.

Axillary temperature is taken by placing the tip of the thermometer into the deepest part of the axilla and lowering the arm to close the axilla over the thermometer.

Tympanic temperature is taken by placing the sensor carefully into the ear. The sensor should be placed as far into the ear as is comfortable. Sensor covers must be changed for each patient.

Norms

LO-3

Normal core temperature is considered to be a range centered at 98.6°F or 37°C. An individual's temperature will fluctuate throughout a 24-hour period, but these fluctuations should not be more than a few degrees. Depending upon time of day, site of measurement, and level of activity, normal temperatures will vary within general ranges.[4] Therapeutic treatments of heat and cold will cause variations of local site temperatures of several degrees Fahrenheit, and may affect core temperatures by 1°F or 2°F. Table 3–3 presents temperature ranges for various situations.

TEMPERATURE RANGES

Hyperthermia greater than 106°F
Normal 98.6°F ± 1 or 2°
Hypothermia less than 94°F

TABLE 3–3. Ranges of Normal Temperatures

	Site			
	Oral		Rectal	
Situation	°F	°C	°F	°C
Usual Normal Range	96.8 to 99.5	36.0 to 37.5	96.8 to 99.7	36.0 to 37.6
Morning/Cold weather	95.0 to 96.8	35.0 to 36.0	95.9 to 97.0	35.3 to 36.1
Hard work/Emotion/ A few normal adults/ Many active children	99.7 to 101.0	37.6 to 38.3	99.7 to 101.5	37.6 to 38.6
Hard exercise			101.2 to 104.0	38.4 to 40.0

LO-4

Patients with a normal core temperature of 98.6°F are considered to be **afebrile** when oral temperature remains below 100°F (37.8°C). When oral temperature in these patients exceeds 100°F, they are considered to be **febrile. Hyperthermia** is defined as a rectal core temperature greater than 106°F (41.1°C). **Hypothermia** is defined as a rectal core temperature less than 94°F (34.4°C).[4]

3.5 REVIEW QUESTIONS

1. What are the four major vital signs?

2. Define pulse and list the common sites at which pulse is measured.

3. What are the normal and abnormal ranges for pulse?

4. How is the accuracy of pulse measurement affected by different methods for computing pulse?

5. How is target heart rate determined?

6. Define blood pressure and list the common sites at which blood pressure is measured.

7. What are the normal and abnormal ranges for blood pressure?

8. Define respiration and list the common sites at which respiration is measured.

9. What are the normal and abnormal ranges of respiration?

10. Define body temperature and list the common sites at which body temperature is measured.

11. What are the normal and abnormal ranges of body temperature?

3.6 SUGGESTED ACTIVITIES

1. Students practice assessing vital signs of classmates with classmate sitting or lying quietly. Students document results as the results would be included in the Objective section of a SOAP note. Students compare results to norms to determine if results are in the normal range or hyper or hypo.

2. Students practice assessing vital signs of classmates before, during, and after activity such as riding a stationary bike, running on a treadmill, or lifting weights. Students document results as the results would be included in the Objective section of a SOAP note. Students compare results to norms.

3.7 References

1. Hollerbach AD and Sneed NV. Accuracy of radial pulse assessment by length of counting interval. *Heart and Lung.* 1990;19:258–264.
2. Jones ML. Accuracy of pulse rates counted for fifteen, thirty, and sixty seconds. *Military Med.* 1970;Dec:1127–1135.
3. Hargest TS. Start your count with zero. *Am J Nursing,* 1974;74:887.
4. Guyton AC. *Textbook of Medical Physiology.* 8th ed. Philadelphia: WB Saunders; 1991.
5. McArdle WD, Katch FI, and Katch VL. *Exercise Physiology: Energy, Nutrition, and Human Performance.* 2nd ed. Philadelphia: Lea and Febiger; 1985;358–359.
6. Kispert CP. Clinical measurements to assess cardiopulmonary function. *Phys Ther.* 1987;67:1886–1890.
7. Humberstone N. Respiratory assessment. In: Irwin S, Tecklin JS, eds. *Cardiopulmonary Physical Therapy.* St. Louis, MO: CV Mosby; 1985; vol 1:209–229.

Chapter

4

Aseptic Techniques

 Learner Objectives

The student will be able to:

1 Use defined terms correctly.
2 Describe universal precautions, including who is responsible for implementation, when to implement, and methods of implementation.
3 Recognize when the guidelines for a sterile field are violated, and act appropriately.
4 Describe the purposes for each of the components of apparel used when implementing aseptic techniques.
5 Describe proper technique for handwashing.
6 Distinguish between procedures for handwashing and scrubbing.
7 Demonstrate proper procedure for donning a sterile gown, sterile gloves while wearing a sterile gown, and sterile gloves while wearing a clean gown.
8 Demonstrate proper procedure for removal of contaminated gloves.
9 Describe the characteristics of wounds that are evaluated, and the purposes and methods of wound dressings.
10 Describe commonly used wound dressing materials and their correct application.
11 Describe methods of sterilization of objects used in medical settings.
12 Describe general principles for disposal of medical waste, managing laundry in a medical setting, and housekeeping in a medical setting.
13 Describe general principles of isolation, and the purposes of steps used in isolation.
14 Distinguish between Category Specific and Disease Specific systems of isolation.

INTRODUCTION

Increased emphasis on the importance of prevention of disease transmission
and the spread of infection through proper patient care techniques has occurred in recent years. Part of this emphasis has occurred because of the increasing incidence of catastrophic diseases, such as acquired immunodeficiency syndrome (AIDS). An expansion of research on techniques that may
prevent the transmission of such diseases has also provided new information concerning cleaning, disinfecting, and sterile technique. Although the
concepts of cleanliness and aseptic technique in patient care have been in
use during the past 2 centuries, changes in these techniques are constantly
occurring because of newly discovered information.

In most cases, health care personnel do not have direct contact with all
steps in the sequence of preparation and use of equipment for patient care.
Those who perform equipment and environment preparation are rarely involved in the use of the equipment with patients, while those who use equipment in the clinical environment during patient care are rarely involved in the
process of equipment and environment preparation. It is important, however,
for personnel involved in patient care to understand the underlying basis for
aseptic techniques, and processes used to achieve the goals of asepsis. Use of
this information makes the requirements of, and rationale for, aseptic technique and isolation precautions easier to understand, and assists in avoiding
errors of omission and commission that can affect patients adversely.

Much of the material in this chapter is taken from publications in the
public domain produced by the **Center for Infectious Diseases** (CID), a
part of the **Centers for Disease Control and Prevention** (CDC) (Public
Health Service, US Department of Health and Human Services). The Center
for Infectious Diseases is continually updating recommendations for cleaning, disinfecting, and sterile technique based on an increasing body of scientific knowledge. While the information in this chapter can provide a starting
point for study in aseptic techniques, it is strongly advised that updated information on specific techniques be sought directly from the Center for Infectious Diseases. Such information can be obtained from:

> US Department of Health and Human Services
> Public Health Service
> Centers for Disease Control and Prevention
> Center for Infectious Diseases
> Hospital Infections Program
> Atlanta, GA 30333
> (404) 639-3311.

Information specific to an institution can be obtained from the appropriate
department within the institution.

LO-1

4.1   DEFINITIONS

Definitions are used by the medical community to standardize terminology.
Several terms utilized in this chapter are defined below. Not all definitions
related to ASEPTIC TECHNIQUES are included.

Aseptic technique: Aseptic techniques consist of the methods and procedures used to create and maintain a sterile field.

Bacterial barrier: A bacterial barrier is a barrier that keeps microorganisms
   from coming in contact with sterile items.

Cleanliness: Three levels of cleanliness—cleaning, disinfection, and sterilization—have been established for equipment use in patient care.[1]

Cleaning is the physical removal of organic material or soil from objects. The process of cleaning is usually performed with water, with or without detergents. Cleaning is the least rigorous of the three levels and is designed to remove microorganisms rather than kill them. Cleaning usually precedes either of the next two levels, disinfection or sterilization.

Disinfection is an intermediate level between cleaning and sterilization. Three levels of disinfection—high, intermediate, and low—have been defined. Disinfection is usually performed using pasteurization or chemical germicides.

Sterilization is the highest level of cleanliness. Sterilization is the destruction of all forms of microbial life by steam under pressure, liquid or gaseous chemicals, or dry heat.

Contaminated: An item, surface, or field is considered to be contaminated whenever it has come into contact with anything that is not sterile.

Nosocomial infection: Infection acquired while hospitalized for treatment of other conditions.

Patient care equipment categories: Three categories of patient care equipment—critical, semicritical, and noncritical[1]—provide a basis for the level of cleanliness deemed necessary.

Critical items are those that are introduced directly into the circulatory system or other normally sterile areas of the body. Surgical instruments, implants, and the blood compartment of a hemodialyzer are examples of critical items.

Semicritical items include, but are not limited to, endotracheal tubes and fiberoptic endoscopes. There is less degree of risk of infection associated with semicritical items.

Noncritical items are items that do not touch the patient, or touch the patient in areas that are normally not sterile, ie, intact areas of skin. Blood pressure cuffs and crutches are examples of noncritical items.

Recommendations ranking scheme: The Center for Infectious Diseases of the CDC has established three categories to indicate the scientific support for their recommendations.[2]

Category I recommendations are strongly supported by well-designed and controlled clinical studies. Recommendations in this category are considered effective, and applicable in most hospitals.

Category II recommendations are supported by highly suggestive clinical studies. Recommendations in this category may not have been adequately studied, but are based on a logical or strong theoretical rationale. Such recommendations are considered to have probable effectiveness, and as practical to implement in most hospitals.

Category III recommendations are proposed by some investigators, authorities, or organizations. At the time of classification in this category, there was a lack of supporting data, strong theoretical rationale, or indication of benefits to be derived on a cost-effective basis. Recommendations in this category are considered important issues to be studied, and may be implemented by some hospitals. Such recommendations are not generally recommended for widespread use.

Shelf life: Shelf life is the length of time an item that has been packaged and sterilized is considered to remain sterile as long as it remains unopened.

Sterile: An item or environment is considered sterile while there is an absence of living microorganisms.

Sterile field: A sterile field is an area in which there are no microorganisms considered to be living.

Unsterile (nonsterile): Any item or environment is considered unsterile when it has not been sterilized, has come into contact with an item that is no longer considered sterile, has entered a field that is not sterile, or has exceeded its shelf life.

LO-2

4.2 UNIVERSAL PRECAUTIONS

Universal precautions is the application to all patients of Blood and Body Fluid Precautions by all health care workers. It is extremely important that universal precautions be implemented by *all* health care workers with *all* patients because of the rising incidence of viruses and diseases, such as human immunodeficiency virus (HIV) and hepatitis. Universal precautions are intended to prevent parenteral, mucous membrane, and nonintact (open) skin exposures of health care workers to pathogens in blood and other body fluids and tissues. The recommendations are that a **protective barrier** exist between a health care worker and potentially infective materials. At a minimum, a protective barrier is considered to be the use of nonsterile gloves. In certain circumstances masks, eye protection, and protective clothing may be required. The context and detail of Blood and Body Fluid Precautions are discussed later in this chapter in the section "Alternative Systems for Isolation Precautions," and specifically the subsection "Blood and Body Fluid Precautions."

> **CLINICAL NOTE**
>
> All health care workers use universal precautions with all patients

> **PROTECTIVE BARRIERS**
>
> Gloves
> Mask
> Eye protection
> Protective clothing

4.3 STERILE FIELD

The primary goal of using aseptic techniques is to prevent infection. One aseptic technique is to provide and maintain a **sterile field.** A sterile field is most commonly required in an operating room. There may be a necessity for a sterile field, however, in patient care areas other than the operating room for the performance of minor procedures. Such procedures may include, but not be limited to, insertion of arterial lines or debridement of burn patients.

There are eight guidelines for providing and maintaining a sterile field. The first four guidelines concern creation of a sterile field. The second four guidelines concern maintenance of the sterile field.

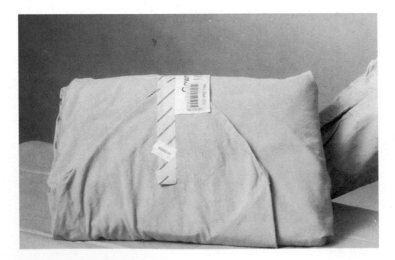

Figure 4.3–1. Sterile package with sterilization indicator tape.

Guideline 1

LO-3

All items used within the boundaries of a sterile field must be sterile. The items must have been properly sterilized and maintained to preserve their sterile state. Once items have been sterilized, they must be used within the allowable shelf life of the item and sterilization process. The **expiration date,** or end of **shelf life** is marked on each sterile package. Certain types of equipment and different types of packaging may affect the shelf life of a sterile package.

Shelf-life date of a sterile package is not

a guarantee that the package is sterile. Packages are only considered to remain sterile when the

1. Initial packaging was performed properly
2. Initial sterilization was performed properly
3. Package was stored in a proper manner
4. Package was not mishandled during distribution
5. Shelf-life date has not been exceeded

Guideline 2

Once a sterile package has been opened, the edges are not considered sterile. Care in opening sterile packages is required to avoid having the edges touch the contents of the package, or having the edges touch the gloved hands or sterile gown. Most sterile packages have enough packaging material around the edges to keep the unsterile edges far enough away from the sterile contents.

Whenever possible, single-use items are preferred. Because single-use items are discarded after use, there is no concern about contamination before they are reused. This does not mean, however, that single-use items cannot become contaminated before the initial use through improper technique or carelessness.

Guideline 3

Once donned properly, sterile gowns are considered to be sterile in the front from shoulder level to table top level, including the sleeves. For this reason, during and after scrubbing, gowning, and gloving, the hands must be held above table top level, in front of the body. Unsterile personnel can only assist with tie ends by using sterile forceps.

Guideline 4

Tables are only considered to be sterile at table top level. **Sterile drapes** cover the top of a surface and descend on all sides of the surface. Such draping may be on a patient or on an instrument table. In all cases, only the top surface is considered sterile. Demarcation of sterile surfaces are fairly easy on tables, but more difficult on patients. A guideline to use for demarcation on a patient that is draped is to consider that a surface above the level of the instrument table, or above waist level, whichever is higher, is a sterile surface as long as it is properly draped. Undraped, improperly draped surfaces, or surfaces below the top level of the instrument table or waist, are considered unsterile.

CLINICAL NOTE

1. Sterile field: Sterile objects only

LO-3

CLINICAL NOTE

2. Open sterile package: Edges not sterile

LO-3

CLINICAL NOTE

3. Sterile gown: Front of gown, shoulder to table top level, including sleeves

LO-3

CLINICAL NOTE

4. Sterile area: Top of table only

LO-3

CLINICAL NOTE

5. Sterile area: Only sterile objects and personnel in sterile attire enter

Guideline 5

Only sterile items and personnel in sterile attire may enter a sterile area. Only sterile items and personnel in sterile attire may touch sterile items without causing contamination. Personnel considered unsterile may not touch any item in a sterile area, or any item to be placed in a sterile area. Transfer of sterile items into a sterile area may be accomplished by using sterile forceps to hold the item as it is passed into the sterile area. The set of forceps is considered contaminated after a single use, and may not be used again until properly sterilized. Unsterile personnel may not reach across or into a sterile area.

LO-3

CLINICAL NOTE

6. Sterile area: All personnel are responsible for ensuring sterile area

Guideline 6

Activity in a sterile area cannot be allowed to render the area unsterile. Sterile personnel may not leave and re-enter a sterile area without performing the scrubbing and gowning process again. Personnel in sterile attire should not sit on, or lean against, unsterile surfaces. Movements within the sterile area must be measured and careful to avoid contact between sterile and unsterile surfaces.

All personnel, sterile or unsterile, in or around a sterile area must be aware of the boundaries of a sterile area. Any contamination of a sterile area must be pointed out immediately by any personnel present for the protection of the patient.

LO-3

CLINICAL NOTE

7. Examine sterile package for contamination prior to use

Guideline 7

Penetration of a sterile covering or barrier is considered to cause contamination of a sterile field. Liquids are the most likely cause of penetration of a sterile barrier. Liquids spilled within a sterile field may cause penetration of a sterile barrier.

A less noticeable, but highly potential, cause of penetration is air flow. The design of climate control for sterile areas provides for the most purified air possible, and a slightly higher gradient of air pressure in the sterile area. The higher air pressure gradient in the sterile area will cause air flow away from the site of potential infection. The climate control system should also be physically separated from other areas of the institution so that airborne microorganisms picked up in sterile areas do not permeate the atmosphere of the entire institution.

LO-3

CLINICAL NOTE

8. When in doubt, consider it unsterile

Guideline 8

When there is doubt about the sterile quality of an area, a field, or an item, it should be considered unsterile. Improper packaging, sterilization processing, storage, or handling can occur without overt signs. Appropriate use of all items in a sterile environment is the responsibility of the user. Only proper judgment, rigid discipline, and appropriate use provides protection for a patient.

Sterile areas and fields should be prepared as close to the time of use as feasible. They should not be left unattended. Sterile fields should not be prepared and then covered for later use. A delay in using equipment or supplies laid out in a sterile field necessitates the preparation of a new sterile field with new sterile equipment and supplies.

4.4 APPAREL

Scrub Suits

Scrub suits are used by health care personnel to

1. Limit the introduction of infectious agents into patient care environments
2. Provide ease of movement during patient care
3. Avoid soiling clothing

Scrub suits are not sterile.

LO-4

> **CLINICAL NOTE**
> Protection:
> Scrub suits

Masks

Masks are recommended to prevent transmission of infectious agents through the air by acting as a barrier to the dispersal and receipt of infectious material. Masks protect the wearer from inhaling

1. Large-particle aerosols (droplets) that are transmitted by close contact and generally travel only short distances (about 3 feet).
2. Small-particle aerosols (droplet nuclei) that remain suspended in the air and thus travel longer distances.

Masks may prevent transmission of infections spread by direct contact with mucous membranes, because masks block personnel from touching the mucous membranes of their nose and mouth until after they have washed their hands and removed the mask.

Masks are recommended for all persons

1. In close proximity to patients with infections transmitted by large-particle aerosols (droplets).
2. Entering the room of a patient with infections capable of being transmitted over longer distances in the air.

When the use of a mask is indicated, it should be used only once and discarded in an appropriate receptacle. Masks should not be reused because

1. Using the same mask when moving between two or more patients can spread infection
2. Masks become ineffective when moist

Lowering a mask around the neck and placing it over the nose and mouth again is the same as reusing a mask.

Masks should cover both the nose and the mouth. High efficiency disposable masks are more effective than cotton gauze or paper tissue masks in preventing airborne and droplet spread.

LO-4

> **CLINICAL NOTE**
> Masks: Protect
> wearer and others
> in environment

Eye Protection

Shields, glasses, or goggles are worn to protect the eyes from contact with infected material or airborne contaminants. Shields and goggles are usually constructed of clear plastic. They provide a barrier in front and on the sides

LO-4

of the eyes. Glasses are usually used when the personnel involved require prescription vision correction. In most cases, glasses only provide a barrier in front of the eyes. Glasses with side shields provide an additional barrier. When prescription glasses are necessary, shields or goggles that can be worn over prescription glasses provide the best degree of protection.

LO-4

Gowns

Gowns are used to

1. Prevent soiling and contamination by infectious materials
2. Prevent transmission of infection
3. Create a sterile field

In most cases, unsterile gowns may be worn. Unsterile gowns can be constructed of either paper or cloth. Paper gowns are disposable. Sterile gowns are constructed of cloth and must be laundered when they are used as unsterile gowns, or laundered and sterilized when they are used as sterile gowns. Gowns of any type, and in any situation, should be worn only once and then removed and placed in an appropriate receptacle.

LO-4

Gloves

Gloves are now worn as a universal precaution. Gloves are worn to prevent transmission of infection from personnel to patient, and patient to personnel. Nonsterile gloves are worn when hands are likely to become contaminated with potentially infective material, ie, body fluids or excretions, since it is often not known which patient's body fluids or excretions contain infectious agents. Sterile gloves are required when certain invasive procedures are performed, or when open wounds are touched. Handwashing is required after gloves are removed because gloves can become perforated during use, and because bacteria can multiply rapidly on gloved hands.

When gloves are required, disposable single-use gloves should be worn. Used gloves should be removed properly and discarded into an appropriate receptacle.

Accessories

Additional apparel, including caps, beard covers, and shoe covers, must be worn as necessary to maintain clean or sterile fields.

LO-5

4.5   HANDWASHING

Introduction

Handwashing is the single most important means of preventing the spread of nosocomial infection. Hands must be washed between all patient contacts. Handwashing is defined as a vigorous and brief rubbing together of all surfaces of lathered hands, followed by rinsing under a flowing stream of water.

Although handwashing is considered the most important single procedure for preventing nosocomial infections, two reports showed poor compliance with handwashing protocols by personnel in medical intensive care units, especially by physicians[3] and personnel taking care of patients that are on isolation precautions.[4] Failure to wash hands is a complex problem that may be caused by lack of motivation or lack of knowledge about the importance of handwashing.

The circumstances that require handwashing are frequently found in high-risk units, because patients in these units are often infected or colonized with virulent or multiply resistant microorganisms, and are highly susceptible to infection because of wounds, invasive procedures, or diminished immune function. Handwashing in these units is indicated between direct contact with different patients and is often indicated more than once in the care of one patient, ie, after touching excretions or secretions and before going on to another care activity for the same patient.

CDC Recommendations (PB85-923404)

1. Indications
   a. In the absence of a true emergency, personnel should always wash their hands
      (1) before performing invasive procedures; *Category I*
      (2) before taking care of particularly susceptible patients, such as those who are severely immunocompromised and newborns; *Category I*
      (3) before and after touching wounds, whether surgical, traumatic, or associated with an invasive device; *Category I*
      (4) after situations during which microbial contamination of hands is likely to occur, especially those involving contact with mucous membranes, blood or body fluids, secretions, or excretions; *Category I*
      (5) after touching inanimate sources that are likely to be contaminated with virulent or epidemiologically important microorganisms; these sources include urine-measuring devices or secretion-collection apparatuses; *Category I*
      (6) after taking care of an infected patient or one who is likely to be colonized with microorganisms of special clinical or epidemiologic significance, eg, multiply resistant bacteria; *Category I*
      (7) between contacts with different patients in high-risk units. *Category I*
   b. Most routine, brief patient care activities involving direct patient contact other than that discussed in 1.a. above, eg, taking a blood pressure, do not require handwashing. *Category II*
   c. Most routine hospital activities involving indirect patient contact, eg, handling patient medications, food, or other objects, do not require handwashing. *Category I*
2. Handwashing Technique—For routine handwashing, a vigorous rubbing together of all surfaces of lathered hands for at least 10 seconds, followed by thorough rinsing under a stream of water, is recommended. *Category I*
3. Handwashing With Plain Soap
   a. Plain soap should be used for handwashing unless otherwise indicated. *Category II*
   b. If bar soap is used it should be kept on racks that allow drainage of water. *Category II*

c. If liquid soap is used the dispenser should be replaced or cleaned and filled with fresh product when empty; liquids should not be added to a partially full dispenser. *Category II*

4. Handwashing With Antimicrobial-Containing Products (Health Care Personnel Handwashing)

   a. Antimicrobial handwashing products should be used for handwashing before personnel care for newborns and when otherwise indicated during their care, between patients in high-risk units, and before personnel take care of severely immunocompromised patients. *Category III* (Hospitals may choose from products in the product category defined by the FDA as health care personnel handwashes. Persons responsible for selecting commercially marketed antimicrobial health care personnel handwashes can obtain information about categorization of products from the Center for Drugs and Biologics, Division of OTC Drug Evaluation, FDA, 5600 Fishers Lane, Rockville, MD 20857.)

   b. Antimicrobial-containing products that do not require water for use, such as foams or rinses, can be used in areas where no sinks are available. *Category III*

5. Handwashing Facilities

   a. Handwashing facilities should be conveniently located throughout the hospital. *Category I*

   b. A sink should be located in or just outside every patient room. More than one sink per room may be necessary if a large room is used for several patients. *Category II*

   c. Handwashing facilities should be located in or adjacent to rooms where diagnostic or invasive procedures that require handwashing are performed, eg, cardiac catheterization, bronchoscopy, sigmoidoscopy, etc. *Category I*

LO-5

LO-6

CLINICAL NOTE

Lather, and rub all surfaces: At least 10 seconds each

4.6   PROCEDURES

Handwashing

The ideal duration of handwashing is not known. For most activities, a vigorous, brief rubbing together of all surfaces of lathered hands for a minimum of 10 seconds, followed by rinsing under a stream of water is recommended. When hands are visibly soiled, more time may be required for handwashing.

The absolute indications for handwashing with plain soaps and detergents versus handwashing with antimicrobial-containing products are not known because of the lack of well-controlled studies comparing infection rates when such products are used. For most routine activities, handwashing with plain soap appears to be sufficient, since soap will allow most transient microorganisms to be washed off.[5-7]

Scrubbing

LO-6

Scrubbing must be performed before entering a sterile field. Scrubbing is a series of specific steps of hand cleaning using scrub brushes and nail cleaners, and is of longer duration than handwashing. Two classifications of scrubbing are recommended prior to entering a sterile field. The long scrub requires approximately 7 to 10 minutes. The short scrub requires approximately 3 to 5 minutes. Requirements for each type of scrub may vary from institution to institution, and institutional policy should be confirmed before it becomes necessary to scrub. Whenever there is doubt as to environmental conditions and institutional policy, assume that the long scrub is necessary.

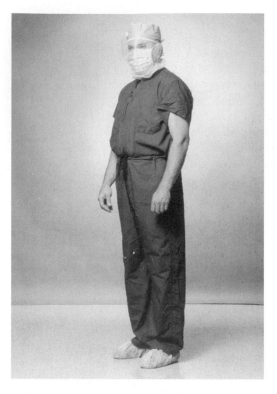

Figure 4.6–1. Scrub suit and accessories.

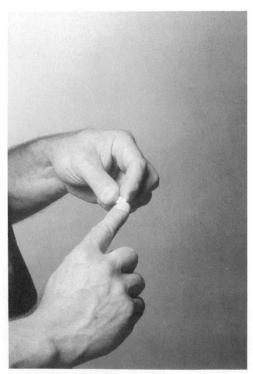

Figure 4.6–2. Using nail cleaner.

Prior to beginning the scrubbing procedure, a freshly laundered scrub suit (pants and shirt or dress), scrub cap, and a new mask are donned. The scrub suit is fastened completely and properly. All head hair must be covered by a scrub cap. Facial hair, when present, must be covered by a mask, and beard cover when necessary. The mask is formed to fit tightly but comfortably over the nose and mouth. Eye shields are worn to protect the eyes.

Water at the scrub sink is turned on using the knee or foot control. The temperature of the water should be warm and the flow moderate. A preliminary wash to remove surface dirt mechanically is performed by wetting and lathering both hands and arms to approximately 3 inches above the elbow. After rinsing the hands and arms, a nail cleaner from the nail cleaner dispenser is used to clean each nail on both hands. During nail cleaning, the hands are kept under the running water. In the illustration the hands are not in a flow of water to permit the use of the nail cleaner to be observed without distortion.

Following completion of nail cleaning, a prepackaged scrub sponge and brush are used. The sponge is wetted and squeezed gently to release lather. In this portion of the scrub, cleaning starts at the fingertips and moves proximally along each arm. A sponge is used to lather the specified areas, and each area is scrubbed with a brush. The illustrations for this section demonstrate the use of a brush only. The number of brush strokes listed for each segment is the minimum number, with each brush stroke consisting of one forward and one backward motion. Brush strokes should be as vigorous as tolerable for the area being cleansed. Each hand and arm must undergo the same sequence.

The fingernails of one hand are held to-gether and given 30 strokes for a long scrub (short scrub, 20 strokes).

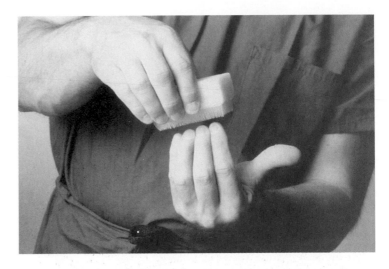

Figure 4.6–3. Position for fingernail scrub.

Each of the four long surfaces of each finger receives 15 strokes for a long scrub (short scrub, 10 strokes) using the narrow width of the brush. Starting at one side of one hand, each finger is cleaned in order.

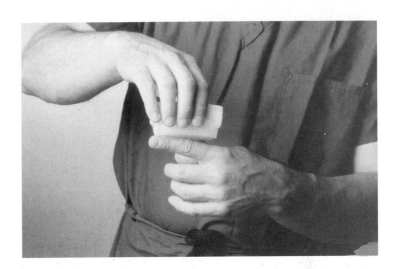

Figure 4.6–4. Position for lateral aspect finger scrub.

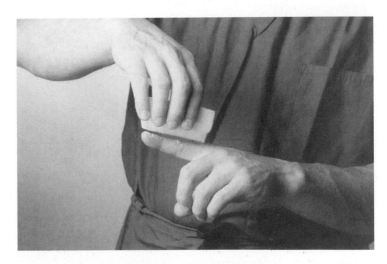

Figure 4.6–5. Position for dorsal aspect finger scrub.

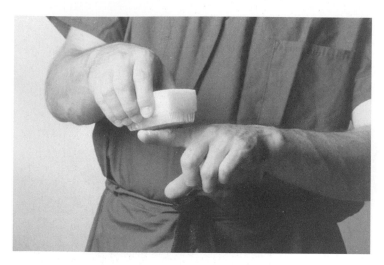

Figure 4.6–6. Perpendicular scrub across knuckles.

Several additional strokes are performed across each web space as the adjacent finger surfaces are cleansed. When all fingers of one hand are completed, several additional strokes across each set of knuckles are performed.

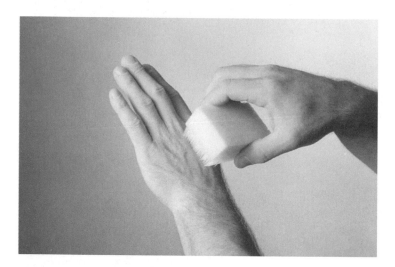

Figure 4.6–7. Position for hand scrub.

Each hand is considered to have six surfaces: the two narrow sides, a dorsal surface to the radial side, a dorsal surface to the ulnar side, a distal palmar surface, and a proximal palmar surface. Each surface receives 15 strokes for a long scrub (short scrub, 10 strokes).

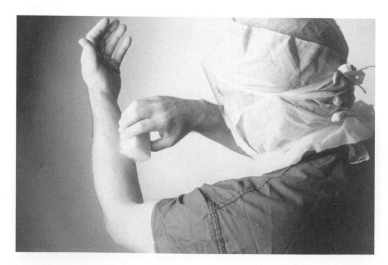

Figure 4.6–8. Position for forearm scrub.

The forearm has four surfaces. The entire length of the forearm is not scrubbed at one time. Starting at the wrist, scrub each of the four surfaces one third of the way along the forearm, one forearm at a time. When the forearm scrub has been completed, several horizontal strokes across the elbow and antecubital fossa are performed. The four surfaces of the upper arm are scrubbed with 15 strokes for a long scrub (short scrub, 10 strokes) to approximately 3 inches above the elbow.

Without rinsing the first scrubbed arm, scrub the second arm. After the second arm has been scrubbed, the scrub brush and sponge are discarded.

One arm at a time is rinsed from fingertips to elbow.

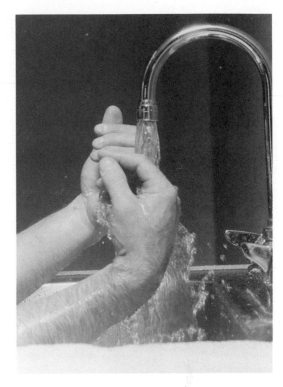

Figure 4.6–9. Position for scrub rinse.

When both arms have been rinsed, the arms are held in a V position, with the hands at shoulder height and the elbows at the lowest point. In this way, water will drop from the point of the elbows.

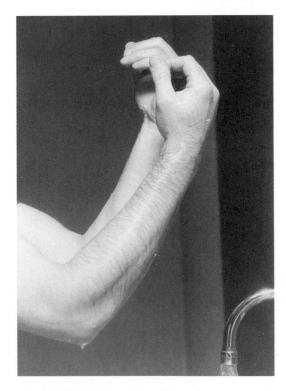

Figure 4.6–10. "V" position of arms for water run-off.

Having finished scrubbing and rinsing, the hands and arms must be protected from any contact. The water is turned off using the knee or foot control. When necessary, doors are opened by backing into them and pushing through the doorway proceeding to the area in which the sterile pack has been opened.

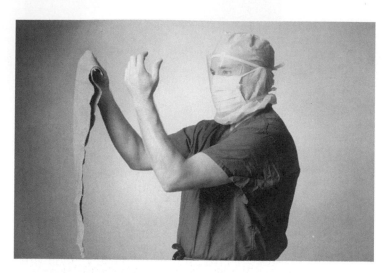

Without touching the sterile field, a towel from a sterile pack is grasped and lifted directly upward. The towel is held away from the body to avoid contamination from the scrub suit. Stepping back from the sterile pack, the towel is permitted to open lengthwise, remaining folded across the width of the towel.

Figure 4.6–11. Opening sterile towel for drying following scrub.

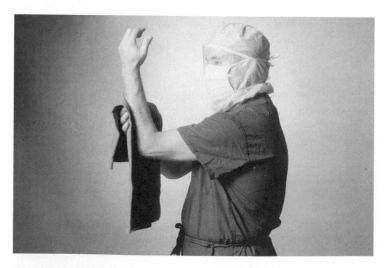

Using one end of the folded towel, one hand and arm are dried from distal to proximal. Each finger, and then the hand, is dried by a patting motion. The forearm and arm are dried using a slow, circular motion. Do not return to an area that has already been dried. When one arm has been completed, the unused portion of the towel is used to dry the other hand and arm. When both arms have been completely dried, discard the towel into the appropriate laundry hamper without touching any other equipment or clothing.

Figure 4.6–12. Using sterile towel for drying following scrub.

Gowning

LO-7

The gown is part of a sterile pack like the one containing the towel used for drying following the scrub process. The part of the gown facing you as you look at an open sterile pack is the inside, or unsterile side.

To gown, grasp the gown firmly and lift it up and away from the sterile field. Move away from the table on which the sterile pack rests, keeping hands above waist height at all times. Shake open the gown so it unfolds. Holding the inside of the gown only, locate the neck and armholes of the gown.

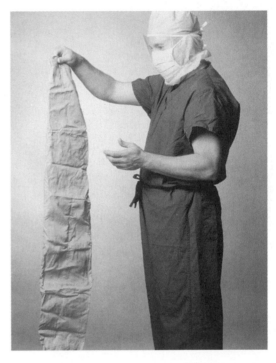

Figure 4.6–13. Lifting sterile gown from sterile pack in preparation for gowning.

Without touching the outside, or sterile side of the gown, work both arms into the sleeves at the same time. Stop when the hands reach the stockinette cuff.

The gown is tied at the back and neck closures by a circulating nurse or other unsterile personnel.

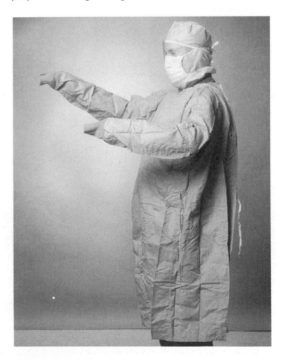

Figure 4.6–14. Inserting arms into armholes of sterile gown.

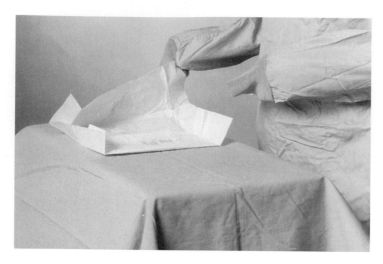

Figure 4.6–15. Opening inner wrapper of sterile glove set.

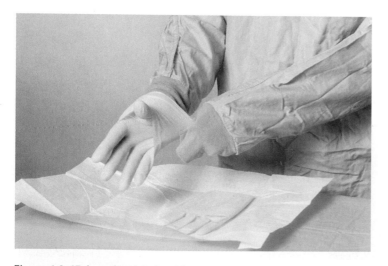

Figure 4.6–16. Inserting right thumb into thumb hole.

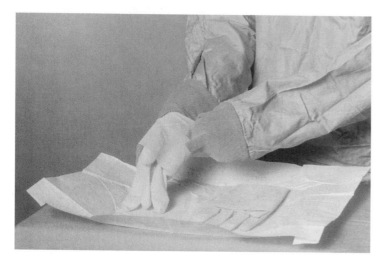

Figure 4.6–17. Inserting right hand into glove.

Gloving

With Sterile Gown

LO-7

To glove, both hands must be kept inside the gown sleeves just proximal to the stockinette cuff. Using the gown sleeves as "mittens," approach the sterile field without allowing the gown to touch the table, and open the sterile portion of the glove pack.

Gloves are packaged with the wrist end of the glove turned back onto the palm, creating a cuff. The exposed side of the cuff is the inside, or unsterile side, of the glove. The portion of the cuff facing into the palm of the glove is the outside, or sterile side, of the glove.

With the hands inside the gown sleeves and using the gown sleeves as "mittens," grasp the right glove with the left hand. With the right hand palm up, insert the thumb of the right hand (still inside the gown sleeve) into the thumb hole of the right-hand glove.

Holding the glove securely with the right thumb, work the remainder of the glove over the open end of the gown sleeve.

With the right glove stretched over the open end of the right gown sleeve, the right hand is worked through the stockinette cuff and into the glove as if the glove and sleeve were one piece.

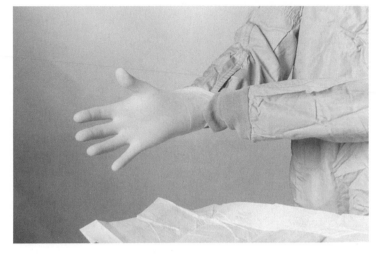

Figure 4.6–18. Completing insertion of right hand into glove.

The first two or three fingers of the gloved right hand are now slipped down inside the sterile side of the cuff of the left glove, starting at the palm of the glove, and pointing toward the crease of the cuff at the wrist.

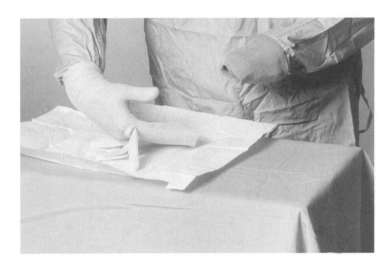

Figure 4.6–19. Position to lift left glove.

The left glove is lifted using the fingers inside the cuff only. The thumb of the gloved right hand cannot be used to grasp the left glove. While holding the left glove by the first two or three fingers on the inside (sterile side) of the cuff, the left hand is worked into the left glove.

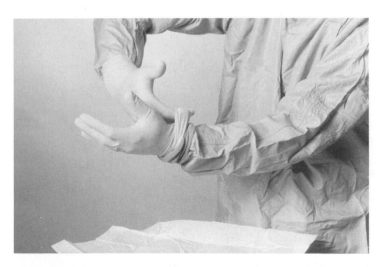

Figure 4.6–20. Inserting left hand into glove.

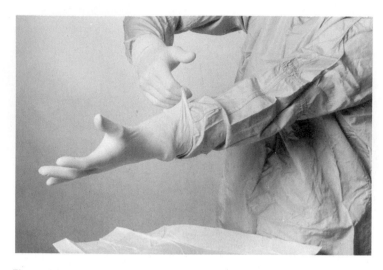

Figure 4.6–21. Unfolding cuff of left glove over gown sleeve.

With the fingers of the left hand in the proper position inside the left glove, the fingers of the right hand can unfold the cuff by pulling the cuff up over the sleeve of the gown,

and letting the wrist portion of the glove snap into place.

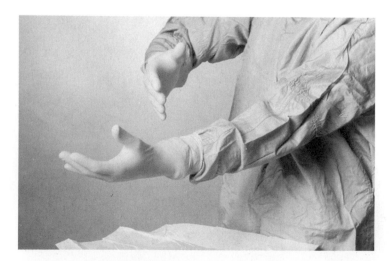

Figure 4.6–22. Completed gloving of left hand.

The gloved fingers of the left hand can now be placed on the inside (sterile side) of the right glove cuff.

The gloved left hand can then unfold the right cuff over the right sleeve.

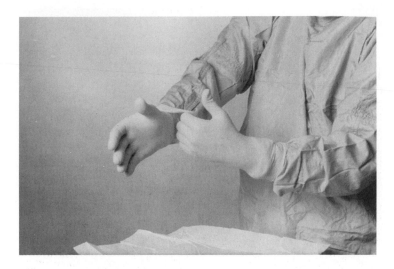

Figure 4.6–23. Unfolding cuff of right glove over gown sleeve.

Once both glove cuffs have been properly placed, the gloves can be adjusted on the fingers.

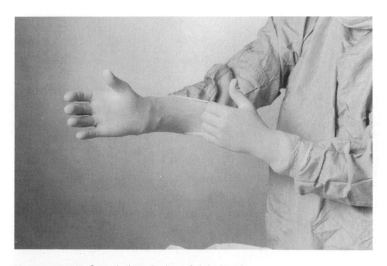

Figure 4.6–24. Completing gloving of right hand.

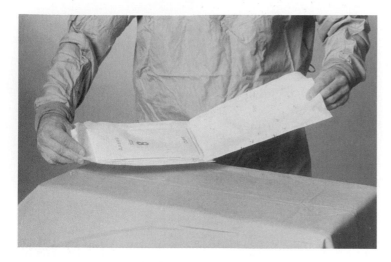

Figure 4.6–25. Opening outer wrapper of sterile glove package.

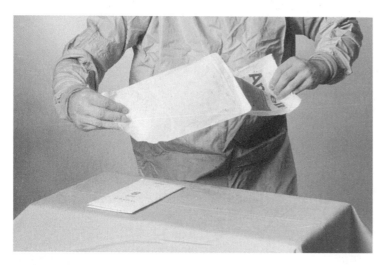

Figure 4.6–26. Placing inner package with sterile gloves on table.

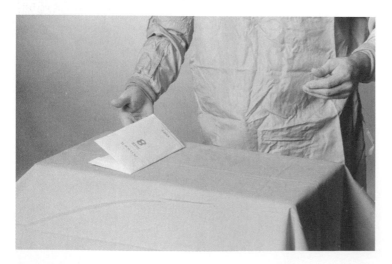

Figure 4.6–27. Opening inner wrapper of sterile glove set.

With Clean Gown

LO-7

An alternative method of gloving is used when only the gloved hands need to be sterile.

When gowning, the arms can be pushed all the way through the cuffs of the gown. The sterile portion of the glove pack is then opened without touching the gloves.

The wrist end of each glove has been turned back on itself, creating a cuff where the inside, or unsterile side, is now outward. Grasping the left glove by its cuff on the unsterile portion with a bare right hand, the left hand can be worked into the left glove.

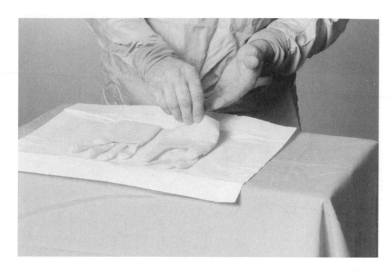

Figure 4.6–28. Grasping left glove with right hand.

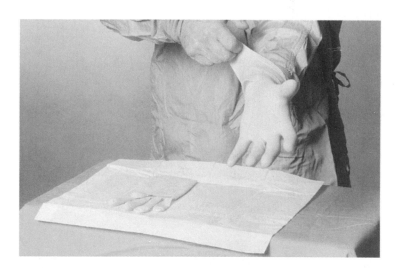

Figure 4.6–29. Inserting left hand into glove.

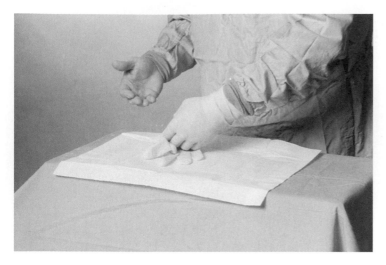

Figure 4.6–30. Lifting right glove with left hand.

Once the left glove is in place, it is now a sterile surface. The first two or three fingers of the gloved left hand are now slipped down inside the sterile side of the cuff of the right glove, starting at the palm of the right glove and pointing toward the crease of the cuff at the wrist.

The right glove is then lifted using the fingers inside the cuff only. The thumb of the gloved left hand cannot be used to grasp the right hand glove. As the right glove is held by the first two or three fingers on the inside (sterile side) of the cuff, the right hand is worked into the right glove.

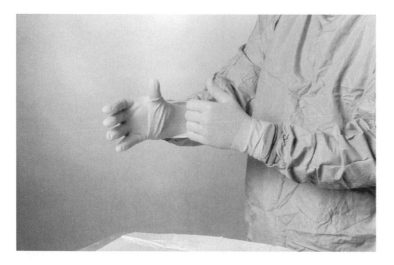

Figure 4.6–31. Inserting right hand into glove.

Once the fingers of the right hand are in the proper position inside the right glove, the fingers of the left hand can unfold the cuff by pulling the cuff up over the sleeve of the gown and letting the wrist portion of the glove snap into place.

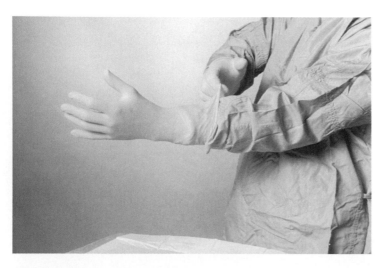

Figure 4.6–32. Completing gloving of left hand.

The fingers of the right hand, now sterile, can now be placed on the inside (sterile side) of the left glove cuff. The fingers of the gloved right hand can then unfold the cuff in the same manner as was done for the right glove. Once both glove cuffs have been properly placed, the gloves can be adjusted on the fingers.

For both methods of glove use, once gloved, both hands must remain above waist level, or the level of draping that defines the sterile field, whichever is appropriate. When a glove becomes torn or punctured during a sterile procedure, it no longer provides proper protection. Such a glove must be removed and discarded as soon as is feasible, and another sterile glove donned. This may require interruption of a procedure provided that the interruption does not threaten the patient's welfare.

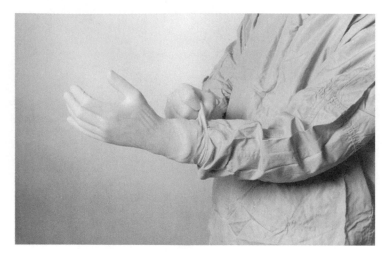

Figure 4.6–33. Grasping cuff of first glove for removal.

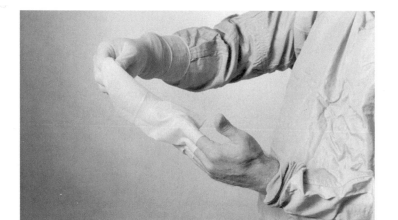

Figure 4.6–34. Removing first glove by turning glove inside out.

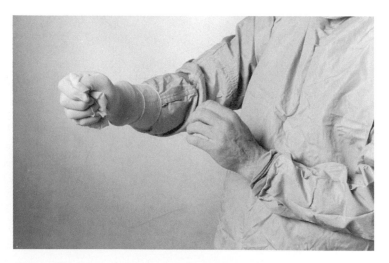

Figure 4.6–35. Compacted first glove held in gloved other hand.

Removal of Contaminated Gloves

LO-8 Contaminated gloves are removed in a manner that prevents the spread of contaminants. One hand grasps the cuff of the other glove.

The glove that has been grasped at the cuff is turned inside out as it is removed.

The glove that has been removed is compacted into the palm of the hand that still is gloved.

The thumb of the ungloved hand is hooked inside the remaining glove.

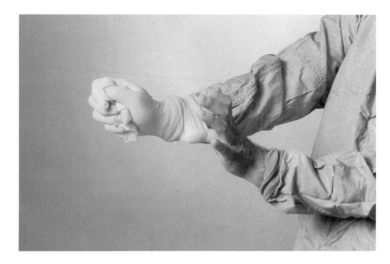

Figure 4.6–36. Hooking thumb inside remaining glove.

The thumb pulls the remaining glove toward the fingers, turning it inside out over the compacted glove. When removing gloves, the material should not be permitted to snap in order to avoid dislodging material that has accumulated on the gloves.

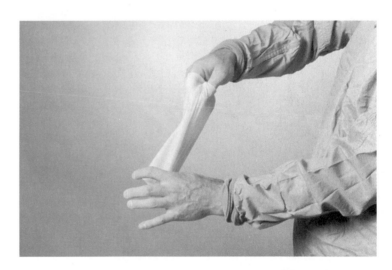

Figure 4.6–37. Removing remaining glove by turning glove inside out.

The second glove is now inside out, with the inside exposed. The first glove is compacted inside the second glove.

The gloves must be disposed of in an appropriate container, and the hands washed.

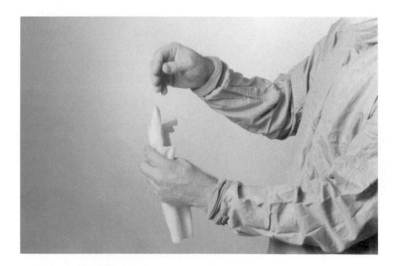

Figure 4.6–38. Gloves removed with first glove inside second glove, and both inside out.

4.7   WOUND DRESSINGS

LO-9

Purpose

The purposes of wound dressings are to

1. Protect physically the site of injury
2. Prevent contamination of a wound
3. Prevent transmission of infection from a wound
4. Promote healing

There is little definitive research concerning specific clinical protocols for wound dressings. Many institutions and health care professionals have preferred methods of caring for specific types of wounds. This section presents basic information concerning wound dressings. Information for a specific institution should be sought from the appropriate departments or practitioners within the institution.

LO-9

Evaluation

Documentation of wound characteristics is necessary for appropriate selection of dressing materials and protective agents, and for monitoring progress in wound healing. Evaluation of the wound is necessary to determine

1. The cause of the wound
2. The location, area, and depth of the wound
3. Whether the wound is wet or dry
4. Whether the wound is infected, and when infected, the source, mechanism, and microorganism of infection

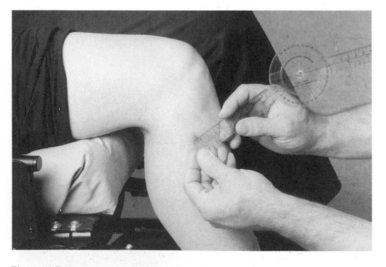

Figure 4.7–1. Measuring width of wound.

Measurement of the wound can be performed using a ruler. There are also specialized clear plastic circular rulers. These rulers should be limited to single patient use. Measurements should include width, length, and depth. The ruler should not make contact with the wound itself.

Another method of documenting the extent of a wound is by photographing the wound.

Preparation

Necessary supplies, such as gauze pads, roll gauze, tape, and topical agents, must be easily accessible during the procedure. Sterile fields, when required, must be set up appropriately.

Protection of the wound from contamination requires the appropriate application of aseptic techniques. Proper preparation for personnel includes handwashing or scrubbing, and masking, gowning, and gloving, when required.

LO-10

CLINICAL NOTE

Prepare needed supplies before starting work with patient

Methods of Application

Five methods of dressing applications generally used for wound management are

1. Dry to dry
2. Wet to wet
3. Wet to dry
4. Occlusive
5. Rigid.

A **dry-to-dry dressing** is the application of a dry absorbent or nonabsorbent dressing to cover the wound. A **wet-to-wet dressing** is the application of a gauze pad soaked in normal saline solution or other similar solution before application. Resoaking of a wet dressing is performed while the dressing remains in place. This prevents the dressing from drying out and becoming embedded in the eschar. The wet-to-wet dressing assists in softening the eschar in preparation for removal. A **wet-to-dry** dressing is the application of a wet dressing that is allowed to dry before removal. The dressing dries embedded in the eschar, and debrides the wound when the dried, embedded dressing is removed. **Occlusive dressings** are applied to provide a semipermeable barrier to air and moisture penetration. **Rigid dressings** provide physical protection to a wound and the adjacent area.

Choice of materials for, and method of application of, dressings may depend on

1. The cause of the wound.
2. Whether the wound is clean or infected, and when infected, the microorganism causing the infection.
3. The type, if any, of an antimicrobial agent to be applied.
4. The site, area, and depth of the wound.
5. Whether a trained professional, the patient, or the patient's family will be responsible for monitoring and changing the dressing.

Identification of the specific microorganism responsible for infection is beneficial in treating any wound. Specific antimicrobial agents may require specific types of dressing materials to ensure that the agent is properly applied to the wound.

When a wound is draining, absorption of exudate can be a consideration requiring a dry dressing. When a wound tends to be dry, and the dryness impedes healing, a wet dressing would be required. Limiting exposure to

LO-10

CLINICAL NOTE

Goal determines method of wound dressing

CLINICAL NOTE

Draining wounds require absorbent dressings

CLINICAL NOTE

Wet dressings soften eschar

air, or maintaining a moist environment within the wound, can require an occlusive dressing.

The location of a wound can dictate the type of dressing applied, or the method of application. Wounds over joints may require rigid dressings to prevent joint motion from disrupting the wound, or the dressings may have to be applied in a way that accommodates joint motion. Wounds can require extensive modification of bedding and seating arrangements, so sleeping and sitting activities do not disrupt the dressing or put pressure on the wound.

The depth of a wound can require additional measures, such as packing the wound with gauze, to ensure that deeper layers of a wound heal before surface layers, avoiding development of an unhealed cavity.

Underlying pathologic conditions may have an impact on the dressings chosen and the application of dressings. No dressing should ever be applied in a manner that impedes circulation. The existence of peripheral vascular disease is a condition that requires special attention to avoid further impairment of circulation.

When long-term care of a wound is required, care may be provided outside an institutional setting. Careful evaluation and consideration must be given to the patient's, or family's, ability to understand and carry out specific instructions. A wound site that cannot be seen easily by the patient is a wound that may not be well cared for by a patient. Physical impairments, such as a stroke impairing manual dexterity, or mental impairment, such as Alzheimer's disease impairing mental faculties, may prohibit a patient from providing wound care. When noninstitutional care is appropriate, the patient or patient's family must be instructed carefully in proper wound care. Whenever possible, simple procedures should be used. Supervision must be provided to ensure that proper techniques are followed.

Materials and Application

LO-10

The size of dressings, whether prepackaged or constructed, should cover the wound site plus some portion of healthy tissue on all sides of a wound. In no case should the adhesive portion of the dressing come in contact with a wound.

The most basic dressing is an adhesive strip of tape with a small gauze center, commonly called by the trademark name Band-Aid. These dressings are available from a number of companies in various shapes and sizes. Topical antimicrobial agents may be applied under the gauze portion of this dressing. The adhesive portion of the dressing may be plastic or paper with a hypoallergenic adhesive to limit skin reaction to the application of the dressing.

Dressings with nonadhering pads that do not stick to wounds or the exudate from wounds are also available. These dressings, commonly called by the trademark name Telfa pads, are available from a number of companies in various shapes and sizes. These basic dressings are usually best for small wounds, although self-made dressings of the same nature can be constructed in any size when the necessary material is available.

Gauze is the most common material used for dressings, and is available in pads and rolls. Sterile and nonsterile gauze is available in several sizes. If sterile gauze is to be used, proper aseptic handling techniques should be used during opening and application. Dressings constructed from gauze can be used with topical antimicrobial agents under the dressing when required.

Gauze pads are secured by tape or a gauze roll. Gauze rolls are applied in a spiral wrap, or in a "figure-of-eight" wrap. The amount of pressure applied by the gauze during wrapping should not be excessive, to avoid impairing circulation.

To apply a **gauze wrap,** lay the portion of the gauze roll that is unwrapping against the limb segment, with the still rolled gauze away from the limb.

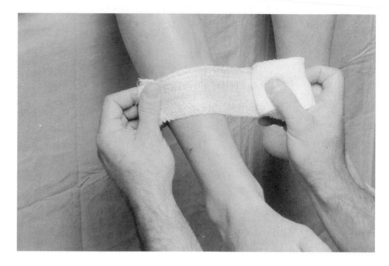

Figure 4.7–2. Holding gauze roll in preparation for wrapping.

A **spiral wrap** is applied by wrapping gauze in a continuous manner around the limb segment. The roll is angled slightly to accommodate for the sloping contour of the limb segment to be wrapped and to avoid creating a tourniquet. The roll of gauze is unrolled around the limb segment, with each successive wrap overlapping the previous wrap by half.

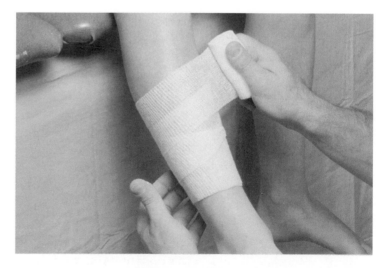

Figure 4.7–3. Spiral wrap (partially completed).

A **figure-of-eight wrap** is started in the same manner as a spiral wrap. Rather than a continuous wrap in the same direction, however, the direction of wrapping changes each time the gauze completes one loop of the figure-of-eight. The illustrations for this section demonstrate a sequence starting in a medial direction on the lower leg. The steps of the sequence are

1. A circumferential anchoring loop around the lower leg
2. In a medial direction across the anterior aspect of the lower leg
3. Around the medial aspect of the lower leg in a descending direction
4. Across the posterior aspect of the lower leg, medial to lateral, in a descending direction
5. Around the lateral aspect of the heel in a descending direction
6. Under the arch, lateral to medial
7. Across the medial aspect of the foot in an ascending direction
8. Across the anterior aspect of the ankle, medial to lateral, in an ascending direction
9. Across the posterior aspect of the heel, lateral to medial
10. Around the medial aspect of the heel in a descending direction
11. Under the arch, medial to lateral
12. Across the anterior aspect of the ankle, lateral to medial, in an ascending direction

These steps are repeated in various combinations. Because each combination ends with the gauze pointing in a different direction, each subsequent combination has different starting and ending points, and intervening directions. Eventually all aspects of the lower leg, ankle, and foot are covered.

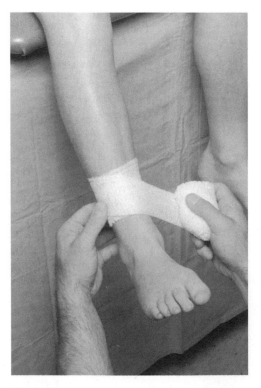

Figure 4.7–4. Anchoring loop for figure-of-eight wrap.

Tape used to secure a dressing can be cloth adhesive tape, or paper tape which has a hypoallergenic adhesive. Tape can be cut to the required length with scissors or torn from the roll. Tape is torn by unrolling the desired amount and firmly grasping the tape between the pad of the thumb and the side of the index finger of each hand, with the hands approximately 1 inch apart.

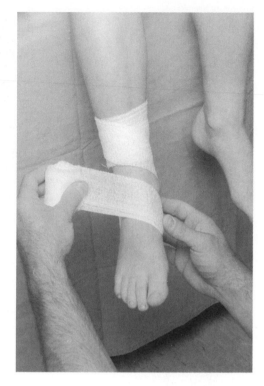

Figure 4.7–5. Step seven of figure-of-eight wrap.

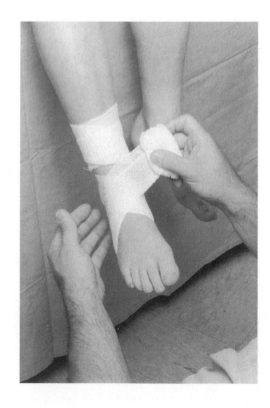

Figure 4.7–6. Step twelve of figure-of-eight wrap.

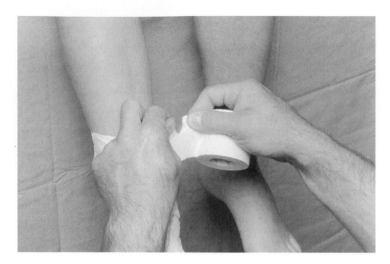

Figure 4.7–7. Tearing tape.

Care should be taken not to roll the edges of the tape over because this makes the tape harder to tear. A quick movement of one hand away from the body and the other hand towards the body will cause the tape to tear between the two hands. Even cloth adhesive tape can be torn in this manner as long as the edges have not been rolled.

CLINICAL NOTE

Do not overlap ends of tape

Because tearing or cutting tape usually takes two hands, it may be more efficient to tear several pieces before applying the wrap or dressing. The pieces can be hung from the edge of a table, cabinet, or bed frame by sticking only a small portion of one end to the object, and letting the remainder of the piece hang free. The pieces should be hung in an accessible place since one hand is usually required to secure the dressing or wrap while the tape is applied. When tape is applied circumferentially on a limb segment, the ends should not overlap. Adhesive and paper tape do not have enough elasticity to avoid impairment of circulation if the ends overlap in this situation.

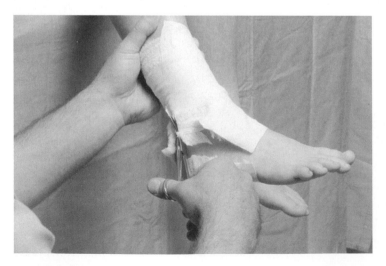

Figure 4.7–8. Removing wrap with bandage scissors.

Removal of a dressing wrapped with cloth adhesive tape requires careful cutting. Bandage scissors, scissors having one flat arm, are used. The flat arm can be slid under the wrap and alongside the limb without cutting the skin. Two cuts must be made to remove an ankle wrap. One cut is made parallel to the lateral border of the foot, distal to the lateral malleolus. A second cut is made parallel to the Achilles tendon, just lateral to the tendon.

Edges of lacerations can be approximated using thin adhesive strips, commonly called by their trademark name of Steri-Strips. The edges of the wound are placed together, and the adhesive strips are placed across the wound. The number of strips required is determined by the open length of the wound.

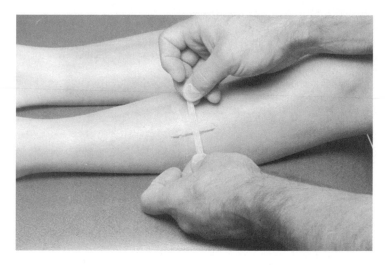

Figure 4.7–9. Application of Steri-Strip.

Compression wraps are applied to control edema in a limb segment, or to provide some support for a joint. Compression wraps are constructed of an elastic material, and are commonly called by the trademark name Ace wrap. Common sizes are 2, 3, 4, 5, and 6-inch widths.

Compression wraps may be applied in spiral or figure-of-eight wraps. When applying compression wraps to control edema, a spiral wrap is used, with more pressure applied distally than proximally. This provides for compression on edematous segments without constricting the flow of fluid towards the core of the body for subsequent elimination. When controlling edema, the entire limb segment distal to the proximal edge of the wrap must be covered by the wrap with appropriately graded pressure. When applying compression wraps for joint support, a figure-of-eight or spiral wrap may be used. When providing support, a compression wrap is applied with even pressure from distal to proximal. Applying a compression wrap for support does not require the entire limb segment distal to the proximal edge of the wrap to be covered. In no case should a wrap be applied with the proximal pressure greater than the distal pressure.

COMPRESSION WRAPS FOR EDEMA

Greatest pressure distally
Decrease pressure proximally

The technique for applying a compression wrap is the same as for applying a gauze wrap.

Frequent examination of compression wraps is necessary to ensure that the amount of compression applied is appropriate, and that the wrap remains in place.

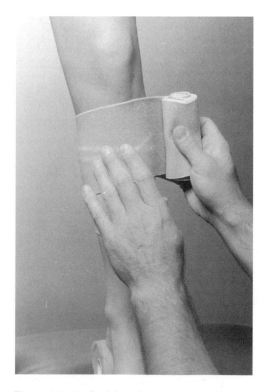

Figure 4.7–10. Applying elastic support wrap.

4.8   CLEANSING AND STERILIZING

General Considerations

LO-11

It is important that all items that will touch normally sterile tissues be sterilized. It is less important that objects touching mucous membranes be sterile. Intact mucous membranes are generally resistant to infection by common bacterial spores but are not resistant to many other microorganisms, such as viruses and tubercle bacilli; therefore, items that touch mucous membranes require a disinfection process that kills all but resistant bacterial spores. In general, intact skin acts as an effective barrier to most microorganisms; thus, items that touch only intact skin need only be clean.

Items must be thoroughly cleaned before processing, because organic material (eg, blood and proteins), may contain high concentrations of microorganisms. Also, such organic material may inactivate chemical germicides and protect microorganisms from the disinfection or sterilization process. For many noncritical items such as blood pressure cuffs or crutches, cleaning can consist only of

CLINICAL NOTE

Cleansing: Wash, rinse, dry

1. Washing with a detergent or a disinfectant–detergent
2. Rinsing
3. Thorough drying

STERILIZATION METHODS

Steam
Gas
Dry heat
Liquid chemicals

Steam sterilization is the most inexpensive and effective method for sterilization. Steam sterilization is unsuitable, however, for processing plastics with low melting points, powders, or anhydrous oils. Items that are to be sterilized but not used immediately need to be wrapped for storage. Sterility can be maintained in storage for various lengths of time, depending on the type of wrapping material, the conditions of storage, and the integrity of the package.

Several methods have been developed to monitor steam sterilization processes. One method is to check the highest temperature that is reached during sterilization and the length of time that this temperature is maintained. In addition, heat and steam-sensitive chemical indicators can be used on the outside of each pack. These indicators do not reliably document sterility, but they do show that an item has not accidentally bypassed a sterilization process. As an additional precaution, a large pack might have a chemical indicator both on the outside and the inside to verify that steam has penetrated the pack.

Because ethylene oxide **gas sterilization** is a more complex and expensive process than steam sterilization, it is usually restricted to objects that might be damaged by heat or excessive moisture. Before sterilization, objects also need to be cleaned thoroughly and wrapped in a material that allows the gas to penetrate. Chemical indicators need to be used with each package to show that it has been exposed to the gas sterilization process. Ethylene oxide gas is toxic and precautions such as local exhaust ventilation, should be taken to protect personnel.[8] All objects processed by gas sterilization also need special aeration according to manufacturers' recommendations before use to remove toxic residues of ethylene oxide.

Powders and anhydrous oils can be sterilized by **dry heat.** Microbiological monitoring of dry-heat sterilizers, and following manufacturers' recommendations for their use and maintenance, usually provides a wide margin of safety for dry-heat sterilization.

Liquid chemicals can be used for sterilization and disinfection when steam, gas, or dry-heat sterilization is not indicated or available. With some formulations, high-level disinfection can be accomplished in 10 to 30 minutes, and sterilization can be achieved if exposure is for significantly longer times. Nevertheless, not all formulations are equally applicable to all items that need to be sterilized or disinfected. No formulation can be considered as an "all purpose" chemical germicide. In each case, more detailed information can be obtained from the EPA, descriptive brochures from the manufacturers, peer-reviewed journal articles, and books.

Gloves may be indicated to prevent skin reactions when some chemical disinfectants are used. Items subjected to high-level disinfection with liquid chemicals need to be rinsed in sterile water to remove toxic or irritating residues and then thoroughly dried. Subsequently, the objects need to be handled aseptically with sterile gloves and towels and stored in protective wrappers to prevent recontamination.

Hot-water disinfection (pasteurization) is a high-level, nontoxic disinfection process that can be used for certain items, for example, respiratory therapy breathing circuits.

In recent years, some hospitals have considered re-using medical devices labeled disposable or single use only. Since there is lack of evidence in dictating increased risk of nosocomial infections associated with re-using all single-use items, a categorical recommendation against all types of re-use is not considered justifiable. Rather than recommending for or against reprocessing and re-use of all single-use items, it appears more prudent to recommend that hospitals consider the safety and efficacy of the reprocessing procedure of each item or device separately and the likelihood that the device will function as intended after reprocessing. In many instances, it may be difficult, if not impossible, to document that the device can be reprocessed without residual toxicity and still function safely and effectively. Few, if any, manufacturers of disposable or single-use medical devices provide reprocessing information on the product label.

Hydrotherapy pools and immersion tanks present unique disinfection problems in hospitals. It is generally not economically feasible to drain large hydrotherapy pools that contain thousands of gallons of water after each patient use. Typically, these pools are used by a large number of patients and are drained and cleaned every 1 to 2 weeks. The water temperature is typically maintained near 37°C. Between cleanings, water can be contaminated by organic material from patients, and high levels of microbial contamination are possible. One method to maintain safe pool water is to install a water filter of sufficient size to filter all the water at least 3 times per day and to chlorinate the water so that a free chlorine residual of approximately 0.5 mg/L is maintained at a pH between 7.2 and 7.6. Local public health authorities can provide consultation regarding alternate halogen disinfectants and hydrotherapy pool sanitation.

HYDROTHERAPY POOLS AND TANKS

Special care to prevent contamination
All surfaces disinfected

Hubbard and immersion tanks have entirely different problems than large pools, since they are drained after each patient use. All inside surfaces need to be cleaned with a disinfectant–detergent, then rinsed with tap water. After the last patient each day, an additional disinfection step is performed. One general procedure is to circulate a chlorine solution (200 to 300 mg/L) through the agitator of the tank for 15 minutes and then rinse it out. It is also recommended that the tank be thoroughly cleaned with a disinfectant–detergent, rinsed, wiped dry with clean cloths, and not filled until ready for use.

An alternative approach to control of contamination in hydrotherapy tanks is to use plastic liners and create the "whirlpool effect" without agitators. Such liners make it possible to minimize contact of contaminated water

TABLE 4–1. Levels of Disinfection According to Type of Microorganism

	Bacteria Tubercle		Fungi[a]		Viruses	
Levels	**Vegetative**	**Bacillus**	**Spores**		**Lipid and Medium Size**	**Nonlipid and Small**
High	+[b]	+	+	+	+	+
Intermediate	+	+	±[c]	+	+	±[d]
Low	+	−	−	±	+	−

[a] Includes asexual spores but not necessarily chlamydospores or sexual spores.
[b] Plus sign indicates that a killing effect can be expected when the normal use-concentrations of chemical disinfectants or pasteurization are properly employed; a negative sign indicates little or no killing effect. ± Only with extended exposure times are high-level disinfectant chemicals capable of actual sterilization.
[c] Some intermediate-level disinfectants can be expected to exhibit some sporicidal action.
[d] Some intermediate-level disinfectants may have limited virucidal activity.

CLINICAL NOTE

Designing procedures: Consult infectious disease control personnel

with the interior surface of the tank and also obviate the need for agitators that may be very difficult to clean and decontaminate.

Different types of microorganisms require different levels of disinfection. Different objects and equipment may be cleansed and stored in different ways, depending upon the level of criticality. Tables 4–1 and 4–2 indicate different levels of disinfection and types of processing required. These charts are reproduced from the Guideline for Handwashing and Hospital Environmental Control, 1985 (PB85-923404), produced by the Center for Infectious Diseases, CDC. For application in clinical settings, information should be sought from the specific institution's infectious disease control personnel.

TABLE 4–2. Methods of Assuring Adequate Processing and Safe Use of Medical Devices

Object and Classification	Example	Method	Comment
		Patient Care Objects	
		Critical	
Sterilized in the hospital	Surgical instruments and devices; trays and sets	1. Thoroughly clean objects and wrap or package for sterilization. 2. Follow manufacturer's instructions for use of each sterilizer or use recommended protocol. 3. Monitor time–temperature charts. 4. Use commercial spore preparations to monitor sterilizers. 5. Inspect package for integrity and for exposure of sterility indicator before use. 6. Use before maximum safe storage time has expired if applicable.	Sterilization processes are designed to have a wide margin of safety. If spores are not killed, the sterilizer should be checked for proper use and function; if spore tests remain positive, discontinue use of the sterilizer until properly serviced. Maximum safe storage time of items processed in the hospital varies according to type of package or wrapping material used; follow manufacturer's instructions for use and storage times.

TABLE 4–2. *(Cont.)*

Object and Classification	Example	Method	Comment
Patient Care Objects			
Critical			
Purchased as sterile	Intravenous fluids; irrigation fluids; normal saline; trays and sets	1. Store in safe, clean area. 2. Inspect package for integrity before use. 3. Use before expiration date if one is given. 4. Culture only if clinical circumstances suggest infection related to use of the item.	Notify the Food and Drug Administration, local and state health departments, and CDC if intrinsic contamination is suspected.
Semicritical			
Should be free of vegetative bacteria. May be subjected to high-level disinfection rather than sterilization process	Respiratory therapy equipment and instruments that will touch mucous membranes	1. Sterilize or follow a protocol for high-level disinfection. 2. Bag and store in safe, clean area. 3. Conduct quality control monitoring after any important changes in the disinfection process.	Bacterial spores may survive after high-level disinfection, but these usually are not pathogenic. Microbiologic sampling can verify that a high-level disinfection process has resulted in destruction of vegetative bacteria; however, this sampling is not routinely recommended.
Non-critical			
Usually contaminated with some bacteria	Bedpans; crutches; rails; ECG leads	1. Follow a protocol for cleaning or, if necessary a low-level disinfection process.	
Water-produced or treated	Water used for hemodialysis fluids	1. Assay water and dialysis fluids monthly. 2. Water should not have more than 200 bacteria/mL and dialysis fluids not more than 2000 bacteria/mL.	Gram-negative water bacteria can grow rapidly in water and dialysis fluids and can place dialysis patients at risk of pyrogenic reactions or septicemia. These water sources and pathways should be disinfected routinely.

CDC Recommendations (PB85-923404)

1. Cleaning
   All objects to be disinfected or sterilized should first be thoroughly cleaned to remove all organic matter (blood and tissue) and other residue. *Category I*
2. Indications for Sterilization and High-Level Disinfection
   a. Critical medical devices or patient-care equipment that enter normally sterile tissue or the vascular system or through which blood flows should be subjected to a sterilization procedure before each use. *Category I*
   b. Laparoscopes, arthroscopes, and other scopes that enter normally sterile tissue should be subjected to a sterilization procedure before each use; if this is not feasible, they should receive at least high-level disinfection. *Category I*
   c. Equipment that touches mucous membranes, eg, endoscopes, endotracheal tubes, anesthesia breathing circuits, and respiratory therapy equipment, should receive high-level disinfection. *Category I*
3. Methods of Sterilization
   a. Whenever sterilization is indicated, a steam sterilizer should be used unless the object to be sterilized will be damaged by heat, pressure, or moisture or is otherwise inappropriate for steam sterilization. In this case, another acceptable method of sterilization should be used. *Category II*
   b. Flash sterilization [270°F (132°C) for 3 minutes in a gravity displacement steam sterilizer] is not recommended for implantable items. *Category II*
4. Biological Monitoring of Sterilizers
   a. All sterilizers should be monitored at least once a week with commercial preparations of spores intended specifically for that type of sterilizer, ie, *Bacillus stearothermophilus* for steam sterilizers and *Bacillus subtilis* for ethylene oxide and dry-heat sterilizers. *Category II*
   b. Every load that contains implantable objects should be monitored. These implantable objects should not be used until the spore test is found to be negative at 48 hours. *Category II*
   c. If spores are not killed in routine spore tests, the sterilizer should immediately be checked for proper use and function and the spore test repeated. Objects, other than implantable objects, do not need to be recalled because of a single positive spore test unless the sterilizer or the sterilization procedure is defective. *Category II*
   d. If spore tests remain positive, use of the sterilizer should be discontinued until it is serviced. *Category I*
5. Use and Preventive Maintenance—Manufacturers' instructions should be followed for use and maintenance of sterilizers. *Category II*
6. Chemical Indicators—Chemical indicators that will show a package has been through a sterilization cycle should be visible on the outside of each package sterilized. *Category II*
7. Use of Sterile Items—An item should not be used if its sterility is questionable, eg, its package is punctured, torn, or wet. *Category I*
8. Reprocessing Single-Use or Disposable Items
   a. Items or devices that cannot be cleaned and sterilized or disinfected without altering their physical integrity and function should not be reprocessed. *Category I*

b. Reprocessing procedures that result in residual toxicity or compromise the overall safety or effectiveness of the items or devices should be avoided. *Category I*

4.9 WASTE DISPOSAL

General Considerations

The most practical approach to infective waste management is to identify those wastes that represent a sufficient potential risk of causing infection during handling and disposal and for which some special precautions appear prudent. Hospital wastes for which special precautions appear prudent include microbiology laboratory waste, pathology waste, and blood specimens or blood products. The risk of either injury or infection from certain sharp items, eg, needles and scalpel blades, contaminated with blood also need to be considered when disposing of such items. While any item that has had contact with blood, exudates, or secretions may be potentially infective, it is not normally considered practical or necessary to treat all such waste as infective. CDC has published general recommendations for handling infective waste from patients on isolation precautions.[9] Additional special precautions may be necessary for certain rare diseases or conditions such as Lassa fever.[10] The EPA has published a draft manual (Environmental Protection Agency, Office of Solid Waste and Emergency Response, Draft Manual for Infectious Waste Management, SW-957, 1982. Washington, 1982) that identifies and categorizes other specific types of waste that may be generated in some research-oriented hospitals. In addition to the above guidelines, local and state environmental regulations may also exist.

Solid waste from the microbiology laboratory can be placed in steam-sterilizable bags or pans and steam sterilized in the laboratory. Alternatively, it can be transported in sealed, impervious plastic bags to be burned in a hospital incinerator. A single bag is probably adequate if the bag is sturdy (not easily penetrated) and if the waste can be put in the bag without contaminating the outside of the bag; otherwise, double-bagging is indicated. All slides or tubes with small amounts of blood can be packed in sealed, impervious containers and sent for incineration or steam sterilization in the hospital. Exposure for up to 90 minutes at 250°F (121°C) in a steam sterilizer, depending on the size of the load and type container, may be necessary to assure an adequate sterilization cycle.[11,12] After steam sterilization, the residue can be safely handled and discarded with all other nonhazardous hospital solid waste. All containers with more than a few milliliters of blood remaining after laboratory procedures and bulk blood may be steam sterilized, or the contents may be carefully poured down a utility sink drain or toilet.

Disposables that can cause injury, such as scalpel blades and syringes with needles, should be placed in puncture-resistant containers. Ideally, such containers are located where these items are used. Syringes and needles can be placed intact directly into the rigid containers for safe storage until terminal treatment. To prevent needle-stick injuries, needles should not be recapped, purposely bent, or broken by hand. When some needle-cutting devices are used, blood may be aerosolized or spattered onto environmental surfaces. However, there is not any data currently available from controlled studies examining the effect, if any, of the use of any of these devices on the incidence of needle-transmissible infections.

LO-12

CLINICAL NOTE

Designing procedures: Consult CDC, local or state environmental agencies

CLINICAL NOTE

Separate wastes with significant potential of risk

CLINICAL NOTE

Use puncture resistance containers for sharp objects such as needles and blades

It is often necessary to transport or store infective waste within the hospital prior to terminal treatment. This can be done safely if proper and commonsense procedures are used. The EPA draft manual mentioned contains guidelines for the storage and transport of infective waste, both on-site and off-site.

CDC Recommendations (PB85-923404)

1. Identification of Infective Waste
   a. Microbiology laboratory wastes, blood and blood products, pathology waste, and sharp items (especially needles) should be considered as potentially infective and handled and disposed of with special precautions. *Category II*
   b. Infective waste from patients on isolation precautions should be handled and disposed of according to the current edition of the "Guideline for Isolation Precautions in Hospitals." (This recommendation is not categorized since the recommendations for isolation precautions are not categorized.)
2. Handling, Transport, and Storage of Infective Waste
   a. Personnel involved in the handling and disposal of infective waste should be informed of the potential health and safety hazards and trained in the appropriate handling and disposal methods. *Category II*
   b. If processing and/or disposal facilities are not available at the site of infective waste generation, ie, laboratory, etc, the waste may be safely transported in sealed impervious containers to another hospital area for appropriate treatment. *Category II*
   c. To minimize the potential risk for accidental transmission of disease or injury, infective waste awaiting terminal processing should be stored in an area accessible only to personnel involved in the disposal process. *Category III*
3. Processing and Disposal of Infective Waste
   a. Infective waste, in general, should either be incinerated or should be autoclaved prior to disposal in a sanitary landfill. *Category III*
   b. Disposable syringes with needles, scalpel blades, and other sharp items capable of causing injury should be placed intact into puncture-resistant containers located as close to the area in which they were used as is practical. To prevent needle-stick injuries, needles should not be recapped, purposely bent, broken, or otherwise manipulated by hand. *Category I*
   c. Bulk blood, suctioned fluids, excretions, and secretions may be carefully poured down a drain connected to a sanitary sewer. Sanitary sewers may also be used for the disposal of other infectious wastes capable of being ground and flushed into the sewer. *Category II* (Special precautions may be necessary for certain rare diseases or conditions such as Lassa fever.[9])

4.10   LAUNDRY

General Considerations

LO-12

Although soiled linen has been identified as a source of large numbers of pathogenic microorganisms, the risk of actual disease transmission seems to be negligible. Therefore, rigid rules and regulations for hygienic storage and processing of clean and soiled linen are not required or recommended.

Soiled linen can be transported in the hospital by cart or linen chute. If linen chutes are used, bagging of linen is necessary. Improperly designed linen chutes can be a means of transmission of microorganisms throughout an institution if bagging of linen is not done.[13]

Soiled linen may or may not be sorted in the laundry before being loaded into washer/extractor units. Sorting before washing protects both machinery and linen from the effects of objects in the linen and reduces the potential for recontamination of clean linen that sorting after washing requires. Sorting after washing minimizes the direct exposure of laundry personnel to infective material in the soiled linen and reduces airborne microbial contamination in the laundry. Protective apparel and appropriate ventilation can minimize these exposures.

The microbicidal action of the normal laundering process is affected by several physical and chemical factors.[14] Although dilution is not a microbicidal mechanism, it is responsible for the removal of significant quantities of microorganisms. Soaps or detergents loosen soil and also have some microbicidal properties. Hot water provides an effective means of destroying microorganisms, and a temperature of at least 71°C (160°F) for a minimum of 25 minutes is commonly recommended for hot-water washing. Chlorine bleach provides an extra margin of safety. A total available chlorine residual of 50 to 150 ppm is usually achieved during the bleach cycle. The last action performed during the washing process is the addition of a mild acid to neutralize any alkalinity in the water supply, soap, or detergent. The rapid shift in pH from approximately 12 to 5 also may tend to inactivate some microorganisms.

Satisfactory reduction of microbial contamination can be achieved at lower water temperatures of 22 to 50°C when the cycling of the washer, the wash formula, and the amount of chlorine bleach are carefully monitored and controlled.[15,16] Instead of the microbicidal action of hot water, low-temperature laundry cycles rely heavily on the presence of bleach to reduce levels of microbial contamination. Regardless of whether hot or cold water is used for washing, the temperatures reached in drying and especially during ironing provide additional significant microbicidal action.

CLINICAL NOTE

Keep all non-linen objects out of laundry

LAUNDRY DISINFECTION

Removing soil
Heat
Chemicals

CDC Recommendations (PB85-923404)

1. Routine Handling of Soiled Linen
   a. Soiled linen should be handled as little as possible and with minimum agitation to prevent gross microbial contamination of the air and of persons handling the linen. *Category II*
      (1) All soiled linen should be bagged or put into carts at the location where it was used; it should *not* be prerinsed in patient care areas. *Category II*
      (2) Linen soiled with blood or body fluids should be deposited and transported in bags that prevent leakage. *Category II*

b. If laundry chutes are used, linen should be bagged, and chutes should be properly designed. *Category II*
2. Hot-Water Washing—If hot water is used, linen should be washed with a detergent in water at least 71°C (160°F) for 25 minutes. *Category II*
3. Low-Temperature Water Washing—If low temperature (<70°C) laundry cycles are used, chemicals suitable for low-temperature washing at proper-use concentration should be used. *Category II*
4. Transportation of Clean Linen—Clean linen should be transported and stored by methods that will ensure its cleanliness. *Category II*

4.11   HOUSEKEEPING

LO-12

General Considerations

CLINICAL NOTE

Routine cleaning: Adequate for most areas

Although microorganisms are a normal contaminant of walls, floors, and other surfaces, these environmental surfaces rarely are associated with transmission of infections to patients or personnel. Therefore, extraordinary attempts to disinfect or sterilize these environmental surfaces are rarely indicated. Routine cleaning and removal of soil, however, are recommended.

Cleaning schedules and methods vary according to the area of the hospital, type of surface to be cleaned, and the amount and type of soil present. Horizontal surfaces, eg, bedside tables and hard-surfaced flooring, in patient care areas are usually cleaned on a regular basis, when soiling or spills occur, and when a patient is discharged. Cleaning of walls, blinds, and curtains is recommended only if they are visibly soiled. Disinfectant fogging is an unsatisfactory method of decontaminating air and surfaces and is not recommended.

There is no epidemiologic evidence to show that carpets influence the nosocomial infection rate in hospitals.[17] Carpets, however, may contain much higher levels of microbial contamination than hard-surfaced flooring and can be difficult to keep clean in areas of heavy soiling or spillage. Therefore, appropriate cleaning and maintenance procedures are indicated.

Disinfectant–detergent formulations registered by the EPA can be used for environmental surface cleaning, but the actual physical removal of microorganisms by scrubbing is probably as important, if not more so, than any antimicrobial effect of the cleaning agent used. Therefore, cost, safety, and acceptability by housekeepers can be the main criteria for selecting any such registered agent. The manufacturers' instructions for appropriate use should be followed.

Special precautions[18] for cleaning incubators, mattresses, and other nursery surfaces with which neonates have contact must be followed, since inadequately diluted solutions of phenolics used for such cleaning and poor ventilation have been associated with hyperbilirubinemia in newborns.[19]

CDC Recommendations (PB85-923404)

1. Choice of Cleaning Agent for Environmental Surfaces in Patient Care Areas—Any hospital-grade disinfectant–detergent registered by the

EPA may be used for cleaning environmental surfaces. Manufacturers' instructions for use of such products should be followed. *Category II*

2. Cleaning of Horizontal Surfaces in Patient Care Areas
   a. Uncarpeted floors and other horizontal surfaces, eg, bedside tables, should be cleaned regularly and if spills occur. *Category II*
   b. Carpeting should be vacuumed regularly with units designed to filter discharged air efficiently, cleaned if spills occur, and shampooed whenever a thorough cleaning is indicated. *Category II*
3. Cleaning Walls, Blinds, and Curtains—Terminal cleaning of walls, blinds, and curtains is not recommended unless they are visibly soiled. *Category II*
4. Disinfectant Fogging—Disinfectant fogging should not be done. *Category I*

4.12 ISOLATION

General Considerations

LO-13

Isolation precautions are designed to prevent the spread of microorganisms among patients, personnel, and visitors. Since agent and host factors are more difficult to control, interruption of the chain of infection in the hospital is directed primarily at transmission. The isolation precautions recommended in this guideline are based on this concept.

> **CLINICAL NOTE**
>
> Isolation interrupts chain of infection

Nevertheless, placing a patient on isolation precautions often presents certain disadvantages to both the hospital and the patient. Some isolation precautions may be time consuming and add to the cost of hospitalization. They may make frequent visits by physicians, nurses, and other personnel inconvenient, and they may make it difficult for hospital personnel to give the prompt and frequent care that is sometimes required. The occasional recommendation of a private room under some circumstances uses valuable space that might otherwise accommodate several patients. Moreover, forced solitude deprives the patient of normal social relationships and may be psychologically injurious, especially for children. In an attempt to balance the disadvantages of placing a patient on isolation precautions against the various hazards posed by transmissible infections, "degrees of isolation" have been designated.

It is safer to "over-isolate" than to "under-isolate," particularly when the diagnosis is uncertain and several diseases are seriously being considered. For the patient who appears to have a disease requiring isolation precautions, it is important to institute appropriate isolation precautions immediately rather than wait for confirmation of the diagnosis. Furthermore, certain general precautions may be required even though the patient does not fully meet the criteria for specific isolation precautions. For example, patients with bacteriuria and indwelling urinary catheters are known to serve as reservoirs of infection for roommates who also have indwelling urinary catheters. Passive carriage on the hands of personnel who provide urinary catheter care transmits these infections. Thus, noninfected patients with catheters should not, *where practical*, share rooms with catheterized patients who have bacteriuria.

> **CLINICAL NOTE**
>
> Institute isolation precautions immediately

Isolation precautions also may have to be modified for a patient who needs constant care or whose clinical condition may require emergency intervention, such as those in intensive care units or nurseries. When such

> **CLINICAL NOTE**
>
> Minimize risk to other patients and personnel

modifications are made, it is essential that the risk to other patients or hospital personnel of acquiring nosocomial infection be minimized.

If a susceptible person has been exposed recently to an infectious disease requiring isolation precautions, the physician should postpone elective admission or prescribe appropriate isolation precautions for a nonelective admission. This situation is most likely to occur with children or young adults.

When used appropriately, prophylactic antimicrobials and active or passive immunization may prevent or ameliorate the course of infections to which patients or personnel have been exposed. These measures should be considered as adjuncts to isolation precautions in preventing the spread of disease.

Spread of infection within a hospital requires three elements

1. A source of infecting organisms
2. A susceptible host
3. A means of transmission for the organism

The source of the infecting agent may be patients, personnel, or on occasion, visitors, and may include persons with acute disease, persons in the incubation period of the disease, or persons who are colonized by the infectious agent but have no apparent disease. Another source of infection can be the person's own endogenous flora, or autogenous infection. Other potential sources are inanimate objects in the environment that have become contaminated, including equipment and medications.

Patients' resistance to pathogenic microorganisms varies greatly. Some persons may be immune to or able to resist colonization by an infectious agent; others exposed to the same agent may establish a commensural relationship with the infecting organism and become asymptomatic carriers; still others may develop clinical disease. Persons with diabetes mellitus, lymphoma, leukemia, neoplasia, granulocytopenia, or uremia and those treated with certain antimicrobials, corticosteroids, irradiation, or immunosuppressive agents may be particularly prone to infection. Age, chronic debilitating disease, shock, coma, traumatic injury, or surgical procedures also make a person more susceptible.

CLINICAL NOTE

Patients may be more susceptible to infection

Microorganisms are transmitted by various routes, and the same microorganism may be transmitted by more than one route. For example, varicella-zoster virus can spread either by the airborne route, eg, droplet nuclei, or by direct contact. The differences in infectivity and in the mode of transmission of the various agents form the basis for the differences in isolation precautions that are recommended in the CDC guidelines.

There are four main routes of transmission—contact, vehicle, airborne, and vectorborne.

ROUTES OF TRANSMISSION

Contact
Airborne
Vehicle
Vectorborne

1. Contact transmission, the most important and frequent means of transmission of nosocomial infections, can be divided into 3 subgroups: direct contact, indirect contact, and droplet contact.
   a. Direct contact—This involves direct physical transfer between a susceptible host and an infected or colonized person, such as occurs when hospital personnel turn patients, give baths, change dressings, or perform other procedures requiring direct personal contact. Direct contact can also occur between two patients, one serving as the source of infection and the other as a susceptible host.
   b. Indirect contact—This involves personal contact of the susceptible host with a contaminated intermediate object, usually inanimate, such as bed linens, clothing, instruments, and dressings.

c. Droplet contact—Infectious agents may come in contact with the conjunctivae, nose, or mouth of a susceptible person as a result of coughing, sneezing, or talking by an infected person who has clinical disease or is a carrier of the organism. This is considered "contact" transmission rather than airborne, since droplets usually travel no more than about 3 feet.

2. The vehicle route applies in diseases transmitted through these contaminated items:
   a. food, such as in salmonellosis;
   b. water, such as in legionellosis;
   c. drugs, such as in bacteremia resulting from infusion of a contaminated infusion product;
   d. blood, such as in hepatitis B, or non-A, non-B hepatitis.

3. Airborne transmission occurs by dissemination of either droplet nuclei, ie, residue of evaporated droplets that may remain suspended in the air for long periods of time, or dust particles in the air containing the infectious agent. Organisms carried in this manner can be widely dispersed by air currents before being inhaled or deposited on the susceptible host.

4. Vectorborne transmission is of greater concern in tropical countries, eg, with mosquito-transmitted malaria. It is of little significance in hospitals in the United States.

The hospital is responsible for ensuring that patients are placed on appropriate isolation precautions. Each hospital should designate clearly, as a matter of policy, the personnel responsible for placing a patient on isolation precautions and the personnel who have the ultimate authority to make decisions regarding isolation precautions when conflicts arise.

All personnel—physicians, nurses, technicians, students, and others—are responsible for complying with isolation precautions and for tactfully calling observed infractions to the attention of offenders. Physicians should observe the proper isolation precautions at all times; they must teach by example. The responsibilities of hospital personnel for carrying out isolation precautions cannot be effectively dictated but must arise from a personal sense of responsibility.

CLINICAL NOTE

All personnel must comply with isolation precautions

Patients also have a responsibility for complying with isolation precautions. The appropriate measures should be explained to the patient by physicians and nurses. An important general patient responsibility is handwashing after touching infective material and potentially contaminated articles.

Infractions of the isolation protocol by some are sufficient to negate the conscientious efforts of others. The maxim, "The chain is no stronger than its weakest link," is certainly true.

CLINICAL NOTE

Patients and their visitors require instruction

Methods

Many techniques and recommendations for isolation precautions are appropriate not only for patients with known or suspected infection, but also for routine patient care. It is appropriate to use gowns for patient care when soiling with feces is likely, whether or not the patient is infected with an enteric pathogen. Caution when handling hypodermic needles and syringes is appropriate at all times.

Handwashing is the single most important means of preventing the spread of infection. The rationale and technique have been presented earlier in this chapter in the section on "Handwashing" and the section on "Procedures/handwashing." Other important means of preventing the spread of infection include the use of masks, gowns, and gloves. These means have also been presented earlier in this chapter in the sections on "Masks, Gowns, Procedures/gowning, Gloves," and "Procedures/gloving."

Some institutions use prestocked isolation carts that contain equipment and supplies for isolation precautions. These can be wheeled to the general area where needed but should be placed in a clean area. Carts should be kept adequately stocked with all necessary supplies.

Private Room

In general, a private room can reduce the possibility of transmission of infectious agents in two ways. First, it separates infected or colonized patients from susceptible patients and thus lessens the chance for transmission by any route. Second, it may act as a reminder for personnel to wash their hands before leaving the room and contacting other patients, especially if a sink is available at the doorway. Nevertheless, a private room is not necessary to prevent the spread of many infections.

A private room is indicated for patients with infections that are highly infectious or are caused by microorganisms that are likely to be virulent when transmitted. A private room is also indicated if patient hygiene is poor, for example, if a patient does not wash hands after touching infective material (feces and purulent drainage or secretions), contaminates the environment, or shares contaminated articles. Such patients may include infants, children, and patients who have altered mental status. A private room may also be indicated for patients colonized with microorganisms of special chemical or epidemiologic significance such as multiply resistant bacteria. Finally, a private room may be indicated for patients whose blood is infective, as with hepatitis B, if profuse bleeding is likely to cause environmental contamination.

In addition to handwashing facilities, a private room should contain bathing and toilet facilities if the room is used for patients requiring isolation precautions. Toilet facilities obviate the need for portable commodes or special precautions for transporting commodes, bedpans, and urinals. An anteroom between the room and the hall, especially for rooms housing patients with highly infectious diseases spread by airborne transmission, will help maintain isolation precautions by reducing the possibility of airborne spread of infectious agents from the room into the corridor whenever the door of the room is opened. Anterooms also provide storage space for supplies, such as gowns, gloves, and masks.

For a few infections, a private room with special ventilation is required. Special ventilation results in negative air pressure in the room in relation to the anteroom or hall, when the room door is closed. The ventilation air, which should generally result in 6 air changes per hour, preferably should be discharged outdoors away from intake vents or receive high efficiency filtration before being recirculated to other rooms.

Roommates for Patients on Isolation Precautions

If infected or colonized patients are not placed in private rooms, they should be placed with appropriate roommates. Generally, infected patients should not share a room with a patient who is likely to become infected, or if consequences of infection are likely to be severe.

PRIVATE ROOM REQUIRED

Highly infectious patients
Multiply resistant bacteria
Poor hygiene techniques
Blood infections

CLINICAL NOTE

Personnel must take precautions to prevent spread of infection

When an infected patient shares a room with noninfected patients, it is assumed that patients and personnel will take measures to prevent the spread of infection. For example, a patient whose fecal material is infective may be in a room with others as long as that patient is cooperative, washes hands carefully, and does not have severe diarrhea or fecal incontinence that will cause either roommates, or objects used by them, to become contaminated. Likewise, personnel need to wear gloves and wash hands when indicated and ensure that contaminated articles are discarded or returned for decontamination and reprocessing. When these conditions cannot be met, a private room is advisable.

In general, patients infected by the same microorganism may share a room. Also, infants and young children with the same respiratory clinical syndrome, for example, croup, may share a room. Such grouping, or cohorting, of patients is especially useful during outbreaks when there is a shortage of private rooms.

Disposal of Articles

Used articles may need to be enclosed in an impervious bag before they are removed from the room or cubicle of a patient on isolation precautions. Such bagging is intended to prevent inadvertent exposures of personnel to articles contaminated with infective material and prevent contamination of the environment. Most articles do not need to be bagged unless they are contaminated, or likely to be contaminated, with infective material. A single bag is probably adequate if the bag is impervious and sturdy, ie, not easily penetrated, and if the article can be placed in the bag without contaminating the outside of the bag; otherwise, double bagging should be used. Bags should be labeled or be a particular color designated solely for contaminated articles or infectious wastes.

CLINICAL NOTE

Label, or use color coded, disposal bags

Disposal of Equipment

A variety of disposable patient care equipment is available and should be considered for patients on isolation precautions. Use of these disposable articles reduces the possibility that equipment will serve as a fomite, but they must be disposed of safely and adequately. Equipment that is contaminated, or likely to be contaminated, with infective material should be bagged, labeled, and disposed of in accordance with the hospital's policy for disposal of infectious wastes. Local regulations may call for incineration or disposal in an authorized sanitary landfill without the bag being opened. No special precautions are indicated for disposable patient care equipment that is not contaminated, or likely to be contaminated, with infective material.

CLINICAL NOTE

Use disposable (single-use only) equipment when available

Reusable Equipment

Ideally, such equipment should be returned to a central processing area for decontamination and reprocessing by trained personnel. When contaminated with infective material, equipment should be bagged and labeled before being removed from the patient's room or cubicle and remain bagged until decontaminated or sterilized. Special procedure trays should be separated into component parts and handled appropriately (some components can be discarded; others may need to be sent to the laundry or central services for reprocessing).

CLINICAL NOTE

Reusable equipment: Decontaminated or sterilized

Needles and Syringes

In general, personnel should use caution when handling all used needles and syringes because it is usually not known which patient's blood is contaminated with hepatitis virus or other microorganisms. Specific recommendations are included in this chapter in the section "Waste disposal/General considerations." If the patient's blood is infective, disposable syringes and needles are preferred. If reusable syringes are used, they should be bagged and returned for decontamination and reprocessing.

Sphygmomanometer and Stethoscope

No special precautions are indicated unless the equipment is contaminated, or likely to be contaminated, with infective material. If contaminated, the equipment should be disinfected in the manner appropriate to the object and to the etiologic agent that necessitated isolation precautions.

Thermometers

Thermometers from patients on isolation precautions should be sterilized or receive high-level disinfection before being used by another patient.

Linen

In general, soiled linen should be handled as little as possible and with a minimum of agitation to prevent gross microbial contamination of the air and of persons handling the linen. Soiled linen from patients on isolation precautions should be put in a laundry bag in the patient's room or cubicle. The bag should be labeled or be a particular color, eg, red, specifically designated for such linen so that whoever receives the linen knows to take the necessary precautions. Linens will require less handling if the bag is hot-water soluble because such bags can be placed directly into the washing machine. However, a hot-water soluble bag may need to be double bagged because they are generally easily punctured or torn or may dissolve when wet. Linen from patients on isolation precautions should not be sorted before being laundered. If mattresses and pillows are covered with impervious plastic, they can be cleaned by wiping with a disinfectant–detergent.

Dishes

No special precautions are necessary for dishes unless they are visibly contaminated with infective material, eg, with blood, drainage, or secretions. Disposable dishes contaminated with infective material can be handled as disposable patient care equipment. Reusable dishes, utensils, and trays contaminated with infective material should be bagged and labeled before being returned to the food service department. Food service personnel who handle these dishes should wear gloves, and they should wash their hands before handling clean dishes or food.

Clothing

Clothing soiled with infective material should be bagged before being sent home or to the hospital laundry; it should be washed with a detergent and, if possible, hot water and bleach.

Books, Magazines, Personal Articles

In general, any of these articles visibly soiled with infective material should be disinfected or destroyed. A child with an infection that can be spread by fomites or by contact transmission should not share toys with other children.

Drinking Water

No special precautions are indicated for drinking water. Containers used to hold water for patients on isolation precautions and glasses should be handled as dishes.

Dressings and Tissues

All dressings, paper tissues, and other disposable items soiled with infective material (respiratory, oral, or wound secretions) should be bagged, labeled, and disposed of in accordance with the hospital's policy for disposal of infectious wastes. Local regulations may call for incineration or disposal in an authorized sanitary landfill without being opened.

Urine and Feces

Urine and feces from patients on isolation precautions can be flushed down the toilet if the hospital uses a municipal or other safe sewage treatment system. A urinal or bedpan from a patient on isolation precautions should be cleaned and disinfected or sterilized before being used by another patient.

Laboratory Specimens

In general, each specimen should be put in a well-constructed container with a secure lid to prevent leaking during transport. Care should be taken when collecting specimens to avoid contamination of the outside of the container. If the outside of the container is visibly contaminated, it should be cleaned, disinfected, or placed in an impervious bag. Specimens from patients on isolation precautions may need to be placed in an impervious bag and labeled before being removed from the room or cubicle; bagging is intended to prevent inadvertent exposures of laboratory or transport personnel to infective material and prevent contamination of the environment. Specimens from patients on isolation precautions may need to be bagged before being sent to the laboratory. This will depend on the kind of specimen and container, the procedures for collecting specimens, and the methods for transporting and receiving specimens in the hospital laboratory.

Patient's Chart

The chart should not be allowed to come into contact with infective material or objects that may be contaminated with infective material.

Visitors

Instruction cards have been designed to give concise information about isolation precautions. These cards are displayed conspicuously in the immediate vicinity of the patient on isolation precautions. Some facilities use color-coded cards that indicate specific conditions and precautions, while other facilities use only a sign indicating that visitors must see a nurse before entering. Visitors should be instructed in the appropriate use of gown, mask, gloves, or other special precautions.

Transporting Patients

Patients infected with virulent or epidemiologically important microorganisms should leave their room only for essential purposes. Appropriate barriers (masks, impervious dressings, etc.) to prevent transmission should be used by the patient and transport personnel. Personnel in the area to which the patient is to be taken should be notified of the impending arrival of the patient and of precautions to be used to prevent transmission of infection. Patients should be alerted to the potential spread of their disease and informed as to how they can assist in maintaining a barrier against transmission of their infection to others.

Routine Cleaning

The same routine daily cleaning procedures used in other hospital rooms should be used to clean rooms or cubicles of patients on isolation precautions. Cleaning equipment used in rooms of patients whose infection requires a private room should be disinfected before being used in other patient rooms. For example, dirty water should be discarded, wiping cloths and mop heads should be laundered and thoroughly dried, and buckets should be disinfected before being refilled. If cleaning cloths and mop heads are contaminated with infective material or blood, they should be bagged and labeled before being sent to the laundry.

Terminal Cleaning

When isolation precautions have been discontinued, the remaining infection control responsibilities relate to the inanimate environment. Therefore, certain epidemiologic aspects of environmental transmission should be kept in mind by personnel involved with terminal cleaning, or cleaning after the patient has been taken off isolation precautions or has ceased to be a source of infection. Although microorganisms may be present on walls, floors, and table tops in rooms used for patients on isolation precautions, these environmental surfaces, unless visibly contaminated, are rarely associated with transmission of infection to others. In contrast, microorganisms on contaminated patient care equipment are frequently associated with transmission of infections to other patients when such equipment is not appropriately decontaminated and reprocessed. Therefore, terminal cleaning should primarily be directed toward those items that have been in direct contact with the patient or in contact with the patient's infective material (excretions, secretions, blood, or body fluids). Disinfectant–detergent solutions used during terminal cleaning should be freshly prepared. Terminal cleaning of rooms or cubicles consists of the following:

1. Generally, housekeeping personnel should use the same precautions to protect themselves during terminal cleaning that they would use if the patient were still in the room. However, masks are not needed if they had been indicated previously only for direct or close patient contact.

2. All nondisposable receptacles (drainage bottles, urinals, bedpans, flowmeter jars, thermometer holders, etc.) should be returned for decontamination and reprocessing. Articles that are contaminated, or likely to be contaminated, with infective material should be bagged and labeled before being sent for decontamination and reprocessing.

3. All disposable items should be discarded. Articles that are contaminated, or likely to be contaminated, with infective material should be bagged, labeled, and disposed of in accordance with the hospital's policy on disposal of infectious wastes. Local regulations may call for the bag's incineration or disposal in an authorized sanitary landfill without being opened. No special precautions are indicated for disposal of items that are not contaminated, or not likely to be contaminated, with infective material.

4. All equipment that is not sent to central services or discarded should be cleaned with a disinfectant–detergent solution.

5. All horizontal surfaces of furniture and mattress covers should be cleaned with a disinfectant–detergent solution.

6. All floors should be wet-vacuumed or mopped with a disinfectant–detergent solution.

7. Routine washing of walls, blinds, and curtains is not indicated; however, these should be washed if they are visibly soiled. Cubicle curtains should be changed if visibly soiled.

8. Disinfectant fogging is an unsatisfactory method of decontaminating air and surfaces and thus should not be used.

9. Airing a room from which a patient has been discharged is not an effective terminal disinfection procedure and is not necessary.

10. The State Health Department and the CDC, Hospital Infections Program, should be consulted about cleaning the room of a patient who has suspected smallpox, Lassa fever, Ebola fever, or other hemorrhagic fevers, ie, Marburg disease.

Postmortem Handling of Bodies

Generally, personnel should use the same precautions to protect themselves during postmortem handling of bodies that they would use if the patient were still alive. However, masks are usually not necessary unless aerosols are expected to be generated. Autopsy personnel should be notified about the patient's disease status so that appropriate precautions can be maintained during and after autopsy. State or local regulations may call for additional special precautions for postmortem handling of bodies.

4.13 ALTERNATIVE SYSTEMS FOR ISOLATION PRECAUTIONS

Introduction

Two systems of implementing isolation precautions have been developed. These are the **Category-Specific** and **Disease-Specific systems.** The Category-Specific system groups patients by the type of isolation precautions that must be implemented. The Disease-Specific system groups patients by the specific infectious disease.

Isolation precautions are often most important during the early stages of a patient's treatment, prior to establishing a definitive diagnosis and imple-

LO-14

CLINICAL NOTE

Category-Specific system: Patients grouped by type of isolation precautions required

menting a specific treatment protocol. In these cases, category-specific precautions, which are more general, and thus offer a wider spectrum of protection, may be more practical and easier to implement.

Because the risk of transmission, and the subsequent consequences of infection, are greater in infants and young children than for adults, more stringent isolation precautions for infants and young children are recommended.

For diseases to be grouped into isolation categories, more isolation precautions must be required for some diseases than only those necessary to prevent transmission of those diseases. Such overuse of isolation precautions can be avoided by using the Disease-Specific method. Category-Specific isolation precautions, however, are easier to teach and administer. With Disease-Specific isolation precautions, each infectious disease is considered individually. Therefore, only those precautions specific to the identified disease need to be implemented. The advantage of the disease-specific isolation precautions system is a savings of supplies and expense. Excessive donning of masks, gowns, and gloves is avoided, saving time and inconvenience. This inconvenience may also cause a lack of proper adherence to necessary precautions.

Each institution can choose the system it wishes to implement. Elements of both cannot be combined easily.

CLINICAL NOTE

Disease-Specific system: Identifies isolation procedures for each disease

System A—Category-specific

Category-Specific isolation precautions is one of two isolation systems. Isolation categories are derived by grouping diseases for which similar isolation precautions are indicated.

Seven isolation categories have been developed. Notification of isolation precautions are posted in the immediate vicinity of the patient. The categories are usually indicated by color-coded isolation precaution cards posted on the door of the patient's room. Some institutions post a sign indicating that personnel and visitors must stop and see a nurse before entering. This system is used to avoid stigmatizing patients. The seven isolation categories, and their coded colors are

CLINICAL NOTE

Category-Specific system: Seven categories

1. Strict Isolation; **yellow card**
2. Contact Isolation; **orange card**
3. Respiratory Isolation; **blue card**
4. Tuberculosis (AFB) Isolation; **gray card**
5. Enteric Precautions; **brown card**
6. Drainage/Secretion Precautions; **green card**
7. Blood/Body Fluid Precautions; **violet card**

Strict Isolation

Strict Isolation is an isolation category designed to prevent transmission of highly contagious or virulent infections that may be spread by both air and contact.

Specifications for Strict Isolation

1. Private room is indicated; door should be kept closed. In general, patients infected with the same organism may share a room.
2. Masks are indicated for all persons entering the room.

3. Gowns are indicated for all persons entering the room.
4. Gloves are indicated for all persons entering the room.
5. Hands must be washed after touching the patient or potentially contaminated articles and before taking care of another patient.
6. Articles contaminated with infective material should be discarded or bagged and labeled before being sent for decontamination and reprocessing.

Diseases Requiring Strict Isolation
- Diphtheria, pharyngeal
- Lassa fever and other viral hemorrhagic fevers, ie, Marburg virus disease*
- Plague, pneumonic
- Smallpox*
- Varicella (chickenpox)
- Zoster, localized in immunocompromised patient or disseminated

* A private room with special ventilation is indicated.

Contact Isolation

Contact Isolation is designed to prevent transmission of highly transmissible or epidemiologically important infections, or colonization, that do not warrant Strict Isolation. All diseases or conditions included in this category are spread primarily by close or direct contact. Thus, masks, gowns, and gloves are recommended for anyone in close or direct contact with any patient who has an infection, or colonization, that is included in this category. For individual diseases or conditions, however, one or more of these three barriers may not be indicated. For example, masks and gloves are not generally indicated for care of infants and young children with acute viral respiratory infections, gowns are not generally indicated for gonococcal conjunctivitis in newborns, and masks are not generally indicated for care of patients infected with multiply resistant microorganisms, except those with pneumonia. Therefore, some degree of "over-isolation" may occur in this category.

Specifications for Contact Isolation
1. Private room is indicated. In general, patients infected with the same organism may share a room. During outbreaks, infants and young children with the same respiratory clinical syndrome may share a room.
2. Masks are indicated for those who come close to the patient.
3. Gowns are indicated if soiling is likely.
4. Gloves are indicated for touching infective material.
5. Hands must be washed after touching the patient or potentially contaminated articles and before taking care of another patient.
6. Articles contaminated with infective material should be discarded or bagged and labeled before being sent for decontamination and reprocessing.

Diseases or Conditions Requiring Contact Isolation
- Acute respiratory infections in infants and young children, including croup, colds, bronchitis, and bronchiolitis caused by respiratory syncytial virus, adenovirus, coronavirus, influenza viruses, parainfluenza

viruses, and rhinovirus
- Conjunctivitis, gonococcal, in newborns
- Diphtheria, cutaneous
- Endometritis, group A *Streptococcus*
- Furunculosis, staphylococcal, in newborns
- Herpes simplex, disseminated, severe primary or neonatal
- Impetigo
- Influenza, in infants and young children
- Multiply resistant bacteria, infection or colonization (any site) with any of the following:

1. Gram-negative bacilli resistant to all aminoglycosides that are tested. (In general, such organisms should be resistant to gentamicin, tobramycin, and amikacin for these special precautions to be indicated.)
2. *Staphylococcus aureus* resistant to methicillin (or nafcillin or oxacillin if they are used instead of methicillin for testing).
3. *Pneumococcus* resistant to penicillin.
4. *Haemophilus influenzae* resistant to ampicillin (beta-lactamase positive) and chloramphenicol.
5. Other resistant bacteria may be included if they are judged by the infection control team to be of special clinical and epidemiologic significance.

- Pediculosis
- Pharyngitis, infectious, in infants and young children
- Pneumonia, viral, in infants and young children
- Pneumonia, *Staphylococcus aureus* or group A *Streptococcus*
- Rabies
- Rubella, congenital and other
- Scabies
- Scalded skin syndrome, staphylococcal (Ritter's disease)
- Skin, wound, or burn infection, major (draining and not covered by dressing or dressing does not adequately contain the purulent material) including those infected with *Staphylococcus aureus* or group A *Streptococcus*
- Vaccinia (generalized and progressive eczema vaccinatum)

Respiratory Isolation

Respiratory Isolation is designed to prevent transmission of infectious diseases primarily over short distances through the air (droplet transmission). Direct and indirect contact transmission occurs with some infections in this isolation category but is infrequent.

Specifications for Respiratory Isolation

1. Private room is indicated. In general, patients infected with the same organism may share a room.
2. Masks are indicated for those who come close to the patient.
3. Gowns are not indicated.
4. Gloves are not indicated.
5. Hands must be washed after touching the patient or potentially contaminated articles and before taking care of another patient.
6. Articles contaminated with infective material should be discarded or bagged and labeled before being sent for decontamination and reprocessing.

Diseases Requiring Respiratory Isolation
- Epiglottitis, *Haemophilus influenzae*
- Erythema infectiosum
- Measles
- Meningitis
  Haemophilus influenzae, known or suspected
  Meningococcal, known or suspected
- Meningococcal pneumonia
- Meningococcemia
- Mumps
- Pertussis (whopping cough)
- Pneumonia, *Haemophilus influenzae,* in children (any age)

Tuberculosis (AFB) Isolation

Tuberculosis (AFB) Isolation is an isolation category for patients with pulmonary TB who have a positive sputum smear or a chest x-ray that strongly suggests current (active) TB. Laryngeal TB is also included in this isolation category. In general, infants and young children with pulmonary TB do not require isolation precautions because they rarely cough, and their bronchial secretions contain few AFB, compared with adults with pulmonary TB. On the instruction card, this category is called AFB (for acid-fast bacilli) isolation to protect the patient's privacy.

Specifications for Tuberculosis (AFB) Isolation

1. Private room with special ventilation is indicated; door should be kept closed. In general, patients infected with the same organism may share a room.
2. Masks are indicated only if the patient is coughing and does not reliably cover mouth.
3. Gowns are indicated only if needed to prevent gross contamination of clothing.
4. Gloves are not indicated.
5. Hands must be washed after touching the patient or potentially contaminated articles and before taking care of another patient.
6. Articles are rarely involved in transmission of TB. However, articles should be thoroughly cleaned and disinfected, or discarded.

Enteric Precautions

Enteric Precautions are designed to prevent infections that are transmitted by direct or indirect contact with feces. Hepatitis A is included in this category because it is spread through feces, although the disease is much less likely to be transmitted after the onset of jaundice. Most infections in this category primarily cause gastrointestinal symptoms, but some do not. For example, feces from patients infected with "poliovirus" and coxsackie viruses are infective, but these infections do not usually cause prominent gastrointestinal symptoms.

Specifications for Enteric Precautions

1. Private room is indicated if patient hygiene is poor. A patient with poor hygiene does not wash hands after touching infective material, contaminates the environment with infective material, or shares

contaminated articles with other patients. In general, patients infected with the same organism may share a room.

2. Masks are not indicated.
3. Gowns are indicated if soiling is likely.
4. Gloves are indicated if touching infective material.
5. Hands must be washed after touching the patient or potentially contaminated articles and before taking care of another patient.
6. Articles contaminated with infective material should be discarded or bagged and labeled before being sent for decontamination and reprocessing.

Diseases Requiring Enteric Precautions

- Amebic dysentery
- Cholera
- Coxsackievirus disease
- Diarrhea, acute illness with suspected infectious etiology
- Echovirus disease
- Encephalitis (unless known not to be caused by enteroviruses)
- Enterocolitis caused by *Clostridium difficile* or *Staphylococcus aureas*
- Enteroviral infection
- Gastroenteritis caused by
  Campylobacter species
  Cryptospordium species
  Dientamoeba fragilis
  Escherichia coli (enterotoxic, enteropathogenic, or enteroinvasive)
  Giardia lamblia
  Salmonella species
  Shigella species
  Vibrio parahaemolyticus
  Viruses—including Norwalk agent and rotavirus
  Yersinia enterocolitica
  Unknown etiology but presumed to be an infectious agent
- Hand, foot, and mouth disease
- Hepatitis, viral, type A
- Herpangina
- Meningitis, viral (unless known not to be caused by enteroviruses)
- Necrotizing enterocolitis
- Pleurodynia
- Poliomyelitis
- Typhoid fever *(Salmonella typhi)*
- Viral pericarditis, myocarditis, or meningitis (unless known not to be caused by enteroviruses).

Drainage and Secretion Precautions

Drainage and Secretion Precautions are designed to prevent infections that are transmitted by direct or indirect contact with purulent material or drainage from an infected body site. This isolation category includes many infections formerly included in Wound and Skin Precautions, Discharge (lesion), and Secretion (oral) Precautions, which have been discontinued. Infectious diseases included in this category are those that result in the production of infective purulent material, drainage, or secretions, unless the disease is included in another isolation category that requires more rigorous precautions. For example, minor or limited skin, wound, or burn infections are included in this category, but major skin, wound, or burn infections are included in Contact Isolation.

Specifications for Drainage and Secretion Precautions

1. Private room is not indicated.
2. Masks are not indicated.
3. Gowns are indicated if soiling is likely.
4. Gloves are indicated for touching infective material.
5. Hands must be washed after touching the patient or potentially contaminated articles and before taking care of another patient.
6. Articles contaminated with infective material should be discarded or bagged and labeled before being sent for decontamination and reprocessing.

Diseases Requiring Drainage and Secretion Precautions

The following infections are examples of those included in this category provided they are *not*

1. Caused by multiply resistant microorganisms.
2. Major (draining and not covered by a dressing *or* dressing does not adequately contain the drainage) skin, wound, or burn infections, including those caused by *Staphylococcus aureus* or group A *Streptococcus*.
3. Gonococcal eye infections in newborns.

See "Contact Isolation" if the infection is one of these three.

- Abscess, minor or limited
- Burn infection, minor or limited
- Conjunctivitis
- Decubitus ulcer, infected, minor or limited
- Skin infection, minor or limited
- Wound infection, minor or limited

Blood and Body Fluid Precautions

Blood and Body Fluid Precautions are designed to prevent infections that are transmitted by direct or indirect contact with infective blood or body fluids. Infectious diseases included in this category are those that result in the production of infective blood or body fluids, unless the disease is included in another isolation category that requires more rigorous precautions, for example, strict isolation. For some diseases included in this category, such as malaria, only blood is infective; for other diseases, such as hepatitis B (including antigen carriers), blood and body fluids (saliva, semen, etc.) are infective.

Specifications for Blood and Body Fluid Precautions

1. Private room is indicated if patient hygiene is poor. A patient with poor hygiene does not wash hands after touching infective material, contaminates the environment with infective material, or shares contaminated articles with other patients. In general, patients infected with the same organism may share a room.
2. Masks are not indicated.
3. Gowns are indicated if soiling of clothing with blood or body fluids is likely.

4. Gloves are indicated for touching blood or body fluids.
5. Hands must be washed immediately if they are potentially contaminated with blood or body fluids and before taking care of another patient.
6. Articles contaminated with blood or body fluids should be discarded or bagged and labeled before being sent for decontamination and reprocessing.
7. Care should be taken to avoid needle-stick injuries. Used needles should not be recapped or bent; they should be placed in a prominently labeled, puncture-resistant container designed specifically for such disposal.
8. Blood spills should be cleaned up promptly with a solution of 5.25% sodium hypochlorite diluted 1:10 with water.

Diseases Requiring Blood and Body Fluid Precautions
- Acquired immunodeficiency syndrome (AIDS)
- Arthropodborne viral fevers, eg, dengue, yellow fever, and Colorado tick fever
- Babesiosis
- Creutzfeldt–Jakob disease
- Hepatitis B (including HBsAg antigen carrier)
- Hepatitis, non-A, non-B
- Leptospirosis
- Malaria
- Rat-bite fever
- Relapsing fever
- Syphilis, primary and secondary, with skin and mucous membrane lesions

System B—Disease-specific

Disease-Specific isolation precautions is one of two isolation systems. The Disease-Specific system groups patients by the specific infectious disease. With Disease-Specific isolation precautions, each infectious disease is considered individually, so that only those precautions (private room, mask, gown, and gloves) that are indicated to interrupt transmission for the specific disease are recommended.

An instruction card has been designed to give concise information about Disease-Specific isolation precautions. When isolation precautions are imposed, information required to complete the cards should be filled in completely and legibly. Cards are conspicuously posted in the immediate area of the patient. Some institutions post a sign indicating that personnel and visitors must stop and see a nurse before entering. This system is used to avoid stigmatizing patients.

This information, including complete listings for Systems A and B is available in the CDC Guideline for Isolation Precautions in Hospitals (PB85–923401), produced by the Center for Infectious Diseases, CDC. For application in clinical settings, updated information from the CDC, and information specific to the institution, should be sought.

Modification of Isolation Precautions

Intensive Care

Patients requiring intensive care are usually at higher risk than other patients of becoming colonized or infected with organisms of special clinical or epidemiologic significance. This occurs because patients in intensive care have frequent contact with personnel, are clustered in a confined area, and are unusually susceptible to infection. Moreover, critically ill patients are more likely to have multiple invasive procedures performed on them. Because there is ample opportunity for cross-infection in the Intensive Care Unit (ICU), infection control precautions must be performed scrupulously. Frequent in-service training and close supervision to ensure adequate application of infection control and isolation precautions are particularly important for ICU personnel.

Most ICUs pose special problems for applying isolation precautions. Modifications that will neither compromise patient care nor increase the risk of infection to other patients or personnel may be necessary. The isolation precaution that is modified most frequently is the use of a private room. Ideally, private rooms should be available in ICUs, but some ICUs do not have them or do not use them for patients who are critically ill if frequent and easy accessibility by personnel is crucial. When a private room is not available or is not desirable because of the patient's critical condition, and if airborne transmission is not likely, an isolation area can be defined within the ICU by curtains, partitions, or an area marked off on the floor with tape. Instructional cards can be posted to inform personnel and visitors about the isolation precautions in use.

> **CLINICAL NOTE**
>
> ICU requires special attention to infection control measures

Patients with infections that can cause serious illness, for example chickenpox, if transmitted in hospitals, should be put in a private room even when the ICU does not have one. Because the risk of these highly contagious or virulent infections to patients and personnel is great, the inconvenience and expense associated with intensive care in a private room outside the ICU must be accepted.

One isolation precaution that should never be modified in intensive care units is frequent and appropriate handwashing. Hands should be washed between patients and may need to be washed several times during the care of a patient so that microorganisms are not transmitted from one site to another on the same patient; eg, from urinary tract to wound. Antiseptics, rather than soap, should be considered for handwashing in intensive care units.

Infants and Newborns

Isolation precautions for newborns and infants may have to be modified from those recommended for adults because

1. Usually only a small number of private rooms are available for newborns and infants.
2. During outbreaks, it is frequently necessary to establish cohorts of newborns and infants.

Moreover, a newborn may need to be placed on isolation precautions at delivery because its mother has an infection.

It has often been recommended that infected newborns or those suspected of being infected (regardless of the pathogen and clinical manifestations) should be put in a private room. This recommendation was based on the assumptions that a geographically isolated room was necessary to protect uninfected newborns and that infected newborns would receive closer scrutiny and better care in such a room. Neither of these assumptions is completely correct.

Separate isolation rooms are seldom indicated for newborns with many kinds of infection if the following conditions are met:

1. An adequate number of nursing and medical personnel are on duty and have sufficient time for appropriate handwashing.
2. Sufficient space is available for a 4 to 6-foot aisle or area between newborn stations.
3. An adequate number of sinks for handwashing are available in each nursery room or area.
4. Continuing instruction is given to personnel about the mode of transmission of infections.

When these criteria are not met, a separate room with handwashing facilities may be indicated.

Another incorrect assumption regarding isolation precautions for newborns and infants is that forced-air incubators can be substituted for private rooms. These incubators may filter the incoming air but not the air discharged into the nursery. Moreover, the surfaces of incubators housing newborns or infants can easily become contaminated with organisms infecting or colonizing the patient, or personnel working with the patient through portholes may have their hands and forearms colonized. Forced-air incubators, therefore, are satisfactory for limited "protective" isolation of newborns and infants but should not be relied on as a major means of preventing transmission from infected patients to others.

Isolation precautions for an infected or colonized newborn or infant, or for a newborn of a mother suspected of having an infectious disease can be determined by the specific viral or bacterial pathogen, the clinical manifestations, the source and possible modes of transmission, and the number of colonized or infected newborns or infants. Other factors to be considered include the overall condition of the newborn or infant and the kind of care required, the available space and facilities, the nurse-to-patient ratio, and the size and type of nursery services for newborns and infants.

In addition to applying isolation precautions, cohorts can be established to keep to a minimum the transmission of organisms or infectious diseases among different groups of newborns and infants in large nurseries. A **cohort** usually consists of all well newborns from the same 24 or 48-hour birth period; these newborns are admitted to and kept in a single nursery room and, ideally, are taken care of by a single group of personnel who do not take care of any other cohort during the same shift. After the newborns in a cohort have been discharged, the room is thoroughly cleaned and prepared to accept the next cohort.

Cohorting is not practical as a routine for small nurseries or in neonatal intensive care units or graded care nurseries. It is useful in these nurseries, however, as a control measure during outbreaks or for managing a group of infants or newborns colonized or infected with an epidemiologically important pathogen. Under these circumstances, having separate rooms for each

CLINICAL NOTE

Cohort: Grouping of all newborns born within specific time period

cohort is ideal, but not mandatory. For many kinds of infections, if cohorts can be kept separate within a single large room, and if personnel are assigned to take care of only those in the cohort, separate rooms are not necessary.

During outbreaks, newborns or infants with overt infection or colonization and personnel who are carriers, if indicated, should be identified rapidly and placed in cohorts; if rapid identification is not possible, exposed newborns or infants should be placed in a cohort separate from those with disease and from unexposed infants and newborns and new admissions. The success of cohorting depends largely on the willingness and ability of nursing and ancillary personnel to adhere strictly to the cohort system and to meticulously follow patient care practices.

Severely Compromised Patients

Patients with certain diseases, such as cancer or burns, and patients who are receiving certain therapeutic regimens, such as total body irradiation or steroids, are highly susceptible to infection. Such patients are considered to be severely compromised because the basic disease process from which they suffer, or the therapeutic regimen for treatment, makes them more susceptible to the transmission of infection.

The use of protective isolation does not appear to reduce this risk any more than strong emphasis on appropriate handwashing during patient care. Protective isolation may fail to reduce the risk of infection because compromised patients are often infected by their own (endogenous) microorganisms or are colonized and infected by microorganisms transmitted by the inadequately washed hands of personnel or by nonsterile items used in routine protective isolation. Such items may include patient care equipment, food, water, and air. Vigorous efforts to exclude all microorganisms by using patient-isolator units, eradicating endogenous flora, and sterilizing food, water, and fomites may prevent or delay onset of some infections; thus, these procedures have been recommended by some for use with very high-risk patients who have a predictable temporary period of high susceptibility. However, these extraordinary and expensive precautions do not appear warranted for most compromised patients.

In general, compromised patients should be taken care of by using precautions that are no different from routine good patient-care techniques, but for these patients, routine techniques must be emphasized and enforced. All personnel must frequently and appropriately wash their hands before, during, and after patient care. Compromised patients should be kept separate from patients who are infected or have conditions that make infection transmission likely. Private rooms should be used whenever possible.

Patients With Burns

Burn wounds are classified as major or minor according to several risk factors for burn-associated complications. Only the infectious complications of burns are considered here. Major burn wounds are classified as those that cannot be covered effectively, or those with drainage that cannot be contained effectively by use of dressings. The drainage from a minor burn can be covered and contained by dressings.

Most major burn wounds and many minor ones have become infected by the second or third day after the burn occurs. Care of burn patients, therefore, involves efforts to prevent colonization and infection of the wound,

> **COMPROMISED PATIENTS AND PATIENTS WITH BURNS**
>
> Highly susceptible to infection
> Strict adherence to routine patient-care procedures essential

and isolation precautions to prevent transmission to other patients. Other important methods of care include use of topical and systemic antimicrobials, vaccines, and general supportive measures. Burn wounds have been grouped under the subheading "skin, wound, or burn infection."

Isolation precautions and infection control techniques for major burn wounds vary among burn centers. These precautions may involve the use of strictly enforced frequent handwashing, sterile gowns, sterile gloves, and masks. Because it is not possible to "isolate" a major wound by use of dressings, a private room or a special burn center is indicated for such patients.

4.14 REVIEW QUESTIONS

1. What federal agency is responsible for developing and issuing guidelines for aseptic techniques and isolation systems?

2. Describe the eight guidelines for providing and maintaining a sterile field.

3. What apparel is necessary for aseptic techniques?

4. What is the most important procedure for preventing transmission of nosocomial infections?

5. List, in proper sequence, and describe the steps performed during a) scrubbing, b) gowning, c) gloving, d) removal of contaminated gloves.

6. List the four purposes of wound dressing.

7. Describe five methods of dressing applications.

8. List five factors affecting selection of wound dressing materials.

9. How are Hubbard tanks and immersion hydrotherapy tanks properly disinfected?

10. How are contaminated needles, scalpel blades, clothing, and linen properly discarded?

11. What are the four main routes of microorganism transmission?

12. Who is responsible for implementing and monitoring isolation procedures?

13. How do the two isolation systems differ?

4.15 SUGGESTED ACTIVITIES

1. Students practice skills presented: handwashing, gowning, gloving, wound assessment, and application of wound dressings.

2. Students observe other students performing wound dressings using a sterile field and make note of any violation of the guidelines for maintaining a sterile field.

3. Students role-play wound assessment and application of dressings.

4. Students document wound dressing procedures, including the appropriate portions of a SOAP note.

4.16 References

1. Favero MS. Chemical disinfection of medical and surgical materials. In: Block SS, ed. *Disinfection, Sterilization, and Preservation.* 3rd ed. Philadelphia: Lea and Febiger; 1983;469–492.
2. Centers for Disease Control. Guideline for Handwashing and Hospital Environmental Control, 1985. PB85-923404, 1985;2.
3. Albert RK, Condie F. Handwashing patterns in medical intensive care units. *N Engl J Med.* 1981;304:1465–1466.
4. Larson E. Compliance with isolation techniques. *Am J Infect Control.* 1983;11:221–225.
5. Lowbury EJL, Lilly HA, Bull JP. Disinfection of hands: Removal of transient organisms. *Br Med J.* 1964;2:230–233.
6. Sprunt K, Redman W, Leidy G. Antibacterial effectiveness of routine handwashing. *Pediatrics.* 1973;52:264–271.
7. Ojajarvi J. The importance of soap selection for routine hygiene in hospitals. *J Hyg* (Lond). 1981;86:275–283.
8. Occupational exposure to ethylene oxide. *Federal Register.* June 22, 1984; 29 CFR 1910.
9. Garner JS, Simmons BP. Guideline for isolation precautions in hospitals. *Infect Control.* 1983;4:245–325.
10. Centers for Disease Control. Viral hemorrhagic fever: Initial management of suspected and confirmed cases. *MMWR.* 1983;32(Suppl):275–405.
11. Rutala WA, Stiegel MM, Sarubbi FA. Decontamination of laboratory microbiological waste by steam sterilization. *Appl Environ Microbiol.* 1982;43:1311–1316.
12. Lauer JL, Battles DR, Vesley D. Decontaminating infectious laboratory waste by autoclaving. *Appl Environ Microbiol.* 1982;44:690–694.
13. Hughes HG. Chutes in hospitals. *J Can Hosp Assn.* 1964;41:56–57.
14. Walter WG, Schillinger JE. Bacterial survival in laundered fabrics. *Appl Environ Microbiol.* 1975;29:368–373.
15. Christian RR, Manchester JT, Mellor MT. Bacteriological quality of fabrics washed at lower-than-standard temperatures in a hospital laundry facility. *Appl Environ Microbiol.* 1983;45:591–597.
16. Blaser MJ, Smith PF, Cody HJ, et al. Killing of fabric-associated bacteria in hospital laundry by low-temperature washing. *J Infect Dis.* 1984:149:48–57.
17. Anderson RL, Mackel DC, Stoler BS, et al. Carpeting in hospitals: An epidemiological evaluation. *J Clin Microbiol.* 1982;15:408–415.
18. American Academy of Pediatrics, American College of Obstetricians and Gynecologists. Guidelines for perinatal care. Evanston, IL and Washington, DC. AAP, ACOG, 1983.
19. Wyowski DK, Flynt JW, Goldfield M, et al. Epidemic neonatal hyperbilirubinemia and use of a phenolic disinfectant detergent. *Pediatrics.* 1978; 61:165–170.

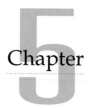

Chapter 5

Turning and Positioning

 Learner Objectives

The student will be able to:

1 Describe the goals of proper positioning.
2 Describe how to determine how much time a patient can spend in a position.
3 Describe the general procedures used to turn and position a patient properly.
4 Describe the specific procedures used to turn a patient to, and position in, supine, prone, sidelying, and sitting.

LO-1

LO-2

INTRODUCTION

Patients are sometimes unable to change their position in bed independently. The goals of proper positioning are to

1. Make the patient as comfortable as possible
2. Prevent development of deformities and pressure sores
3. Provide the patient access to the environment
4. Provide proper positioning for certain treatment procedures

To achieve these goals, the patient and environment must be properly managed. Proper patient turning and positioning is the responsibility of all health care providers who have contact with a patient.

The first time a patient is placed in a new position, the patient's skin should be checked after 5 to 10 minutes, and frequently thereafter, to determine tolerance for the position. A patient must be repositioned at least every 2 hours. More frequent repositioning is required for a patient who has problems such as poor circulation, fragile skin, or decreased sensation.

When a patient is repositioned, the skin over the area on which he or she was lying should be inspected and observed for color and integrity. Special attention should be paid to areas of skin that cover bony protrusions, such as the greater trochanter. Redness of the skin should have resolved before pressure is placed on that area of skin again. When recovery from pressure on the skin is delayed, the patient should be repositioned more frequently than every 2 hours. Excessive or prolonged redness may indicate tissue damage.

When sitting, a patient must relieve pressure on the buttocks and sacrum at least every 10 minutes. Sitting pushups, using the arm rests of a chair, leaning first to one side and then to the other, and leaning forward are methods to relieve pressure on the buttocks in the sitting position.

5.1 GENERAL PROCEDURES

LO-3

When turning and positioning a patient, the patient must be lifted, rather than dragged, across the sheets. This will prevent skin irritation, sometimes called sheet burn. Wrinkles in the sheets, blankets, and personal clothing should be avoided because they increase pressure on a small area of skin and cause skin irritation. Such pressure points are uncomfortable for a patient who is unable to move independently.

Pillows, rolled blankets, or towels are used to support body parts, and to avoid strain or pressure on ligaments, nerves, and muscles. Pillows or towels can be used to provide relief to bony protrusions, or areas of skin breakdown. Sometimes a sensitive area must be relieved of all pressure by supporting the limb segments just proximal and just distal to the sensitive area. This type of positioning is termed **bridging the gap.** To "bridge the gap," the pillows or towels are placed just proximally and distally to the involved area, preventing contact of the involved area with the supporting surface. When an area is "bridged," the time in this position should be reduced because the pillows or towels may increase pressure and decrease circulation on adjacent areas.

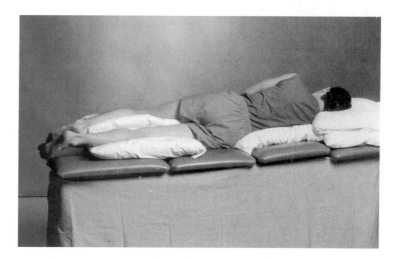

Figure 5.1–1. Positioning to bridge greater trochanter.

When sheets or blankets are used for draping or as bed linen, they should not be tucked in tightly at the foot of the bed. Doing so forces the ankle into a position of plantar flexion. Footboards are occasionally used to maintain the foot in the neutral, or anatomical, position. Footboards are usually ineffective because the patient pushes against the board, forcing his body toward the head of the bed. This permits the ankle to move into a position of plantar flexion. For some patients, stimulation to the sole of the foot causes a reflex that also results in ankle plantar flexion. Footboards, however, can be used to keep sheets and blankets from forcing the foot into plantar flexion as a result of the weight of the bedding. This is accomplished by placing the bedding over the top edge of the footboard.

Whenever possible, the patient should participate actively. For simple procedures, all explanations and directions should be given before initiation of the procedure. For multistep procedures, a general explanation should be given prior to the start of the procedure. As possible at each step, additional directions should be given. The patient may not be able to remember all steps for an entire procedure when they are concentrating on the first few steps.

In this chapter, descriptions of turning and positioning procedures are given as if the patient is unable to assist, or is able to assist only minimally. The illustrations in this chapter demonstrate a patient on a treatment table or mat. The same procedures are used when turning or positioning a patient in bed.

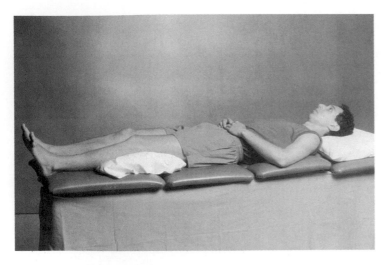

Figure 5.2–1. Supine position with pillow under knees.

5.2   SUPINE POSITION

In the supine position the patient is positioned with the shoulders parallel to the hips, and the spine straight. Many people are more comfortable with a small pillow supporting the head. A pillow can be placed under the knees to relieve strain on the lower back. This position, however, can lead to decreased hip and knee extension range of motion as a result of prolonged positioning in hip and knee flexion.

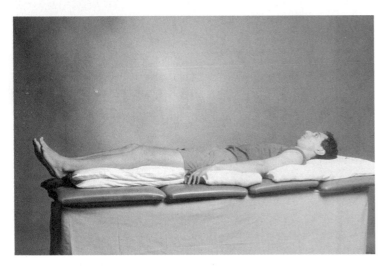

Figure 5.2–2. Supine position with pillow lengthwise.

A pillow placed lengthwise under the legs will reduce knee flexion and relieve pressure on the heels.

5.3   TURNING FROM SUPINE TO PRONE

The patient's initial position is supine. The patient must be removed far enough to one side of the treatment table to allow a full rolling movement to the prone position without coming too near the opposite edge. To roll to the left, the patient is first moved to the right side of the treatment table. When segmental movement of the trunk and lower extremities is possible, the patient is moved in stages. When the patient cannot tolerate such movement, more than one person, or specialized beds, will be needed.

The patient is moved to the edge of the treatment table in stages. First the upper trunk,

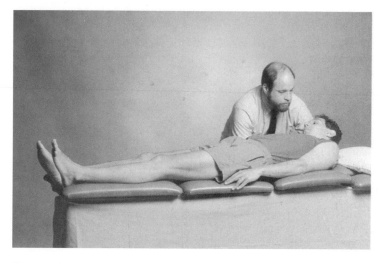

Figure 5.3–1. Moving upper trunk.

then the lower trunk,

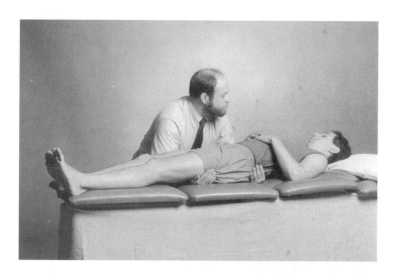

Figure 5.3–2. Moving lower trunk.

and finally the lower extremities are moved.

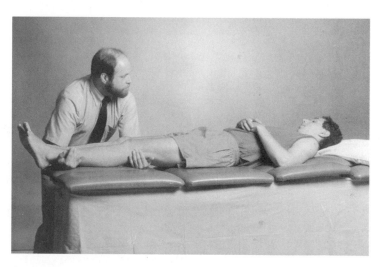

Figure 5.3–3. Moving lower extremities.

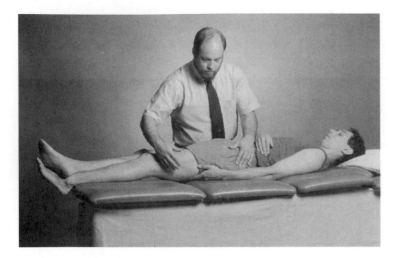

Figure 5.3–4. Position of extremities prior to turning.

The right lower extremity is crossed over the left lower extremity, with the right ankle resting on top of the left ankle. The patient's left upper extremity is adducted, placing the hand under the left hip, palm against the hip.

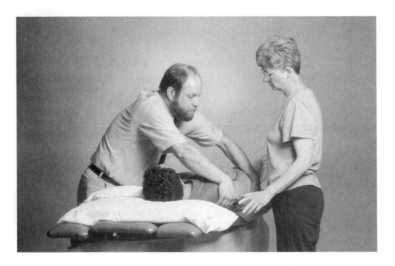

Figure 5.3–5. Position of therapist and assistant at start of turning.

The therapist should be positioned on the side to which the patient will be turned. When the treatment table is narrow, an assistant stands next to the patient to prevent the patient from falling while the therapist moves from one side of the treatment table to the other side. The assistant can help with positioning pillows and turning the patient. When a pillow will be under the patient while the patient is in the prone position, position the pillow in the proper orientation before the patient is rolled. The right upper extremity is adducted, placing the hand at the right hip, palm against the hip.

When a patient has head and neck control, he can assist in turning his head and neck in the direction of the roll as turning is initiated. When a patient does not have head and neck control, the therapist must be aware that the patient's face may be subject to some rubbing on the mattress or mat during the turn. When the therapist is ready to initiate the movement, he should indicate that to the patient, give a preparatory count, and a specific verbal command.

As the therapist initiates rolling the patient, his hands are on the patient's back. When the patient reaches the half-way point, gravity may cause the patient to finish the roll in an uncontrolled manner. Therefore, the therapist must rotate his hands as the patient reaches the midpoint of the roll, positioning his hands on the anterior surface of the patient to control the second half of the roll.

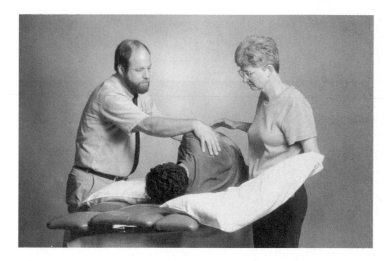

Figure 5.3–6. Therapist's hand position for first part of turning.

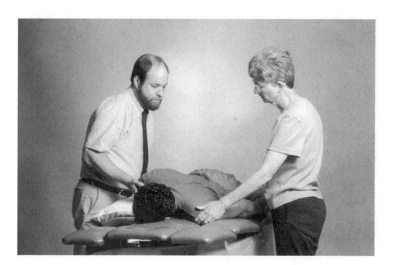

Figure 5.3–7. Therapist's hand position for second part of turning.

When the roll is completed, the first body segment to be repositioned is the head. The head must be placed in a comfortable position facing to one side. There should be no pressure on the eyes, nose, or mouth. The position of the pillow under the trunk is adjusted as needed. The arms should be placed in a position of slight abduction, approximately 20 to 30 degrees. Finally, the feet are uncrossed if they remained crossed after the roll is completed. The feet should be placed approximately 6 to 8 inches apart.

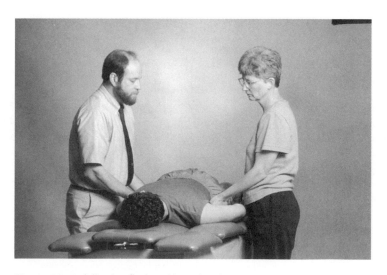

Figure 5.3–8. Adjusting final position of patient.

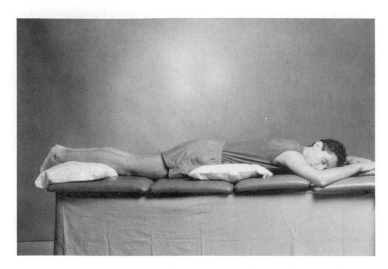

Figure 5.4–1. Prone position with arms overhead.

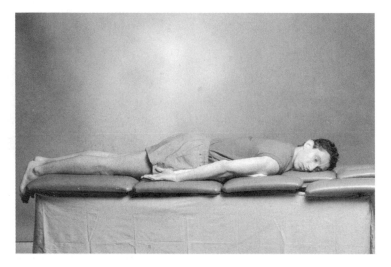

Figure 5.4–2. Prone position with arms at side, pillow lengthwise, and feet over end of table.

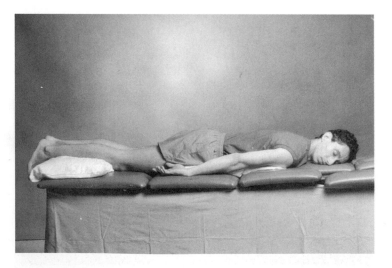

Figure 5.4–3. Prone position with arms at side, pillow lengthwise, and lower legs on pillow.

5.4   PRONE POSITION

LO-4

In the prone position, the patient is positioned with the shoulders parallel to the hips, and the spine straight. The head may be turned to either side, or maintained in the midline, with a small pillow or towel under the forehead to increase comfort.

The patient's arms may be positioned alongside the trunk or alongside the head. In some patients, circulation to the arms is impaired when the arms are placed alongside the head. The arms should be positioned alongside the head only when the patient has sensation in the arms. When the arms are positioned alongside the head, the therapist must check frequently for numbness or tingling in the patient's arms.

A pillow may be placed lengthwise or crosswise under the trunk. The amount of spinal curvature should not be excessive at any segment. The lengthwise position may be more comfortable when the patient has limited neck mobility. The crosswise position of the pillow may be more comfortable for a patient with low back pain. The lordotic curve of the lumbar region generally is reduced by the crosswise position of the pillow. Care with positioning of the pillow to ensure comfort and alignment is particularly important for women with large breasts.

The patient's feet can be positioned over the end of the treatment table. A pillow under the lower legs can also be used to avoid positioning the ankles in plantar flexion. A pillow under the lower leg places the knee in slight flexion, however, and may promote loss of knee extension range of motion.

5.5 TURNING FROM PRONE TO SUPINE

LO-4 In many respects, rolling from prone to supine is the reverse of rolling from supine to prone. The patient's initial position is prone. The preparatory steps of moving to one side of the treatment table, and of placement of the patient's hands, remain the same. The crossing of the lower extremities is usually unnecessary.

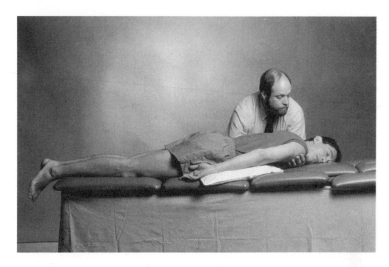

Figure 5.5–1. Moving head and upper trunk.

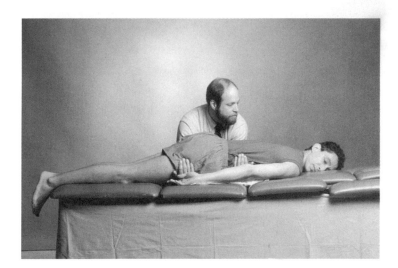

Figure 5.5–2. Moving lower trunk.

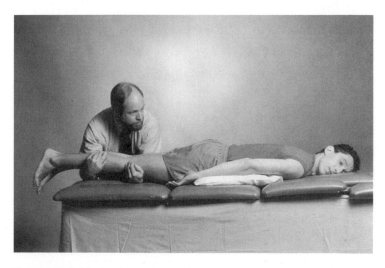

Figure 5.5–3. Moving lower extremities.

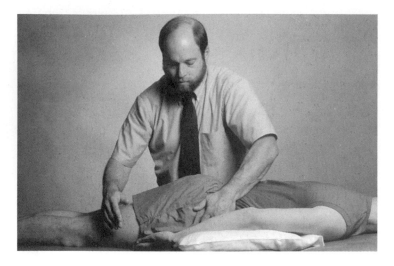

Figure 5.5–4. Positioning patient's hand for turning.

The right upper extremity is adducted, placing the hand under the right hip, palm against the hip.

The therapist is again positioned on the side to which the patient will roll. When the treatment table is narrow, an assistant should guard the patient as the therapist moves from one side of the treatment table to the other side. The assistant can help with positioning of pillows and the patient. When rolling prone to supine, rubbing of the face on the mattress or mat can be avoided by having the patient start by facing away from the therapist. When the patient has head control, he can assist by looking up and over his shoulders as he is turned towards the therapist.

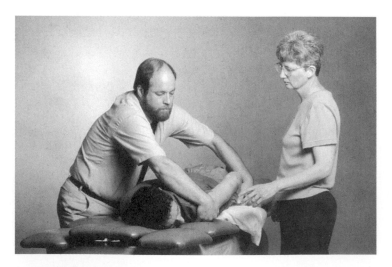

Figure 5.5–5. Position of therapist and assistant at start of turning.

The left upper extremity is adducted, placing the hand at the hip, palm against the hip. The therapist supports the left upper extremity against the patient's body as the patient is rolled.

As in rolling from supine to prone, the therapist must control both phases of the rolling motion. Initially, the therapist reaches over the patient, placing his hands on the patient's anterior surface. When the patient reaches the halfway point, gravity may cause the patient to finish the roll in an uncontrolled manner. Therefore, the therapist must rotate his hands as the patient reaches the midpoint of the roll, positioning his hands on the posterior surface of the patient to control the second half of the roll. Once the turn is completed, the extremities are positioned as for the supine position.

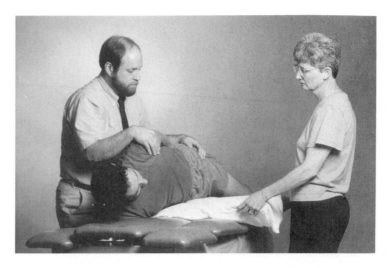

Figure 5.5–6. Therapist's hand position for first part of turning.

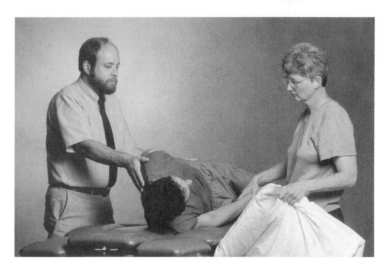

Figure 5.5–7. Therapist's hand position for second part of turning.

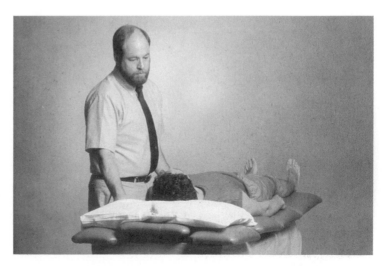

Figure 5.5–8. Adjusting final position of patient.

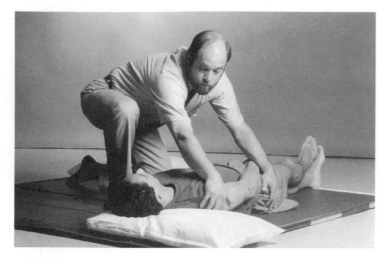

Figure 5.6–1. Starting position for turning on floor mat.

5.6 TURNING ON THE FLOOR MAT

LO-4

When turning a patient on the floor mat, the same steps are followed as when turning a patient on a treatment table. The therapist should be positioned on the side to which the patient will turn. A half-kneeling position should be assumed, with the "down" knee at the level of the patient's hips, and the "up" knee at the level of the patient's shoulders. In the illustrations in this section, the patient will turn to the left.

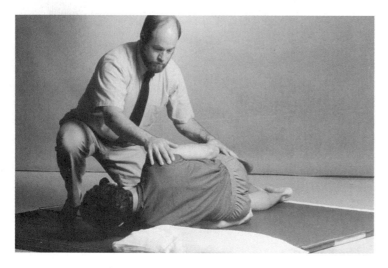

Figure 5.6–2. Therapist's hand position for first part of turning.

The therapist places his left hand on the patient's right hip, holding the patient's right hand on the hip. The therapist's right hand is placed on the patient's right shoulder. The hand position must rotate at the midpoint of the roll, as described earlier.

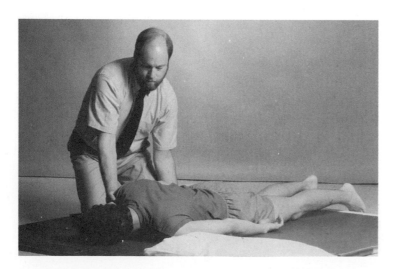

Figure 5.6–3. Therapist's hand position for second part of turning.

The therapist must move out of the patient's way as he is turned, allowing the patient to complete the roll without rolling into the therapist.

5.7 TURNING FROM SUPINE TO SIDELYING

A sidelying position can be attained from either the supine or prone positions. The illustrations in this section demonstrate turning to the left.

LO-4

To position a patient on his left side, the initial position is supine and to the right side of the treatment table, but not on the extreme edge. The left arm is abducted to approximately 45 degrees. The right lower extremity is crossed over the left lower extremity at the ankle.

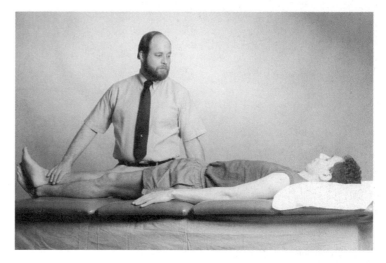

Figure 5.7–1. Starting position to turn to sidelying.

The therapist assumes a position on the side to which the patient is turning. The therapist's left hand grasps the patient's right hip, holding the patient's right hand against the patient's hip. The therapist's right hand grasps the patient's right shoulder. The patient is rolled to the sidelying position.

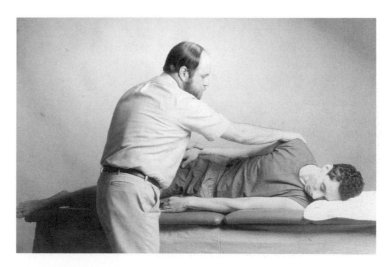

Figure 5.7–2. Turning to sidelying.

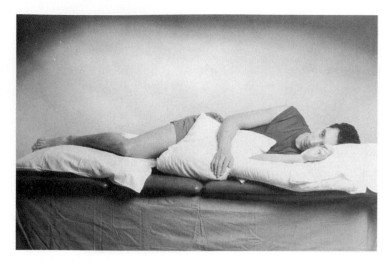

Figure 5.8–1. Sidelying position with upper trunk rotated forward.

5.8   SIDELYING POSITION

LO-4

In the sidelying position, a patient may be positioned with the upper trunk rotated forward or backward. Proper positioning requires a pillow under the head. When a patient is rotated forward, a pillow is placed in front of the patient. The uppermost upper extremity is brought forward to rest on the pillow.

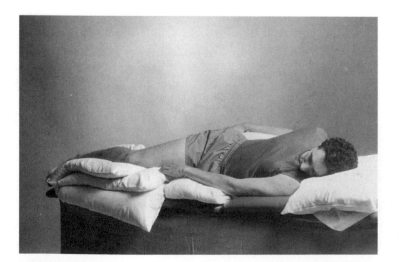

Figure 5.8–2. Sidelying position with upper trunk rotated backward.

When a patient is rotated backward, the pillow is placed behind the patient, and the uppermost upper extremity is extended and supported by the pillow behind the patient.

To avoid excessive pressure on the lowermost lower extremity, the uppermost lower extremity should not lie directly on top of the lowermost lower extremity. In both positions, the uppermost lower extremity is flexed at the hip and knee, and supported on pillows. To avoid excessive pull on the lower trunk the uppermost lower extremity must be supported by a sufficient number of pillows to support the lower extremity in proper alignment with the trunk.

5.9   ASSUMING SITTING

LO-4 There are several methods for a patient to assume a sitting position from supine. The method used depends upon the patient's functional abilities, the medical problem, and starting position. In all cases, a patient should not be left unguarded in the sitting position when he cannot maintain the position safely.

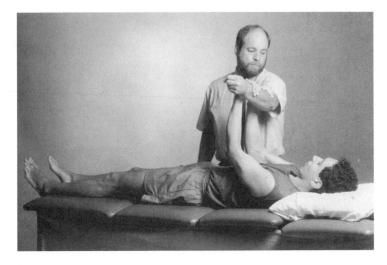

Figure 5.9–1. Starting position to assume long sitting.

Supine to Long Sitting

When a patient has enough strength, he can assume a long sitting position by doing a situp on the treatment table. When minimal assistance is needed, as for a patient with generalized weakness, a trapeze bar can be used. In some cases a patient performs a situp or uses a trapeze bar while the therapist assists at the same time. To assist in the assumption of the sitting position, the therapist can put an arm behind the patient's back to assist the patient. The therapist should be aware of putting too much pressure on a small area of the patient's back.

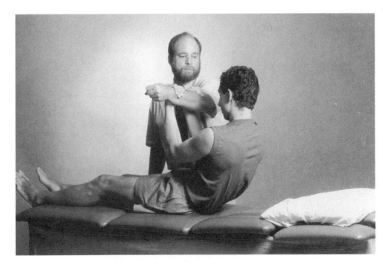

Figure 5.9–2. Patient pulling to long sitting.

When a trapeze bar is not available, the therapist can stabilize his arm in front of the patient and allow the patient to pull himself up by pulling on the therapist's arm. The therapist should not move his arm and do the patient's work. The therapist must move toward the patient's feet, however, to permit the patient to assume the long sitting position.

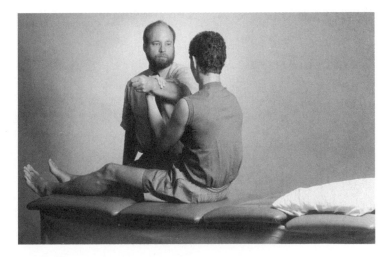

Figure 5.9–3. Therapist moves to permit assumption of long sitting.

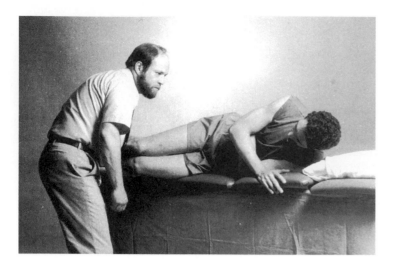

Figure 5.9–4. Initial sidelying position to assume sitting.

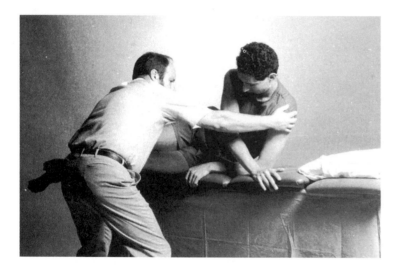

Figure 5.9–5. Using lower legs as counterweights to assume sitting.

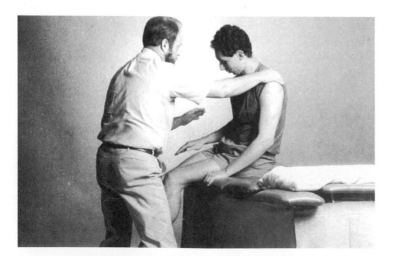

Figure 5.9–6. Completing assumption of sitting on side of treatment table.

Sidelying to Side of Treatment Table

To assist a patient to assume sitting on the side of a treatment table, the patient's lower extremities can be lowered over the edge of the treatment table to act as counterweights.

The patient assumes a sidelying position to the side of the treatment table where the patient wants to sit. In the sidelying position, flexing the hips and knees 60 to 90 degrees moves the lower legs off the treatment table. As the lower legs move off the treatment table, they act to rotate the patient into a sitting position. With the legs acting as counterweights, the patient uses his upper extremities to assume sitting. The therapist can assist by controlling the lowering of the legs and lifting the upper trunk as necessary.

Supine to Side of Treatment Table

This method also uses the lower legs as counter-weights, and is necessary for patients who require more assistance.

The therapist places one arm behind the patient's shoulders, and his other arm under the patient's thighs. The therapist pivots the patient so that the patient's lower legs are past the side of the treatment table. At the same time, the therapist begins to lift the patient's trunk. The lower legs are lowered completely as the patient's trunk is brought into an upright position. Lifting the patient's trunk is easier for the therapist because the lower legs serve as a counterweight.

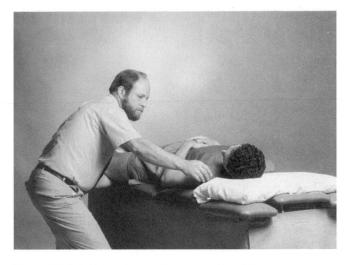

Figure 5.9–7. Initial supine position to assume sitting.

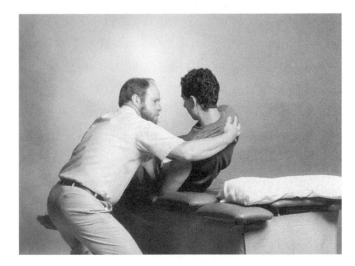

Figure 5.9–8. Pivoting and assisting patient into sitting.

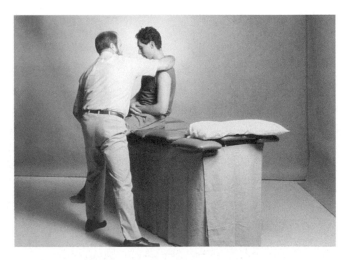

Figure 5.9–9. Completing assumption of sitting on side of treatment table.

5.10 REVIEW QUESTIONS

1. How often does a patient need to be repositioned?

2. Describe how to "bridge a gap."

3. Describe how to position a patient properly in the supine, prone, and sidelying positions.

4. Describe how to turn a patient properly from supine to prone, supine to sidelying, sidelying to prone, sidelying to supine, and prone to supine.

5. Describe how to assist a patient to sitting from supine.

5.11 SUGGESTED ACTIVITIES

1. Demonstrate to students the specific procedures presented.

2. Students practice the specific procedures presented working in groups of three (role-playing patient, therapist, and assistant).

3. Students practice performing turning and positioning while other partners role-play various diagnoses (see case studies below). The student role-playing the patient can add "character" to the role by using such examples as being cooperative, noncooperative, in pain, hard of hearing, or faint to enhance the activity. The "patient" must role-play the diagnosis and character consistently.

4. Students monitor vital signs and check for signs of skin irritation as appropriate.

5. Students practice teaching "family and patients" and other health care providers how to perform turning and positioning.

6. Students document treatment using the SOAP note format.

CASE STUDIES

1. The patient is a 67-year-old female who has left hemiplegia (stage 1 of recovery).

2. The patient is a 23-year-old male with C3 complete quadriplegia.

3. The patient is a 4-year-old with cerebral palsy, presenting with severe spastic quadriplegia.

4. The patient is an 81-year-old female with a fractured right hip (intertrochanteric fracture).

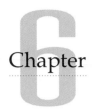

Chapter

Range-of-Motion Exercise

 Learner Objectives

The student will be able to:

1 Distinguish between joint range of motion (ROM) and muscle ROM.
2 Indicate when passive ROM (PROM), active-assisted ROM (AAROM), and active ROM (AROM) exercises are appropriate.
3 Describe different joint end feels.
4 Describe differences in movement when a patient has normal muscle tone, spasticity, rigidity, and pain.
5 Describe the general methods used to perform ROM exercises properly.
6 Describe the anatomical position.
7 Define the terms used to describe movements in the anatomical planes.
8 Describe the benefits of using diagonal patterns of motion.
9 Describe the combining components of motion used in proprioceptive neuromuscular facilitation (PNF).
10 Describe, and correctly perform, the specific procedures used to perform ROM exercises in the anatomical planes and diagonal patterns of motion.

INTRODUCTION

LO-1

Range-of-motion exercises are movements of each joint and muscle through the available range of motion. Range-of-motion exercises are performed to prevent the development of contractures, muscle shortening, and tightness in capsules, ligaments, and tendons that can limit mobility. Range-of-motion exercises also provide sensory stimulation that is beneficial to patients.

Each joint must have range of motion performed in two different ways. First, range of motion must be performed with respect only to actual joint surface movements; this type is called **joint range of motion.** Second, range of motion must be performed with respect to the length of the muscles that cross a joint; this type is called **muscle range of motion.** The therapist must differentiate between range-of-motion exercises that use only the available range of motion and stretching exercises, which are designed to increase the available range of motion.

LO-2

Joint and muscle range-of-motion (ROM) exercises may be performed as **passive (PROM), active assisted (AAROM),** and **active (AROM)** range-of-motion exercises. Passive exercise is usually performed when the patient is unable to move the body segment, such as paralysis. Other indications for the performance of passive range of motion include cases in which active participation results in increased muscle tone, pain, excessive cardiopulmonary stress, or when patients lack safe control of movements. During passive exercise, the patient is relaxed and the therapist moves the body segment. Active assisted range-of-motion exercise is performed when the patient needs assistance in moving because of paresis, weakness, pain, cardiopulmonary problems, or increased muscle tone. During active assisted exercise, the therapist assists the patient to move through the available range of motion. Active range-of-motion exercises are performed independently by the patient, although they may be supervised by the therapist to ensure correct performance.

CLINICAL NOTE

Indications for ROM

The limit of a range of motion is achieved when the body segment cannot be moved further because of restriction by tissues or patient reports of pain. When the limit of a range of motion is attained, the quality of the restriction felt by the therapist which limits further motion is described as **end feel.** Normal end feels vary depending on the reason for the limitation of further motion. When further motion is limited by bone abutting bone, the end feel is hard, and is called a bony end feel. An example of bony end feel is when complete elbow extension is attained, and the humerus and ulna make contact with each other. When further motion is limited by soft tissue approximation, the end feel is soft. An example of soft end feel is when elbow flexion is limited by forearm soft tissue approximating the muscle bulk of elbow flexors on the anterior surface of the upper arm. A firm end feel with minimal give is a result of a taut capsule or ligament. Therefore this is known as a capsular end feel. An example of soft end feel is when complete elbow flexion is attained. When further motion is limited by pain, there is no tissue limitation to motion and the end feel is described as empty. This is called an empty end feel.

LO-3

CLINICAL NOTE

Types of end feel

In some patients, involuntary muscle contractions may interfere with range of motion. This can occur in patients with upper motor neuron lesions, or when a patient involuntarily contracts muscles to avoid pain. Mus-

LO-4

cle tone is altered in upper motor neuron lesions, and usually presents as spasticity or rigidity. **Spasticity** presents as gradually increasing resistance to movement. A point may be reached where further movement is prevented temporarily, and then followed by a sudden reduction of tone if resistance is maintained (clasp-knife phenomenon). Following the sudden reduction of tone, movement through the remaining range of motion is possible. Spasticity usually occurs in antigravity muscles. **Rigidity** usually presents as resistance to passive movement in any direction. The resistance of rigidity is the same throughout the range of motion. Rigidity occurs in both antigravity and progravity muscles. Cogwheel rigidity, as observed in Parkinsonian patients, is a pattern of alternating resistance and lack of resistance throughout a range of motion. In the presence of spasticity or rigidity, slow maintained movement will usually permit movement through the complete range of motion without eliciting interference.

6.1   METHOD

Range-of-motion exercises are performed by moving body segments through each anatomic plane of motion separately, or by combining components of motion. When combining components of motion are used, the most commonly used are the diagonal patterns of motion of the **proprioceptive neuromuscular facilitation (PNF)**[1] approach to therapeutic exercise.

When a therapist performs a range-of-motion exercise with a patient, the patient's body segment is held gently and firmly to provide support. Hand placement should allow movement of the body segment through complete range of motion with minimal hand repositioning. Support must be provided for all segments distal to the joint at which the motion is to occur. The speed of movement should be slow to moderate. Joint range-of-motion exercise should encompass all planes of motion available in a joint. Muscle range-of-motion exercise must lengthen a multijoint muscle across all joints over which the muscle acts simultaneously. Several joints may be exercised simultaneously, such as the combinations of hip and knee flexion with ankle dorsiflexion and hip and knee extension with ankle plantar flexion.

Joint range of motion is performed to maintain capsule and ligament length and move synovial fluid in the joint to maintain nutrition of joint cartilage. To ensure moving a joint through its complete joint range of motion, multijoint muscles (muscles that cross more than one joint) must *not* be lengthened simultaneously across all joints over which they act. Muscle range of motion is performed to maintain the length of muscles. To maintain the length of muscles, they *must be* lengthened simultaneously across all joints over which they act. In certain circumstances, a goal of treatment is to allow multijoint muscles to become shortened (not able to be lengthened over all joints at once) to provide a more functional length. An example would be to permit limited shortening of the finger flexors of a quadriplegic patient to provide some grasp and release as the wrist is extended and flexed. This functional use of shortening is called tenodesis action.

To assist the therapist in maintaining proper posture and body mechanics during range-of-motion exercises, an adjustable height table or bed may be used.

LO-5

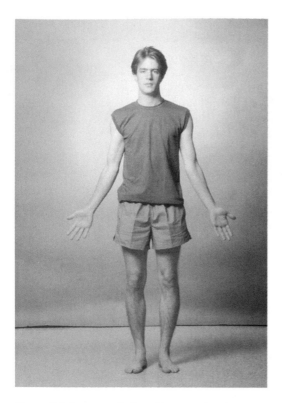

Figure 6.2–1. Anatomical position, anterior view.

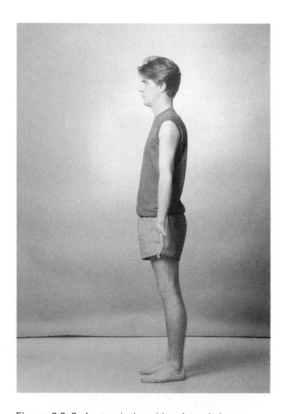

Figure 6.2–2. Anatomical position, lateral view.

6.2 ANATOMICAL PLANES OF MOTION

LO-6

All motions of the body are described in terms of starting from the anatomical position. The anatomical position is described as that position in which a person is standing upright, eyes looking straight ahead, arms at the sides with palms facing forward, and the feet approximately 4 inches apart at the heels with the toes pointing forward.

> **CLINICAL NOTE**
>
> Anatomical planes for full ROM

In the anatomical position, three anatomical (or cardinal) planes are defined. The sagittal plane divides the body into two sides, left and right. The midsagittal plane divides the body exactly into left and right halves. Motions of flexion and extension occur in the sagittal plane. The frontal, or coronal, plane divides the body into front and back portions. Motions of abduction and adduction occur in the frontal plane. The only motions of flexion and extension and abduction and adduction that do not occur in their respective planes are motions of the thumb. Thumb flexion and extension occurs in the frontal plane, and thumb abduction and adduction occurs in the sagittal plane. The transverse plane divides the body into upper and lower portions. All movements of rotation occur in the transverse plane.

The following definitions assume starting in the anatomical position.

LO-7

Flexion: Except for the thumb, flexion is movement in the sagittal plane. For the thumb, flexion is movement in the frontal plane. For the neck, trunk, upper extremities, and lower extremities other than knee and toes, flexion results in approximation of anterior surfaces. For the knee and toes, flexion results in approximation of posterior and plantar surfaces respectively. Dorsiflexion is the movement of the ankle that is considered flexion.

Extension: Except for the thumb, extension is movement in the sagittal plane. For the thumb, extension is movement in the frontal plane. For the neck, trunk, upper extremities, and lower extremities other than knee and toes, extension results in anterior surfaces moving away from each other. For the knee and toes, extension results in posterior and plantar surfaces moving away from each other respectively. Plantar flexion is the movement of the ankle that is considered extension.

Abduction: Except for the thumb, abduction is movement in the frontal plane, and is the result of a limb segment moving away from the midline of the body. For the thumb, abduction occurs in the sagittal plane, and is movement of the thumb away from the palm of the hand.

Adduction: Except for the thumb, adduction is movement in the frontal plane, and is the result of a limb segment moving towards the midline of the body. For the thumb, adduction occurs in the sagittal plane, and is movement into the palm of the hand.

Protraction: Protraction is multiplanar movement of the scapula around the lateral aspect of the ribs toward the anterior aspect of the thorax.

Retraction: Retraction is a multiplanar movement of the scapula around the lateral aspect of the ribs as the scapula returns from protraction to its normal resting position on the posterior aspect of the thorax.

It should be noted that scapular protraction is often termed scapular abduction, and scapular retraction is often termed scapular adduction.

Opposition: Opposition is the approximation of the tips of the thumb and small finger of the same hand.

Internal (medial) rotation: Internal rotation is movement in the transverse plane in which the anterior surface of the limb segment is turned towards the midline of the body.

External (lateral) rotation: External rotation is movement in the transverse plane in which the anterior surface of the limb segment is turned away from the midline of the body.

Supination: Supination is movement that occurs in the transverse plane in the forearm, and as a triplanar motion in the foot and ankle. Supination of the forearm occurs when the upper arm is stabilized, and the forearm is rotated so that the palm faces anteriorly. Supination of the foot occurs when the leg is stabilized and the foot is rotated about the oblique axes of the subtalar and other mid-foot joints, resulting in the triplanar motion that incorporates plantar flexion, forefoot adduction, and inversion of the foot.

Pronation: Pronation is movement that occurs in the transverse plane in the forearm, and as a triplanar motion in the foot and ankle. Pronation of the forearm occurs when the upper arm is stabilized, and the forearm is rotated so that the palm faces posteriorly. Pronation of the foot occurs when the leg is stabilized and the foot is rotated about the oblique axes of the subtalar and other mid-foot joints, resulting in the triplanar motion that incorporates dorsiflexion, forefoot abduction, and eversion of the foot.

Inversion: Inversion is movement of the foot that occurs in the frontal plane about the long axis of the foot. Inversion occurs when the foot is rotated about its long axis so the plantar surface of the foot faces toward the midline of the body.

Eversion: Eversion is movement of the foot that occurs in the frontal plane about the long axis of the foot. Eversion occurs when the foot is rotated about its long axis so the plantar surface of the foot faces away from the midline of the body.

It should be noted that there is confusion concerning the use of the terms supination and pronation or inversion and eversion when describing motion at the foot and ankle. The definitions provided are those used by the majority of clinicians in practice. The clinical definitions are based upon the writing of Root and co-workers.[2] Under the clinical definitions, supination and pronation are terms describing triplanar movement, of which inversion and eversion are uniplanar components. Anatomists,[3] however, describe these terms of foot and ankle motion in the opposite manner. Under the anatomical definitions, inversion and eversion are terms describing triplanar movement, of which supination and pronation are uniplanar components.

The manner in which these terms are used in this text follows the clinical definitions as presented by Root and colleagues[2] as listed in this section.

6.3 DIAGONAL PATTERNS OF MOTION

Two diagonal patterns have been described for the upper and lower extremities.[1,4] Diagonal patterns of motion are achieved by simultaneously combining components of all three cardinal plane motions. Figure 6.3–1 demonstrates the difference between two successive cardinal plane motions on the left, and the simultaneous combining of three cardinal plane motions into a diagonal pattern on the right.

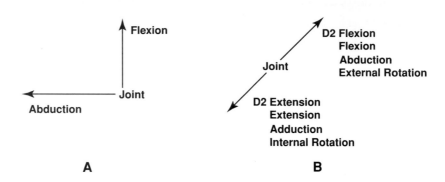

A

B

Figure 6.3–1. Components of motion of the shoulder.
A. Performed in anatomical planes.   B. Performed in diagonal patterns.

LO-8

CLINICAL NOTE

Diagonal patterns for functional ROM

Specific diagonal patterns of motion are described by the combination of motions performed by either the shoulder or the hip joints. These patterns are modified by varying the position or movement of the elbow or knee, providing the ability to perform both joint range of motion and muscle range of motion. The two diagonal patterns are commonly referred to as D1 and D2, where "D" stands for diagonal, and "1" and "2" refers to specific diagonal patterns.

When combining components of motion are performed, joint movements and muscle lengthening may not occur through as much range of motion as when anatomical planes of motion are used. However, the mobility necessary for function is maintained by diagonal patterns. Sensory feedback from movement in diagonal patterns is thought to be closer to the sensory feedback provided by normal active movement than movement in cardinal planes.

Table 6–1 lists the combining components of motion found in the proprioceptive neuromuscular facilitation patterns.

TABLE 6–1. Combining Components of Motion in PNF Diagonals

LO-9

| | Diagonal 1 Upper Extremity | | | Diagonal 1 Lower Extremity | |
	Flexion	Extension		Flexion	Extension
Scapula	Elevation	Depression			
	Abduction	Adduction			
	Upward rotation	Downward rotation			
Shoulder	Flexion	Extension	Hip	Flexion	Extension
	Adduction	Abduction		Adduction	Abduction
	External rotation	Internal rotation		External rotation	Internal rotation
Elbow	Straight	Straight	Knee	Straight	Straight
	or Flexion	or Extension		or Flexion	or Extension
	or Extension	or Flexion		or Extension	or Flexion
Forearm	Supination	Pronation			
Wrist	Flexion	Extension	Ankle	Dorsiflexion	Plantar flexion
	Radial deviation	Ulnar deviation		Inversion	Eversion
Fingers	Flexion	Extension	Toes	Extension	Flexion
	Adduction	Abduction			
Thumb	Flexion	Extension			

| | Diagonal 2 Upper Extremity | | | Diagonal 2 Lower Extremity | |
	Flexion	Extension		Flexion	Extension
Scapula	Elevation	Depression			
	Adduction	Abduction			
	Upward rotation	Downward rotation			
Shoulder	Flexion	Extension	Hip	Flexion	Extension
	Abduction	Adduction		Abduction	Adduction
	External rotation	Internal rotation		Internal rotation	External rotation
Elbow	Straight	Straight	Knee	Straight	Straight
	or Flexion	or Extension		or Flexion	or Extension
	or Extension	or Flexion		or Extension	or Flexion
Forearm	Supination	Pronation			
Wrist	Extension	Flexion	Ankle	Dorsiflexion	Plantar flexion
	Radial deviation	Ulnar deviation		Eversion	Inversion
Fingers	Extension	Flexion	Toes	Extension	Flexion
	Abduction	Adduction			
Thumb	Extension	Opposition			

For each of the following passive range-of-motion procedures, we have indicated the joints for which range of motion is being performed, the movement required to perform that range of motion, and the therapist's hand placement. Where appropriate, precautions have been noted. For those procedures specifically involving multijoint muscles, we have named the muscles involved. **The movements listed are the movements required to lengthen the muscles, and are not the movements that the muscles produce.**

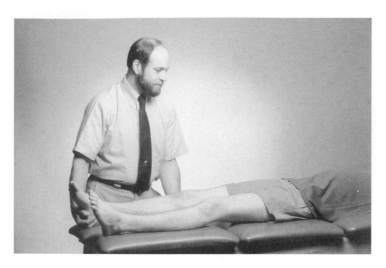

Figure 6.4–1. Hip and knee extension.

6.4   LOWER EXTREMITY

Anatomical Planes

LO-10

Joints: Hip and knee
Motions: Extension and flexion
Position: Supine
Hand Placement: Heel and posterior knee

Precaution: Hip motion is complete when pelvic rotation occurs; anterior pelvic rotation with hip extension, posterior pelvic rotation with hip flexion. Pelvic rotation should not be allowed to occur.

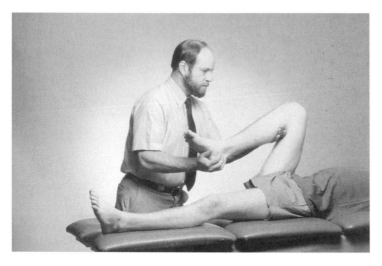

Figure 6.4–2. Hip and knee flexion.

Joints: Hip and knee
Muscles: Semitendinosus, semimembranosus, biceps femoris

LO-10 **Motions:** Hip flexion with knee extension—Straight leg raise (SLR)

Position: Supine

Hand Placement: Heel and posterior knee

Note: This maneuver lengthens the multijoint muscles of the posterior thigh across both joints over which they act.

Precautions: The knee must be kept extended. The hip must not be allowed to rotate, adduct, or abduct. The pelvis must not be allowed to rotate posteriorly.

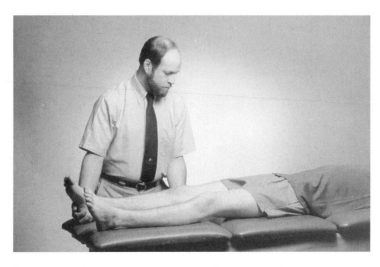

Figure 6.4–3. Starting position for straight leg raise (SLR).

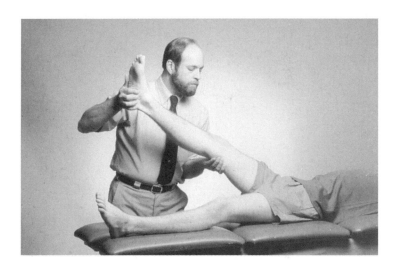

Figure 6.4–4. Hip flexion with knee extended (SLR).

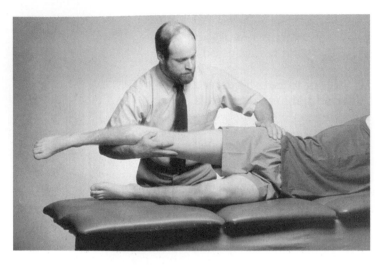

Figure 6.4–5. Hip extension, sidelying.

Joint: Hip
Motion: Extension
Position: Sidelying
LO-10 **Alternative Position:** Prone
Hand Placement: One hand is placed on the pelvis for stabilization. The other hand and forearm supports the patient's lower extremity in the anatomical position.

Note: The knee is maintained in extension.

Precaution: The end of hip extension is achieved when the pelvis starts to rotate anteriorly.

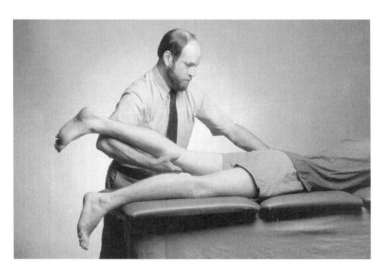

Figure 6.4–6. Hip extension, prone.

Joint: Hip

Motions: Abduction and adduction

LO-10 **Position:** Supine

Hand Placement: Heel and posterior knee

Note: To perform adduction beyond neutral, the opposite lower extremity is abducted.

Precaution: Hip flexion, hip rotation, and pelvic motion must be avoided.

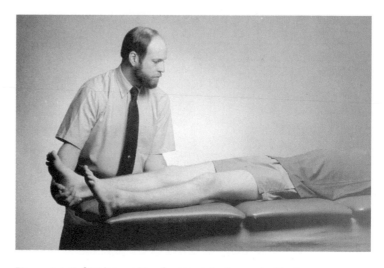

Figure 6.4–7. Starting position for hip abduction and adduction.

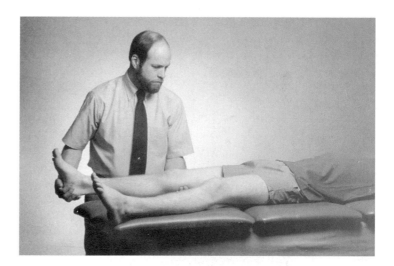

Figure 6.4–8. Hip abduction.

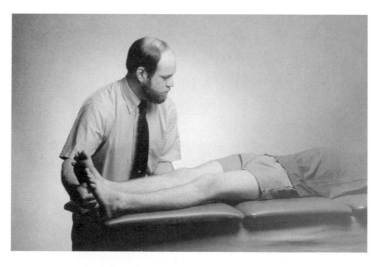

Figure 6.4–9. Hip adduction.

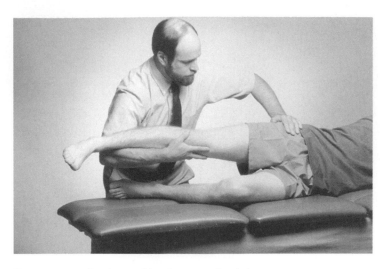

Figure 6.4–10. Starting position for tensor fascia latae.

LO-10

Joint: Hip
Muscle: Tensor fascia latae
Motions: Extension and adduction
Position: Sidelying
Hand Placement: Lower leg and pelvis (In the second picture, the therapist has positioned himself so the position of the lower extremity can be seen.)

Note: The tensor fascia latae flexes and abducts the hip, and may assist in knee extension. Hip extension, adduction, and knee flexion lengthen this muscle.

Precaution: Lateral pelvic motion must not be substituted for hip motion.

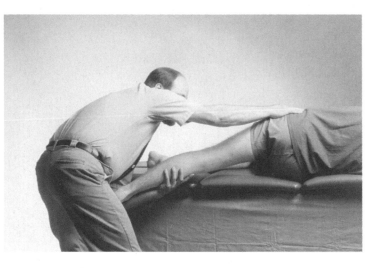

Figure 6.4–11. Ending position for tensor fascia latae.

Joint: Hip

Motions: Internal (medial) and external (lateral) rotation

LO-10 **Position:** Supine with hip and knee flexed to 90 degrees

Alternative Position: Sitting

Hand Placement: Heel and posterior knee

Alternative Hand Placement: Heel and distal anterior thigh

Precautions: Avoid excessive stress on the medial and lateral structures of the knee. Maintain the pelvis flat on the supporting surface.

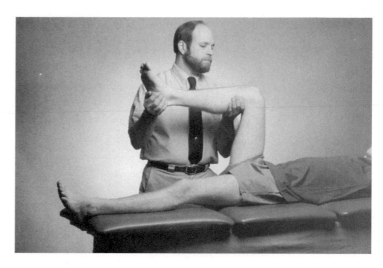

Figure 6.4–12. Starting position for hip rotation.

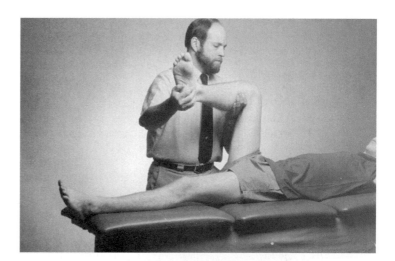

Figure 6.4–13. Hip external rotation.

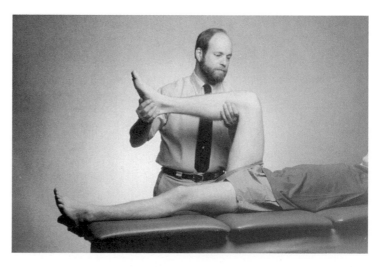

Figure 6.4–14. Hip internal rotation.

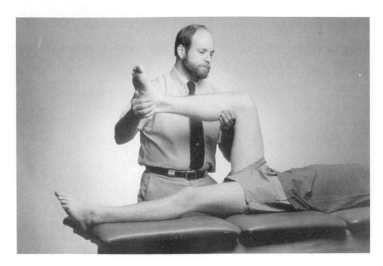

Joint: Knee
Motion: Flexion
Position: Supine with hip flexed to
LO-10 90 degrees
Hand Placement: Heel and poste-
rior knee

Figure 6.4–15. Mid-position for knee flexion.

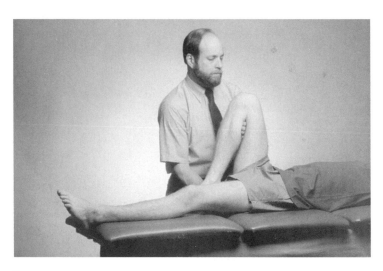

Figure 6.4–16. Ending position for knee flexion.

Joints: Hip and knee

Muscle: Rectus femoris

Motion: Knee flexion

LO-10 **Position:** Prone with hip extended

Alternative Position: Supine with knee at end of table

Hand Placement: One hand stabilizes the pelvis and the other hand flexes the knee.

Precaution: The rectus femoris is a hip flexor and knee extensor. Anterior pelvic rotation or hip flexion should not be allowed to occur.

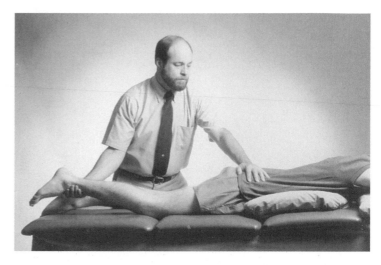

Figure 6.4–17. Starting position for rectus femoris ROM.

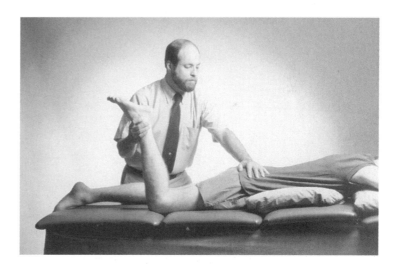

Figure 6.4–18. Ending position for rectus femoris ROM.

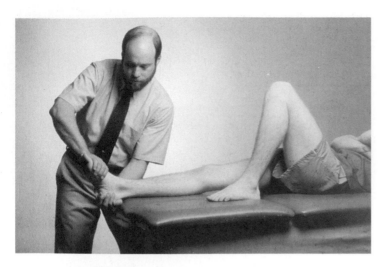

Figure 6.4–19. Starting position for ankle plantar flexion.

Joint: Ankle (talocrural)
Motion: Plantar flexion
Position: Supine
LO-10 **Hand Placement:** Heel and dorsum of foot

Note: Motion should emphasize movement of the talocrural joint, and not the midfoot joints.

Precaution: Force is applied to the heel in the superior direction, and not to the dorsum of the foot.

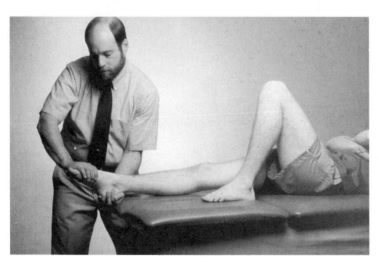

Figure 6.4–20. Ending position for ankle plantar flexion.

Joint: Ankle (talocrural)
Motion: Dorsiflexion
Position: Supine
LO-10 **Hand Placement:** Heel and posterior knee

Note: To stretch the structures of the ankle joint and the one joint soleus muscle, the knee must be flexed so the gastrocnemius muscle does not limit motion.

Precaution: Force is applied to the heel in the inferior direction, and not to the ball of the foot.

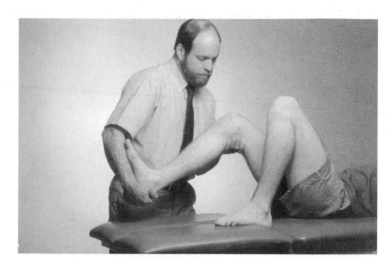

Figure 6.4–21. Ankle dorsiflexion.

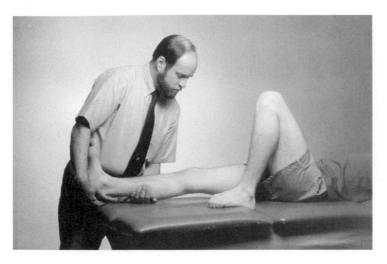

Figure 6.4–22. Position for gastrocnemius ROM.

Joint: Ankle (talocrural)
Muscle: Gastrocnemius
Motion: Dorsiflexion

LO-10 **Position:** Supine with knee in complete extension

Hand Placement: Heel and lower leg

Note: To stretch the gastrocnemius muscle simultaneously across all joints over which it acts, the knee must be kept extended as the ankle is dorsiflexed.

Precaution: The force is applied to the heel in the inferior direction, and not to the ball of the foot.

Joint: Foot (intertarsal)
Motions: Inversion and eversion
Position: Supine
LO-10 **Hand Placement:** One hand stabilizes the lower leg and the other hand grasps the forefoot.

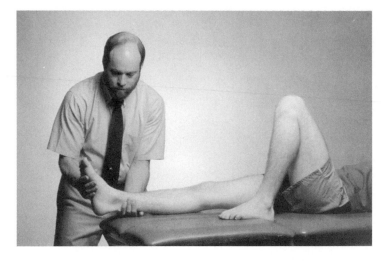

Figure 6.4–23. Starting position for foot inversion and eversion.

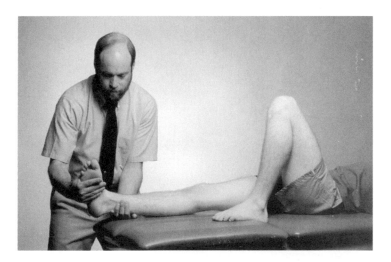

Figure 6.4–24. End position for foot inversion.

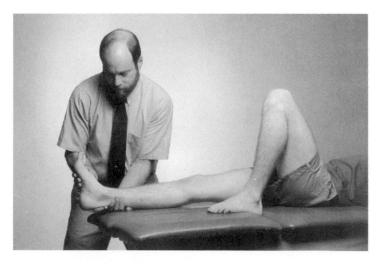

Figure 6.4–25. End position for foot eversion.

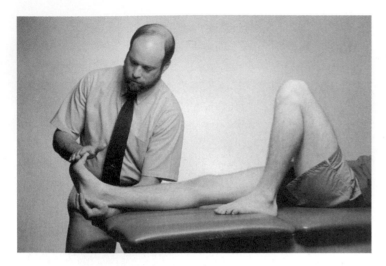

Figure 6.4–26. Toe extension.

Joints: Toes (metatarsophalangeal and interphalangeal)
Motions: Extension and flexion
LO-10 **Positions:** Supine
Hand Placement: One hand stabilizes the foot or lower leg and the other hand grasps the toes.

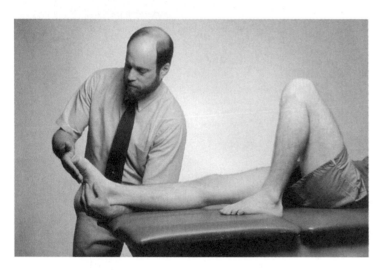

Figure 6.4–27. Toe flexion.

Diagonal Patterns

LO-10

Pattern: PNF diagonal 1 (D1) extension with knee extended

PNF diagonal 1 (D1) flexion with knee extended

Combining Components:

D1 extension with knee straight

hip: extension, abduction, internal rotation

knee: extended

ankle: plantar flexion, eversion

D1 flexion with knee straight

hip: flexion, adduction, external rotation

knee: extended

ankle: dorsiflexion, inversion

Position: Supine

Hand Placement: Heel and posterior thigh

Note: Knee extended (straight) indicates that the knee remains in complete extension throughout the movement of both patterns.

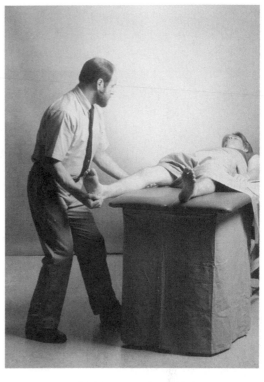

Figure 6.4–28. PNF D1 extension with knee extended.

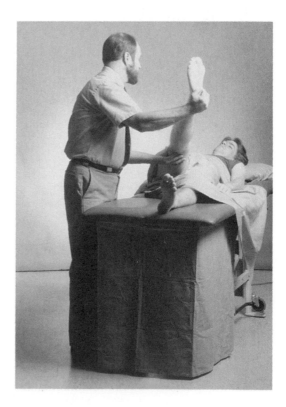

Figure 6.4–29. PNF D1 flexion with knee extended.

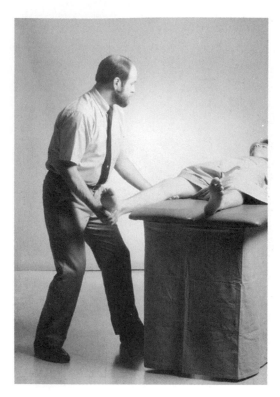

Pattern: PNF D1 extension with knee extension
             PNF D1 flexion with knee flexion
Combining Components:

LO-10
             D1 extension with knee extension
                 hip: extension, abduction, internal
                         rotation
                 knee: extension
                 ankle: plantar flexion, eversion

             D1 flexion with knee flexion
                 hip: flexion, adduction, external
                         rotation
                 knee: flexion
                 ankle: dorsiflexion, inversion

Position: Supine
Hand Placement: Heel and posterior thigh
Note: In these patterns, knee and hip motion occur simul-
         taneously.

Figure 6.4–30. PNF D1 extension with knee
extension.

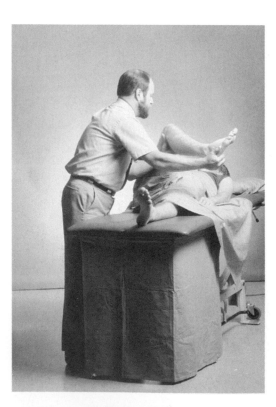

Figure 6.4–31. PFN D1 flexion with knee flexion.

LO-10

Pattern: PNF D1 extension with knee flexion
PNF D1 flexion with knee extension

Combining Components:

D1 extension with knee flexion
    hip: extension, abduction, internal
                rotation
    knee: flexion
    ankle: plantar flexion, eversion
D1 flexion with knee extension
    hip: flexion, adduction, external
                rotation
    knee: extension
    ankle: dorsiflexion, inversion

Position: Supine
Hand Placement: Heel and posterior thigh
Note: In these patterns, the knee and hip motion occur simultaneously.

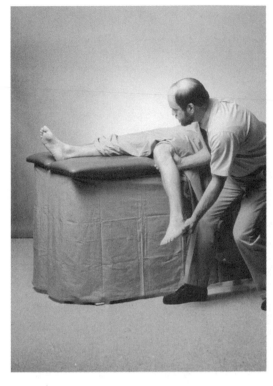

Figure 6.4–32. PNF D1 extension with knee flexion.

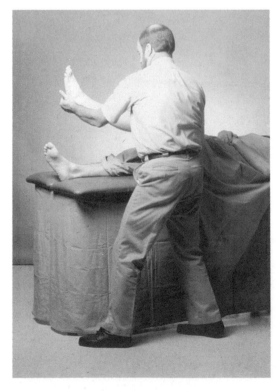

Figure 6.4–33. PNF D1 flexion with knee extension.

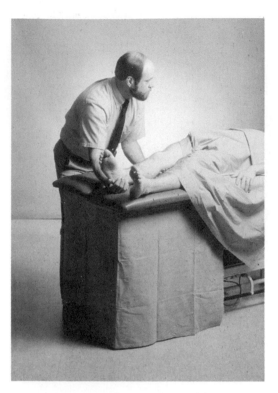

 Pattern: PNF diagonal 2 (D2) extension with knee extended

PNF diagonal 2 (D2) flexion with knee extended

LO-10

Combining Components:

D2 extension with knee straight
hip: extension, adduction, external rotation
knee: extended
ankle: plantar flexion, inversion

D2 flexion with knee straight
hip: flexion, abduction, internal rotation
knee: extended
ankle: dorsiflexion, eversion

Position: Supine

Hand Placement: Heel and posterior thigh

Note: Knee extended (straight) indicates that the knee remains in complete extension throughout the movement of both patterns.

Figure 6.4–34. PNF D2 extension with knee extended.

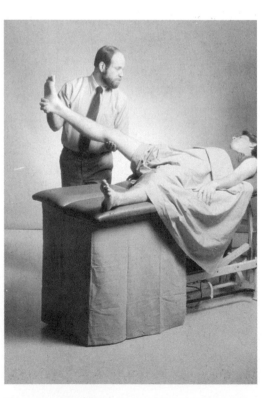

Figure 6.4–35. PNF D2 flexion with knee extended.

Precaution: When performing PNF D2 patterns the therapist must step and move to allow the patient's leg to move through the pattern completely and correctly.

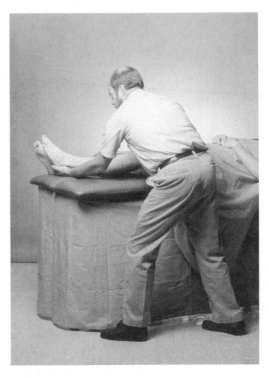

Figure 6.4–36. Starting position for therapist to perform PNF D2 patterns.

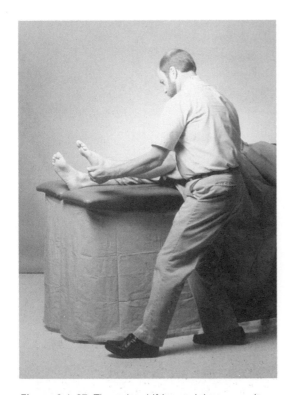

Figure 6.4–37. Therapist shifting weight to permit patient to move.

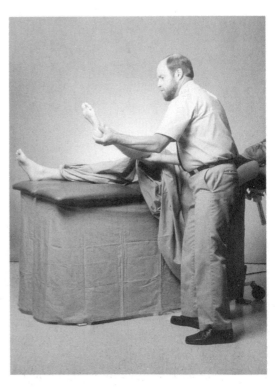

Figure 6.4–38. Therapist steps backward into ending position.

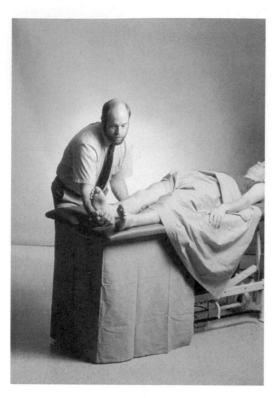

Figure 6.4–39. PNF D2 extension with knee extension.

Pattern: PNF D2 extension with knee extension
               PNF D2 flexion with knee flexion

Combining Components:

LO-10

D2 extension with knee extension

hip:	extension, adduction, external rotation
knee:	extension
ankle:	plantar flexion, inversion

D2 flexion with knee flexion

hip:	flexion, abduction, internal rotation
knee:	flexion
ankle:	dorsiflexion, eversion

Position: Supine

Hand Placement: Heel and posterior thigh

Note: In these patterns, knee and hip motion occur simultaneously.

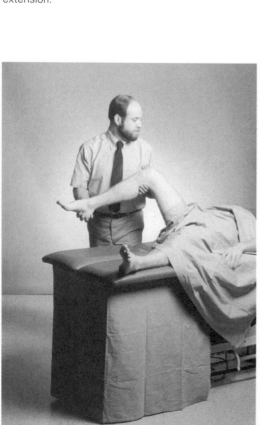

Figure 6.4–40. PNF D2 flexion with knee flexion.

LO-10

Pattern: PNF D2 extension with knee flexion
PNF D2 flexion with knee extension

Combining Components:

D2 extension with knee flexion

hip: extension, adduction, external rotation
knee: flexion
ankle: plantar flexion, inversion

D2 flexion with knee extension

hip: flexion, abduction, internal rotation
knee: extension
ankle: dorsiflexion, eversion

Position: Supine with knees flexed over end of table
Hand Placement: Heel and posterior thigh
Note: In these patterns, knee and hip movements occur simultaneously.

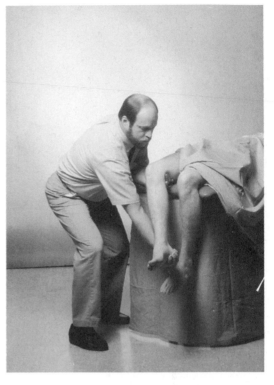

Figure 6.4–41. PNF D2 extension with knee flexion.

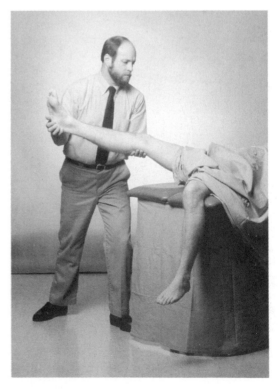

Figure 6.4–42. PNF D2 flexion with knee extension.

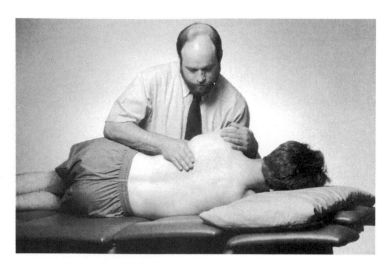

Figure 6.5–1. Scapular protraction.

6.5   UPPER EXTREMITY

Anatomical Planes

LO-10

Joint: Shoulder girdle (scapulothoracic)

Motion: Protraction and retraction
Elevation and depression
Abduction and adduction

Position: Sidelying

Hand Placement: One hand is placed over the acromion and the other hand is placed at the inferior angle of the scapula.

Note: The hand placement for each of the three pairs of motions is the same. The only difference is the direction of force applied to the scapula.

Figure 6.5–2. Scapular retraction.

Joint: Shoulder (glenohumeral)
Motion: Horizontal adduction
Position: Supine with the shoulder abducted to 90 degrees and the elbow flexed to 90 degrees
LO-10
Hand Placement: One hand supports the upper arm and the other hand grasps the hand and forearm.
Note: This motion is referred to as horizontal adduction.

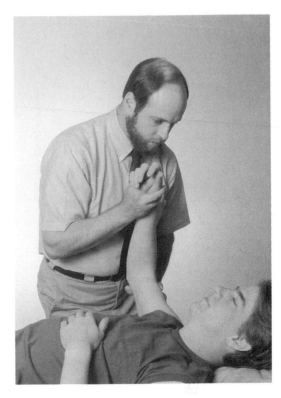

Figure 6.5–7. Starting position for horizontal adduction.

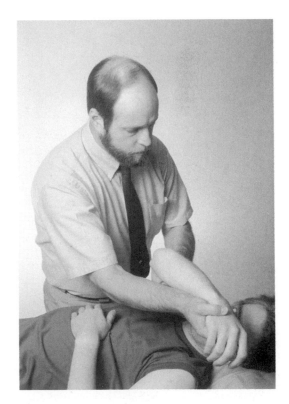

Figure 6.5–8. End position for shoulder horizontal adduction.

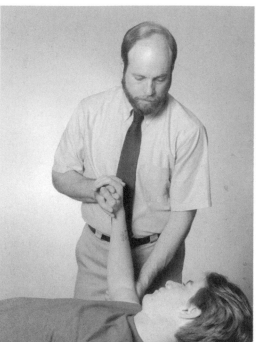

Figure 6.5–9. Starting position for shoulder internal rotation.

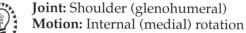

Joint: Shoulder (glenohumeral)
Motion: Internal (medial) rotation
Position: Supine with the shoulder abducted to 90
LO-10 degrees, the elbow flexed to 90 degrees, and the forearm in anatomical position or pronated
Hand Placement: One hand supports the upper arm and the other hand supports the patient's hand and forearm.
Precaution: When the end of the range of internal rotation is reached, the shoulder girdle will start to move into protraction. This should not occur.

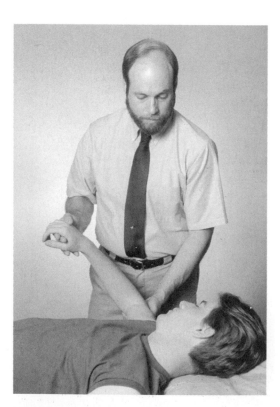

Figure 6.5–10. Partial shoulder internal rotation.

Joint: Shoulder (glenohumeral)

Motion: External (lateral) rotation

Position: Supine with the shoulder abducted to 90 degrees, the elbow flexed to 90 degrees, and the forearm in anatomic position or pronated

Hand Placement: One hand supports the upper arm and the other hand supports the patient's hand and forearm.

Precaution: When the end of the range of external rotation is reached, the shoulder girdle will start to move into retraction. The patient may also extend the trunk when motion is limited. This should not occur.

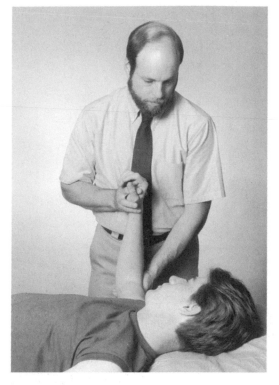

Figure 6.5–11. Starting position for shoulder external rotation.

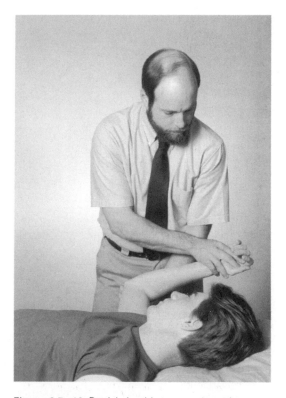

Figure 6.5.–12. Partial shoulder external rotation.

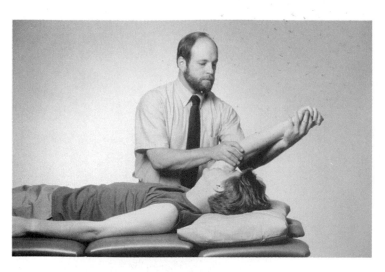

Figure 6.5–13. Starting position for triceps.

LO-10

Joints: Shoulder (glenohumeral) and elbow
Muscle: Triceps brachii
Motion: Flexion
Position: Supine

Hand Placement: One hand supports the wrist and hand while the other hand supports the upper arm.

Note: To lengthen the triceps muscle across both joints over which it acts requires simultaneous flexion of both the shoulder and elbow joints. This lengthening may be achieved by first flexing the shoulder through its available range of motion, and then flexing the elbow through its available range of motion, while the shoulder flexion is maintained.

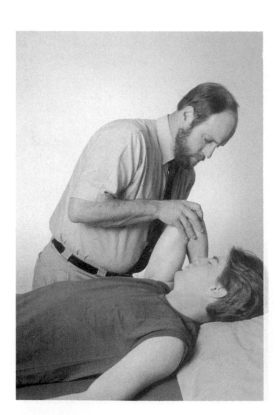

Figure 6.5–14. Ending position for triceps.

Joint: Elbow

Motions: Flexion and extension

Position: Supine with the upper extremity in anatomic position

LO-10

Hand Placement: One hand supports the upper arm and the other hand grasps the hand.

Note: In this illustration the shoulder is slightly flexed to allow visualization of the elbow.

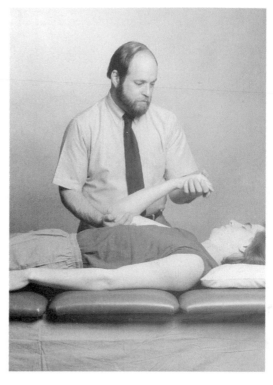

Figure 6.5–15. Elbow flexion.

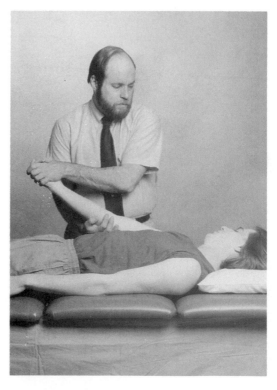

Figure 6.5–16. Elbow extension.

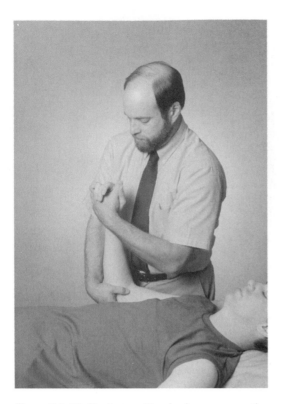

LO-10

Joints: Forearm (radioulnar)
Motions: Pronation and supination
Position: Supine with the elbow flexed to 90 degrees
Alternative Position: Sitting
Hand Placement: One hand grasps the patient's hand and the other hand stabilizes the upper arm.
Precaution: If this hand placement causes excessive stress on the wrist joint, grasp the distal forearm.

Figure 6.5–17. Starting position for forearm pronation and supination.

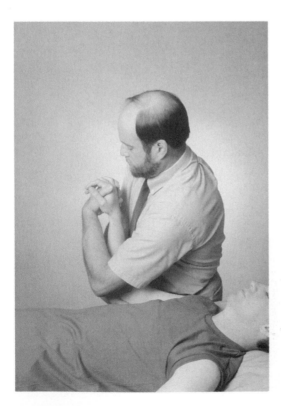

Figure 6.5–18. Forearm pronation.

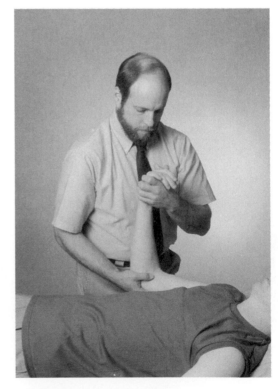

Figure 6.5–19. Forearm supination.

Joints: Wrist (radiocarpal and intercarpal)
Motions: Flexion and extension—finger motion permitted
LO-10 Position: Supine with the elbow flexed, and the fingers free to move
Alternative Position: Sitting
Hand Placement: One hand stabilizes the forearm and upper arm while the other hand grasps the patient's hand.

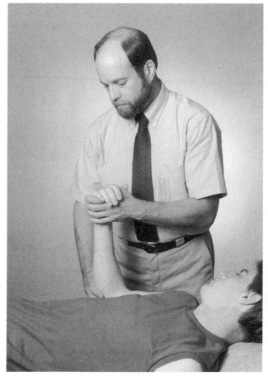

Figure 6.5–20. Starting position for wrist flexion and extension.

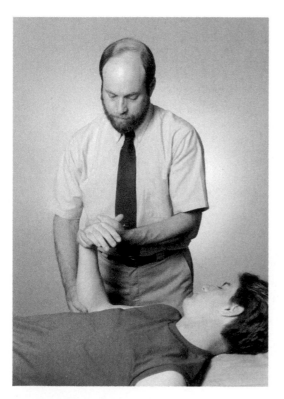

Figure 6.5–21. Wrist flexion.

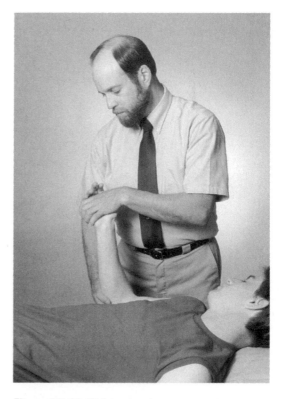

Figure 6.5–22. Wrist extension.

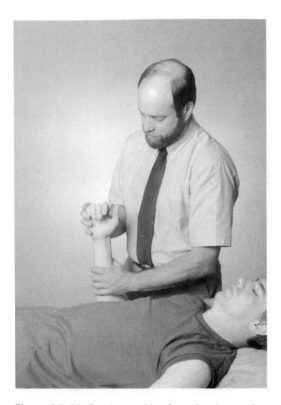

Figure 6.5–23. Starting position for wrist ulnar and radial deviation.

Joints: Wrist (radiocarpal and intercarpal)
Motions: Ulnar and radial deviation
Position: Supine with the elbow flexed

LO-10 **Alternative Position:** Sitting
Hand Placement: One hand stabilizes the forearm while the other hand grasps the patient's hand.
Note: The range of motion for radial deviation is less than ulnar deviation.
Precaution: Avoid wrist flexion and extension while performing ulnar and radial deviation motions.

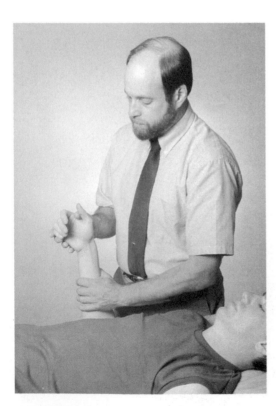

Figure 6.5–24. Wrist ulnar deviation.

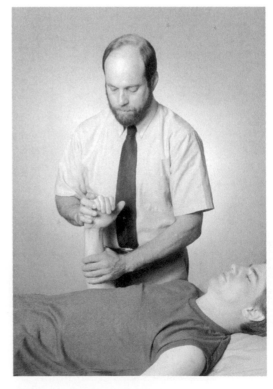

Figure 6.5–25. Wrist radial deviation.

Joints: Fingers (metacarpophalangeal and interphalangeal)

Motions: Flexion and extension

LO-10 **Position:** Supine with the wrist in the neutral position and the elbow flexed to 90 degrees

Alternative Position: Sitting

Hand Placement: One hand stabilizes the forearm and wrist while the other hand grasps the fingers.

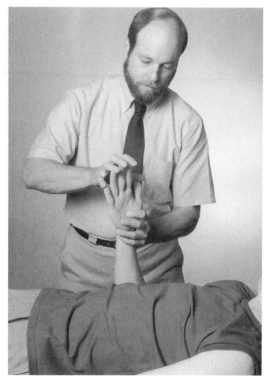

Figure 6.5–26. Starting position for finger flexion and extension.

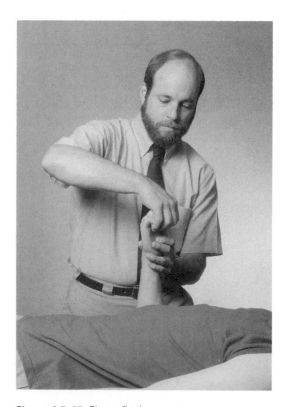

Figure 6.5–27. Finger flexion.

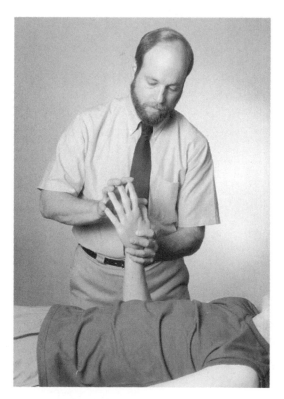

Figure 6.5–28. Finger extension.

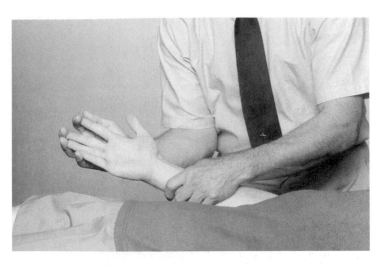

Figure 6.5–29. Starting position for long finger flexors and long finger extensors.

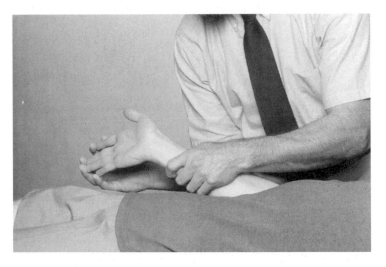

Figure 6.5–30. Ending position for long finger extensors.

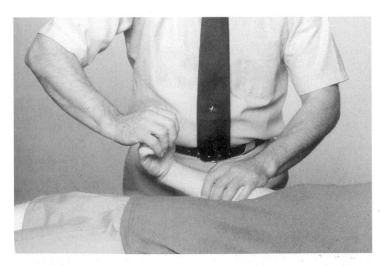

Figure 6.5–31. Ending position for long finger flexors.

Joints: Fingers (metacarpophalangeal and interphalangeal)

LO-10

Muscles: Flexor digitorum superficialis
Flexor digitorum profundus
Palmaris longus
Extensor digitorum
Extensor digiti minimi
Extensor indicis

Motions: Finger extension with wrist flexion
Finger extension with wrist extension
Finger flexion with wrist extension
Finger flexion with wrist flexion

Position: Supine

Alternative Position: Sitting

Hand Placement: One hand stabilizes the forearm and wrist while the other hand grasps the fingers.

Note: These motions lengthen the multijoint muscles that cross the joints of the elbow, wrist, and fingers, to the fullest extent possible. While these muscles cross the elbow joint, the full effect of muscle lengthening can usually be achieved without regard for elbow joint position. The illustrations demonstrate both elbow extended and elbow flexed, but not in all combinations.

Precaution: Some patients should not have the long finger flexors and extensors stretched in this manner. The development of slight tightness in these muscles provides a type of grasp and release called tenodesis. When the wrist extends the fingers flex and when the wrist flexes the fingers extend.

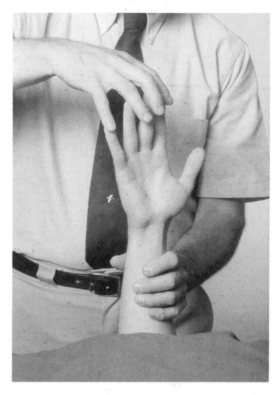

Figure 6.5–32. Starting position for finger flexion with wrist extension and finger extension with wrist flexion.

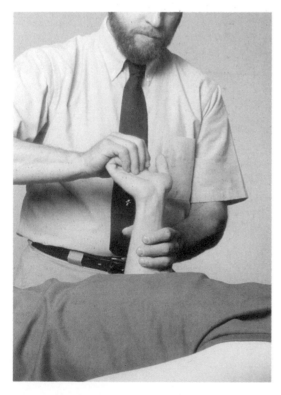

Figure 6.5–33. Ending position for finger flexion with wrist extension.

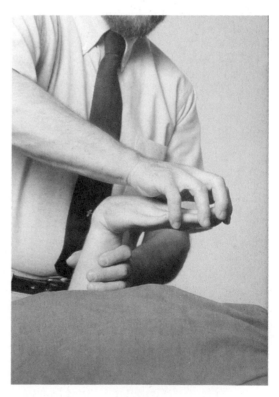

Figure 6.5–34. Ending position for finger extension with wrist flexion.

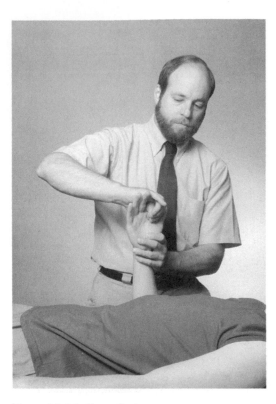

Figure 6.5–35. Finger flexion.

Joints: Fingers (metacarpophalangeal and interphalangeal)

Motions: Flexion and extension

LO-10   **Position:** Supine with elbow flexed and wrist in the neutral position

Alternative Position: Sitting

Hand Placement: One hand stabilizes the forearm and wrist while the other hand grasps the individual digit.

Note: Each digit may be ranged at all its joints and in all directions individually or as a group.

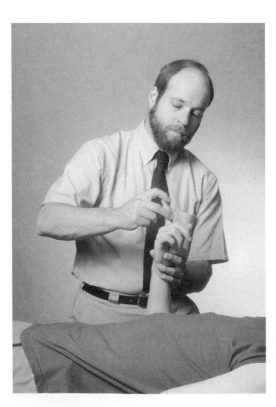

Figure 6.5–36. Finger extension.

Joints: Fingers (metacarpophalangeal)
Motions: Abduction and adduction
Position: Supine with the wrist in the neutral position and the elbow flexed to 90 degrees

LO-10
Alternative Position: Sitting
Hand Placement: One hand grasps the finger to be ranged. The other hand supports the hand and other fingers.
Note: The middle finger is the reference point for abduction and adduction. Movement of the middle finger in both directions is labeled abduction.

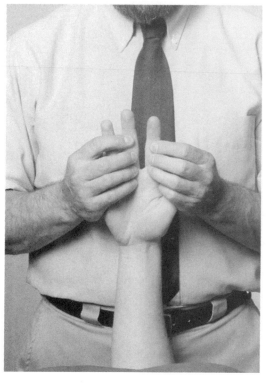

Figure 6.5–37. Starting position for finger abduction and adduction.

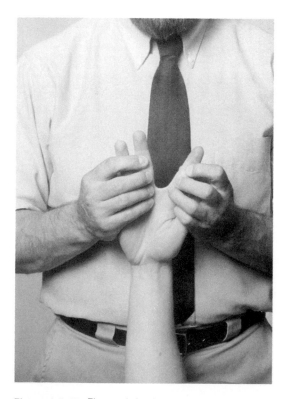

Figure 6.5–38. Finger abduction.

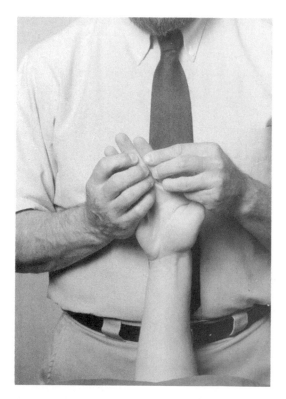

Figure 6.5–39. Finger adduction.

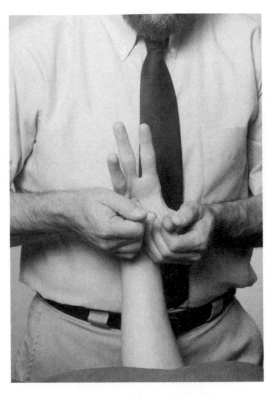

Figure 6.5–40. Opposition of thumb and little finger.

Joints: Thumb (carpometacarpal) and fifth finger
Motion: Opposition
Position: Supine with the wrist in the anatomic
position and the elbow flexed to 90 degrees
LO-10
Alternative Position: Sitting
Hand Placement: One hand grasps the thumb and the
other hand grasps the fifth finger.
Note: To preserve the function of the hand, the arches of
the hand must be maintained. Opposition of the thumb
and fingers can contribute to maintaining the arches of
the hand.

Joint: Thumb (carpometacarpal)

Motions: Abduction and adduction

Position: Supine with the elbow flexed to 90 degrees, the wrist in the neutral position, and the thumb extended

LO-10

Alternative Position: Sitting

Hand Placement: One hand grasps the thumb and the other hand grasps the patient's hand.

Note: Maintaining the "web space" is vital for a functional hand.

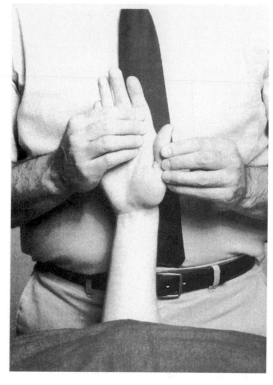

Figure 6.5–41. Thumb adduction.

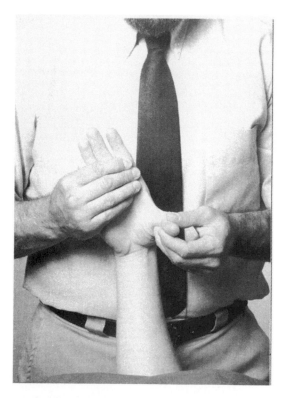

Figure 6.5–42. Thumb abduction.

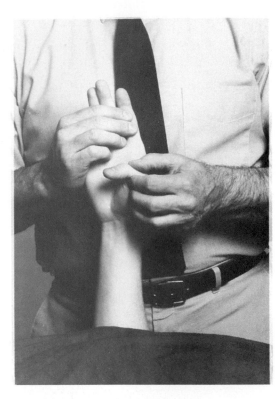

 Joint: Thumb (carpometacarpal and metacarpal phalangeal)
Motions: Flexion and extension
LO-10 **Position:** Supine with the wrist in the neutral position
Alternative Position: Sitting
Hand Placement: One hand grasps the thumb and the other hand grasps the patient's hand.

Figure 6.5–43. Thumb flexion.

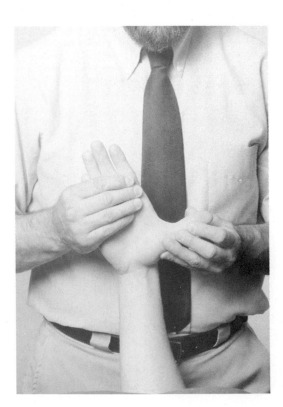

Figure 6.5–44. Thumb extension.

Diagonal Patterns

LO-10

Pattern: PNF diagonal 1 (D1) extension with elbow extended

PNF diagonal 1 (D1) flexion with elbow extended

Combining Components:

D1 extension with elbow extended

shoulder:	extension, abduction, internal rotation
elbow:	extended
forearm:	pronation
wrist:	extension, ulnar deviation
digits:	extension, abduction

D1 flexion with elbow extended

shoulder:	flexion, adduction, external rotation
elbow:	extended
forearm:	supination
wrist:	flexion, radial deviation
digits:	flexion, adduction

Position: Supine

Hand Placement: One hand supports the upper arm and the other hand grasps the patient's hand. When performing range of motion of the patient's right upper extremity, the therapist's left hand controls the patient's wrist and hand.

Note: Elbow extended (straight) indicates that the elbow maintains extension throughout the movement of both patterns.

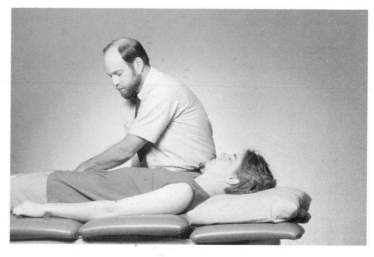

Figure 6.5–45. PNF D1 extension.

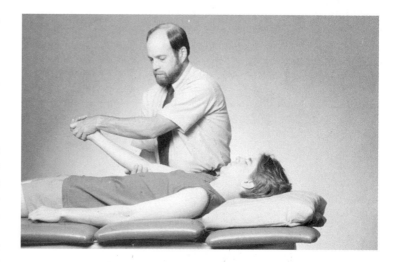

Figure 6.5–46. Mid-position for PNF D1 flexion with elbow extended.

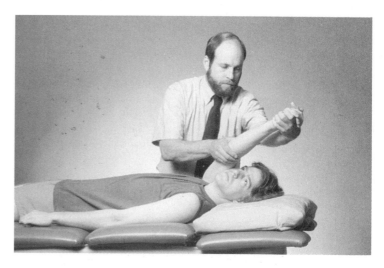

Figure 6.5–47. Ending position for PNF D1 flexion with elbow extended.

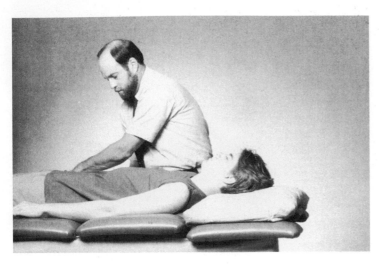

Figure 6.5–48. PNF D1 extension with elbow extension.

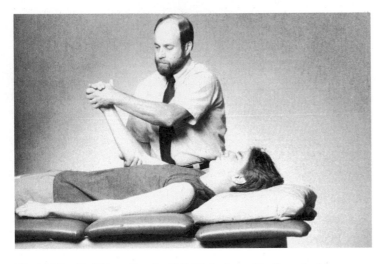

Figure 6.5.–49. Mid-position for PNF D1 flexion with elbow flexion.

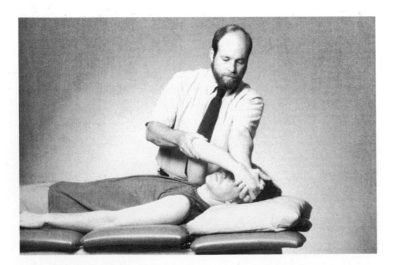

Figure 6.5–50. Ending position for PNF D1 flexion with elbow flexion.

LO-10

Pattern: PNF D1 extension with elbow extension
PNF D1 flexion with elbow flexion

Combining Components:

D1 extension with elbow extension

shoulder:	extension, abduction, internal rotation
elbow:	extension
forearm:	pronation
wrist:	extension, ulnar deviation
digits:	extension, abduction

D1 flexion with elbow flexion

shoulder:	flexion, adduction, external rotation
elbow:	flexion
forearm:	supination
wrist:	flexion, radial deviation
digits:	flexion, adduction

Position: Supine

Hand Placement: One hand supports the upper arm and the other hand grasps the patient's hand. When performing range of motion of the patient's right upper extremity, the therapist's left hand controls the patient's wrist and hand.

Note: In these patterns elbow and shoulder motion occur simultaneously.

LO-10

Pattern: PNF D1 extension with elbow flexion
PNF D1 flexion with elbow extension

Combining Components:

D1 extension with elbow flexion

shoulder:	extension, abduction, internal rotation
elbow:	flexion
forearm:	pronation
wrist:	extension, ulnar deviation
digits:	extension, abduction

D1 flexion with elbow extension

shoulder:	flexion, adduction, external rotation
elbow:	extension
forearm:	supination
wrist:	flexion, radial deviation
digits:	flexion, adduction

Position: Supine

Hand Placement: One hand supports the upper arm and the other hand grasps the patient's hand. When performing range of motion of the patient's right upper extremity, the therapist's right hand controls the patient's wrist and hand.

Note: In these patterns the elbow moves as the shoulder moves.

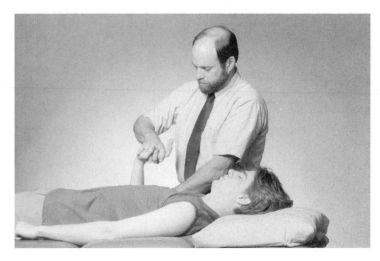

Figure 6.5–51. PNF D1 extension with elbow flexion.

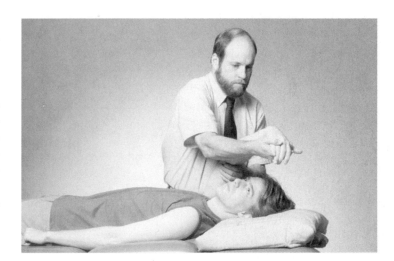

Figure 6.5–52. PNF D1 flexion with elbow extension.

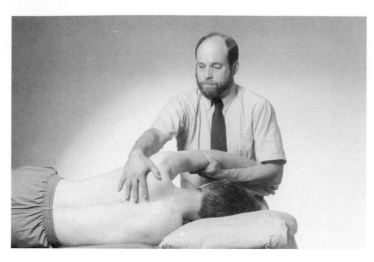

Figure 6.5–53. PNF D1 extension, scapular.

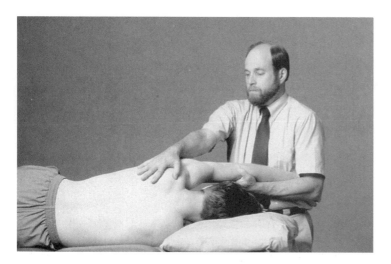

Figure 6.5–54. PNF D1 flexion, scapular.

LO-10

Pattern: PNF D1 extension—scapular

PNF D1 flexion—scapular

Combining Components:

D1 extension

Scapula: depression, adduction, downward rotation

D1 flexion

Scapula: elevation, abduction, upward rotation

Position: Sidelying

Hand Placement: One hand is placed over the scapula, and the other hand and forearm support the patient's upper extremity. When performing range of motion of the patient's left scapula, the therapist's right hand is on the scapula.

LO-10

Pattern: PNF diagonal 2 (D2) extension with elbow extended
PNF diagonal 2 (D2) flexion with elbow extended

Combining Components:

D2 extension with elbow extended

shoulder:	extension, adduction, internal rotation
elbow:	extended
forearm:	pronation
wrist:	flexion, ulnar deviation
digits:	flexion, adduction
thumb:	opposition

D2 flexion with elbow extended

shoulder:	flexion, abduction, external rotation
elboow:	extended
forearm:	supination
wrist:	extension, radial deviation
digits:	extension, abduction

Position: Supine

Hand Placement: One hand supports the upper arm, and the other hand grasps the patient's hand. When performing range of motion of the patient's right upper extremity, the therapist's left hand controls the patient's wrist and hand.

Note: Elbow extended (straight) indicates that the elbow maintains complete extension throughout the movement of both patterns.

Precaution: Patients with limited shoulder flexion may arch their trunk and appear to have more range of motion than actually exists.

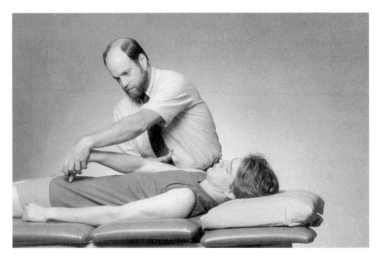
Figure 6.5–55. PNF D2 extension with elbow extended.

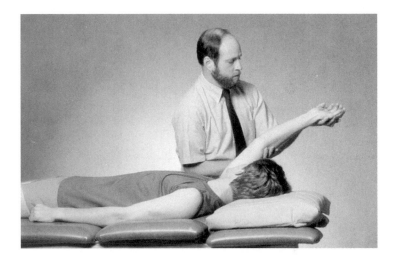
Figure 6.5–56. Mid-position for PNF D2 flexion with elbow extended.

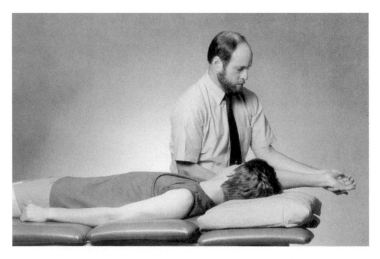
Figure 6.5–57. Ending position for PNF D2 flexion with elbow extended.

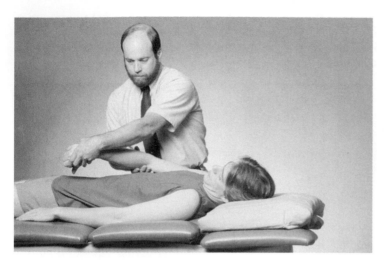

Figure 6.5–58. PNF D2 extension with elbow extension.

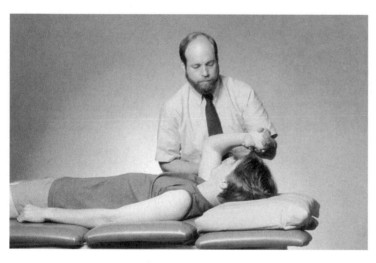

Figure 6.5–59. PNF D2 flexion with elbow flexion.

Pattern: PNF D2 extension with elbow extension
PNF D2 flexion with elbow flexion

LO-10

Combining Components:

D2 extension with elbow extension

shoulder:	extension, adduction, internal rotation
elbow:	extension
forearm:	pronation
wrist:	flexion, ulnar deviation
digits:	flexion, adduction
thumb:	opposition

D2 flexion with elbow flexion

shoulder:	flexion, abduction, external rotation
elbow:	flexion
florearm:	supination
wrist:	extension, radial deviation
digits:	extension, abduction

Position: Supine

Hand Placement: One hand supports the upper arm, and the other hand grasps the patient's hand. When performing range of motion of the patient's right upper extremity, the therapist's left hand controls the patient's wrist and hand.

Note: In these patterns elbow and shoulder motion occur simultaneously.

Pattern: PNF D2 extension with elbow flexion

PNF D2 flexion with elbow extension

LO-10

Combining Components:

D2 extension with elbow flexion

shoulder:	extension, adduction, internal rotation
elbow:	flexion
forearm:	pronation
wrist:	flexion, ulnar deviation
digits:	flexion, adduction
thumb:	opposition

D2 flexion with elbow extension

shoulder:	flexion, abduction, external rotation
elbow:	extension
forearm:	supination
wrist:	extension, radial deviation
digits:	extension, abduction

Position: Supine

Hand Placement: One hand supports the upper arm, and the other hand grasps the patient's hand. When performing range of motion of the patient's right upper extremity, the therapist's left hand controls the patient's wrist and hand.

Note: In these patterns the elbow and shoulder motions occur simultaneously.

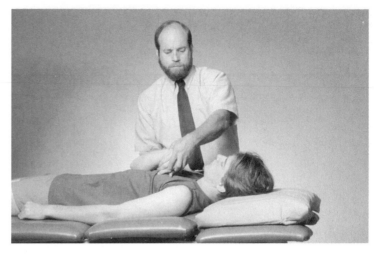

Figure 6.5–60. PNF D2 extension with elbow flexion.

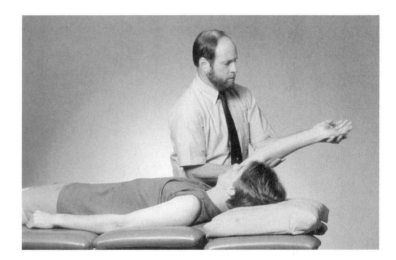

Figure 6.5–61. PNF D2 flexion with elbow extension.

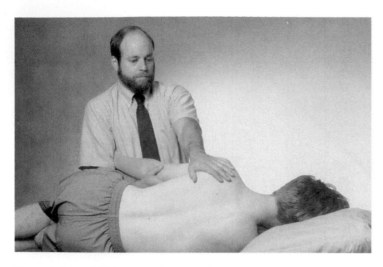

Figure 6.5–62. PNF D2 extension, scapular.

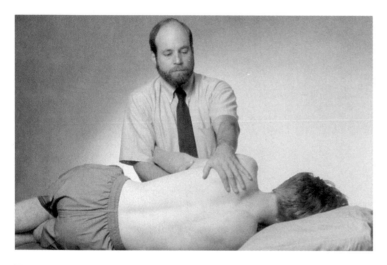

Figure 6.5–63. PNF D2 flexion, scapular.

LO-10

Pattern: PNF D2 extension—scapular

PNF D2 flexion—scapular

Combining Components:

D2 extension
scapula: depression, abduction, downward rotation

D2 flexion
scapula: elevation, adduction, upward rotation

Position: Sidelying

Hand Placement: One hand is placed on the scapula. The other hand and forearm are used to support the arm. When performing range of motion of the patient's left scapula, the therapist's left hand grasps the scapula.

6.6   HEAD, NECK, AND TRUNK

Anatomical Planes

Joints: Head and neck (atlanto-occipital, atlantoaxial, and cervical spine)

LO-10

Motions: Flexion and extension

Position: Supine

Hand Placement: One hand grasps each side of the head without crushing the ear.

Note: When the table does not have a head support that can be lowered, the patient must lie with his head over the end of the table.

Precaution: The patient's head must be carefully supported. The movement must not be forced.

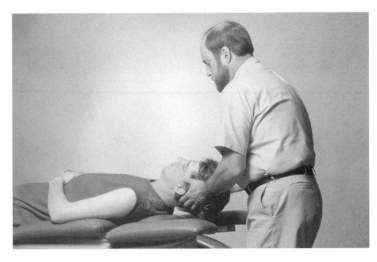

Figure 6.6–1. Starting position for head and neck flexion and extension.

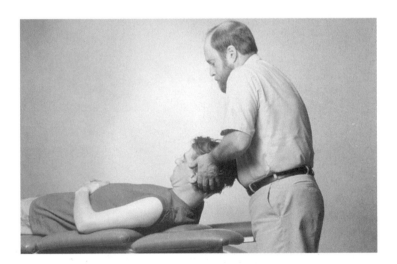

Figure 6.6–2. Head and neck flexion.

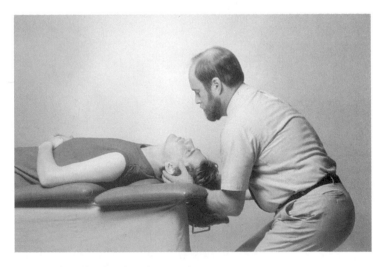

Figure 6.6–3. Head and neck extension.

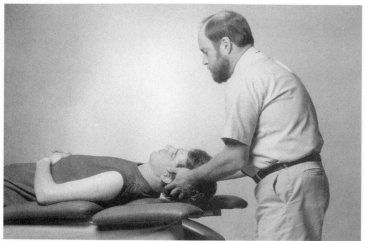

Figure 6.6–4. Starting position for neck rotation.

Joints: Neck (atlantoaxial and cervical spine)
Motion: Rotation
LO-10   Position: Supine
Hand Placement: One hand grasps each side of the head without crushing the ear.
Precaution: The patient's head must be carefully supported. The movement must not be forced.

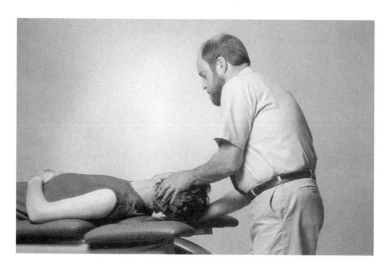

Figure 6.6–5. Neck rotation to right.

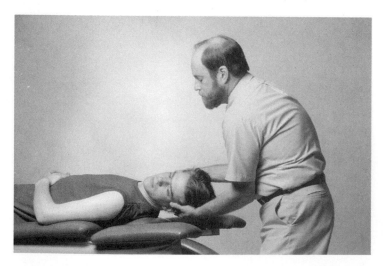

Figure 6.6–6. Neck rotation to left.

Joint: Lower trunk (lumbar spine) and hip

Motion: Lower trunk rotation

LO-10 **Position:** Supine, with hips and knees flexed so the patient's feet are resting flat on the supporting surface close to the buttocks

Hand Placement: One hand grasps the patient's knees and the other grasps the pelvis.

Alternative Hand Placement: One hand grasps both knees of the patient.

Precaution: The patient's shoulders remain on the supporting surface. When the patient's upper trunk begins to roll, the end of lower trunk rotation in that direction has been reached.

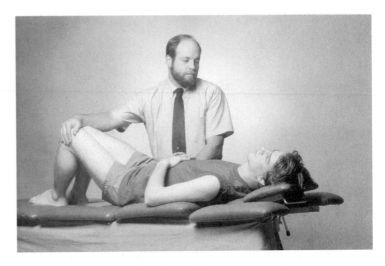

Figure 6.6–7. Lower trunk rotation to left.

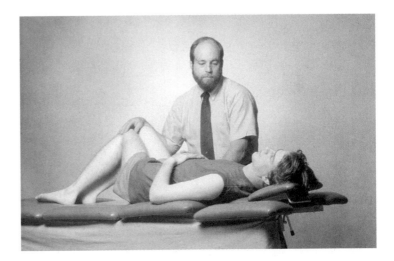

Figure 6.6–8. Lower trunk rotation to right.

6.7 REVIEW QUESTIONS

1. Define passive, active assisted, and active range of motion.

2. How does a therapist support body segments during range-of-motion exercises?

3. What are the differences between joint range of motion and muscle range of motion?

4. What are the types of end feel and the significance of each?

5. Define flexion, extension, abduction, adduction, opposition, internal rotation, external rotation, supination, pronation, inversion, and eversion.

6. Compare and contrast anatomical plane motion with diagonal patterns of motion.

7. What are the combining components of motion for each diagonal pattern of motion of the upper and lower extremities?

6.8 SUGGESTED ACTIVITIES

1. Demonstrate the specific procedures presented in this chapter to students.

2. Students work in pairs to perform the specific procedures. Students rotate partners periodically during practice sessions.

3. Students practice draping while performing ROM exercises.

4. Students practice ROM exercises for all joints and muscles possible in each position—prone, supine, sidelying, and sitting.

5. Students practice performing ROM exercises with the patient on a treatment table, bed, mat table, and mat on the floor.

6. Students practice performing ROM exercises while partners role-play various diagnoses (see Case Studies for suggestions). The student role-playing the patient can add "character" to the role by being cooperative, noncooperative, in pain, hard of hearing, or lacking ROM to enhance the activity. The "patient" must role-play the diagnosis and character consistently.

7. Students practice teaching "family and patients" and other health care providers how to perform ROM exercises.

8. Students document treatment using the SOAP note format.

CASE STUDIES

1. Patient is a 2-year-old female with cerebral palsy, presenting with severe spastic diplegia.

2. Patient is a 16-year-old male with a complete C5 spinal cord injury, presenting with moderate spasticity in the lower extremities.

3. Patient is a 72-year-old female with left hemiplegia (stage 1) following a right CVA.

4. Patient is a 44-year-old female with multiple sclerosis, presenting with moderate spasticity in the lower extremities.

5. Patient is a 60-year-old male with parkinsonism, presenting with moderate rigidity in all extremities and trunk.

6.9 References

1. Knott M and Voss DE. *Proprioceptive Neuromuscular Facilitation*, 2nd ed. New York: Harper & Row, 1968.
2. Root ML, Orien WP, and Weed JH. *Normal and Abnormal Function of the Foot: Clinical Biomechanics—Volume II.* Los Angeles: Clinical Biomechanics Corporation Publishers, 1977.
3. Warwick R and Williams PL. *Gray's Anatomy*, 37th ed. Philadelphia: WB Saunders Co., 1989.
4. Sullivan PE, Markos PD, and Minor MAD. *An Integrated Approach to Therapeutic Exercise: Theory and Clinical Application.* Virginia: Reston Pub. Co., 1982.

Chapter 7

Wheelchairs

 Learner Objectives

The student will be able to:

1 Name the components of a wheelchair and types of wheelchairs.
2 Describe the purpose or function of wheelchair components and types.
3 Describe and demonstrate how wheelchair components and types are manipulated including brakes, seat belts, wheels, armrests, front rigging, and antitipping components; and types of wheelchairs including standard, folding, reclining-back, tilt-in-space, one-arm drive, and amputee-frame wheelchairs.
4 Describe and demonstrate how to measure an individual to determine correct size and components required for a wheelchair including brakes, seat belts, wheels, armrests, front rigging, and antitipping components; and types of wheelchairs including standard, folding, reclining-back, tilt-in-space, one-arm drive, and amputee-frame wheelchairs.

INTRODUCTION

In many cases, wheelchairs are fabricated to fit a specific individual with specific needs. Careful measurement of the patient and selection of appropriate components help provide each user of a wheelchair with a piece of equipment that best meets the specific needs of the individual. While many wheelchairs may incorporate common features, mechanisms that control the features can vary. This chapter illustrates how to measure a patient for a wheelchair, basic wheelchair components, and selected variations of commonly used components.

7.1 WHEELCHAIR BRAKES

One of the most important safety features is the braking system. Wheelchair brakes are most often based on a lever system with a cam, or in some cases a slot, locking mechanism.

LO-1

A general safety rule is that the brake must be engaged whenever a patient is moving into or out of the wheelchair. Engaging the brake prevents forward and backward movement of the wheelchair. Slight side-to-side movement results because the caster wheels are not secured.

To work properly, brakes must make secure contact with the tire to prevent the wheel from moving. When pneumatic tires are not inflated sufficiently, or entire brake mechanisms become loose or slide forward on the wheelchair frame, effectiveness of the brake is reduced because the brake does not make adequate contact with the tire.

LO-2

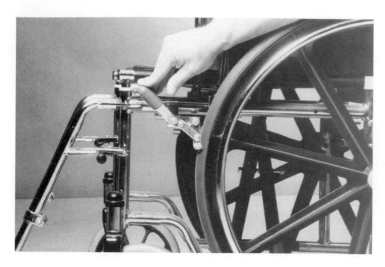

Figure 7.1–1. Engaging brake.

 The direction of the force needed to engage or release the brake can be selected to match the patient's abilities. When the brake is engaged by pushing the brake lever forward,

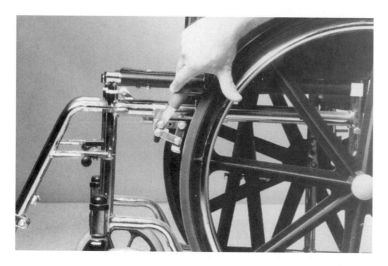

Figure 7.1–2. Releasing brake.

pulling the lever backward releases the brake.

Extensions for brake handles are available. Extensions increase the mechanical advantage of the braking mechanism by increasing the length of the force arm. This decreases the force required for locking or unlocking the brake.

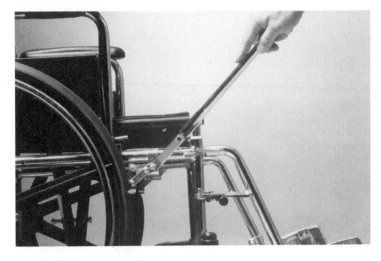

Figure 7.1–3. Using brake extension.

On some reclining back wheelchairs the wheel base enlarges in the anterior/posterior dimension when the back is reclined. When the wheel base is enlarged as the back reclines, the relationship of the brake and wheel is altered, and the brake becomes ineffective. An additional brake is necessary for these wheelchairs. The additional brake is attached to the back upright of the wheelchair.

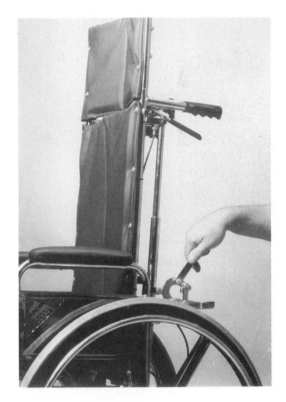

Figure 7.1–4. Additional brake on back upright of reclining back wheelchair.

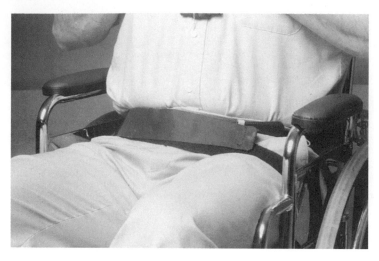

Figure 7.2–1. Velcro seat belt.

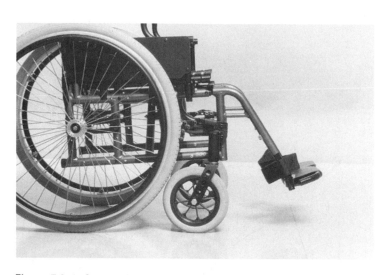

Figure 7.3–1. Caster wheels.

7.2   SEAT BELTS

LO-1

LO-2

LO-3

Another safety feature is a seat belt. Seat belts are used to prevent a patient from falling out of a wheelchair. Seat belts are also used as part of a positioning system designed to provide proper positioning of a patient in a wheelchair.

Seat belts use three mechanisms for fastening. One mechanism is the use of Velcro straps. A second mechanism is the use of latching buckles, such as those used for seat belts in airplanes. A third mechanism is the use of push button buckles, such as those used for seat belts in automobiles.

7.3   CASTER WHEELS

LO-1

LO-2

Caster wheels are the small front wheels of a wheelchair. Two basic styles of tire are available, standard solid rubber, and pneumatic. Pneumatic tires provide some shock absorption, and thus a smoother ride. Pneumatic tires are also wider, making travel easier on soft or uneven surfaces such as sand or gravel.

7.4   DRIVE (PUSH) WHEELS

LO-1

Drive wheels are the large rear wheels of a wheelchair used for propulsion. The large rear tire may be one of two basic types, standard solid rubber or pneumatic. Pneumatic tires may or may not have tread. Treads are used on wheelchairs that are often used outdoors and require improved traction. Pneumatic tires have been modified to reduce the chance of flat tires.

LO-2

Drive wheels have an outer rim used by the patient to propel the wheelchair. Many adaptations of the outer rim, such as projections, are available for use by patients who do not have sufficient grasp for wheelchair propulsion. Projections may add width to the wheelchair making maneuvering in small spaces difficult. Another modification to assist in pushing on the outer rims is a nonslip coating.

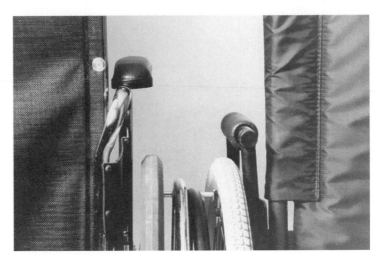

Figure 7.4–1. Two styles of pneumatic tires.

Drive wheels come in two types, standard or "mags." Standard wheels are fabricated with multiple steel or aluminum spokes. The spokes are thin, and are individually adjustable to maintain proper alignment of the wheel. Mag wheels were originally named after their construction using magnesium, a very strong, lightweight metal. Mag wheels have the material strength to maintain their original alignment. Because of the design and type of metal, maintenance of mag wheels is easier than standard wheels.

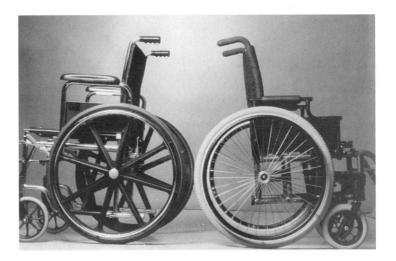

Figure 7.4–2. "Mag" (left) and standard (right) drive wheels.

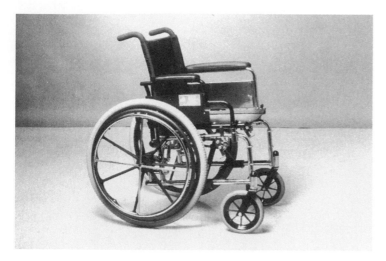

Figure 7.5–1. Desk armrest (front) and full length armrest (rear).

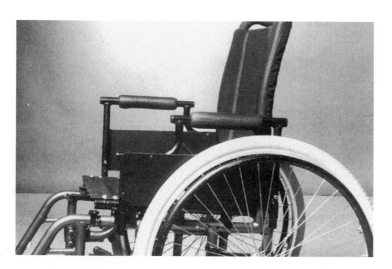

Figure 7.5–2. Desk armrest in standard (front) and reverse (rear) position.

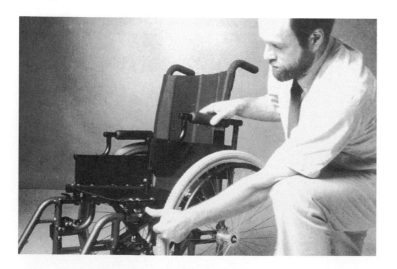

Figure 7.5–3. Releasing lock and removing armrest.

7.5 ARMRESTS

LO-1

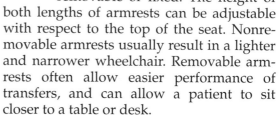

LO-2

Several configurations of armrests are available. Armrests are either full length or desk length. In full-length armrests, the armrests are full height along the entire length of the armrest. In desk armrests, one portion of the armrest length is lower than the remaining portion so a wheelchair can be partially rolled under a table or desk. Both lengths of armrests can be either removable or fixed. The height of both lengths of armrests can be adjustable with respect to the top of the seat. Nonremovable armrests usually result in a lighter and narrower wheelchair. Removable armrests often allow easier performance of transfers, and can allow a patient to sit closer to a table or desk.

Lap trays are secured to, and rest on, armrests. Full length armrests offer more support for a lap tray.

Most desk-length armrests can be removed and reversed so the higher part of the armrest is toward the front of the wheelchair. Reversing a desk armrest provides a higher support for patients when pushing to standing or transferring.

LO-3

Armrests are locked in place as a safety precaution. Several types of mechanisms are used to lock armrests in place. The location and type of lock mechanism varies for different wheelchairs. One common type of lock is operated by a lever that is pushed down to release the lock. Once released, the lever remains in a released position. Thus, only one hand is required to remove the armrest.

7.6   FRONT RIGGING

LO-1

The front rigging of a wheelchair provides support for the lower extremities, and consists of a footplate attached to either a footrest or an elevating legrest. The terms footrest and legrest both refer to the portion of the front rigging that supports the leg.

LO-2

Footplates

LO-1

The patient's feet rest on footplates. Footplates are available in several sizes to accommodate different size feet. Heel loops prevent the foot from sliding off the footplate and under the wheelchair. Toe loops can be used to assist with maintaining the foot on the footplate.

LO-3

The footplate is raised to allow the patient to transfer safely in and out of the wheelchair. When raising a footplate, the heel loop must be pushed forward. Pushing the heel loop forward allows the footplate to be raised completely, and prolongs the life of the heel loop by keeping the heel loop material from being crushed.

To raise a footplate, the heel loop is pushed forward,

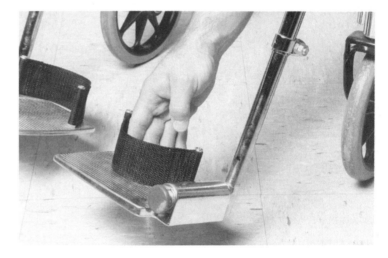

Figure 7.6–1. Heel loop positioned forward in preparation to raise footplate.

and the footplate is raised to a vertical position.

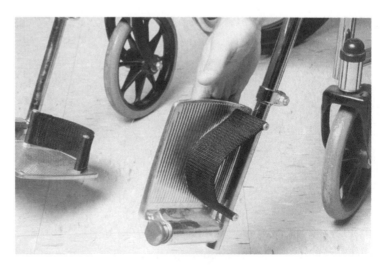

Figure 7.6–2. Footplate raised to vertical position.

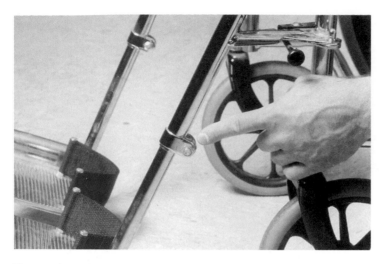

Figure 7.6–3. Adjustment screw for length of front rigging.

The distance from the seat to the footplate for both footrests and elevating legrests can be adjusted to match the length of the lower leg, and to provide proper support for the entire lower extremity. There are several methods for making this adjustment. The method illustrated uses a clamp. Other methods use tension adjustment screws located inside the footrest or legrest tube. Access for the adjustment screws for this method of adjustment are from the underside of the footrest or legrest.

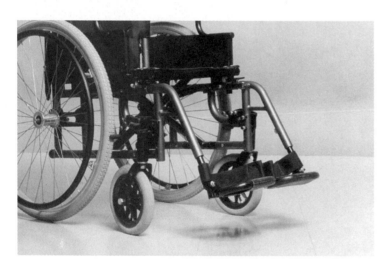

Figure 7.6–4. Footrests.

Footrests

LO-1

Footrests can be fixed or removable. Fixed footrests are generally less expensive, and result in a lighter wheelchair.

LO-3

LO-3   There are two types of removable footrests. One type is removable but does not pivot. The second type is both pivoting and removable. The two types of removable footrests are removed in different ways. The nonpivoting type is removed by unlocking the footrest and sliding the footrest from the frame.

Several types of locks are used to secure pivoting footrests. Pivoting footrests use pivot pins as the center of rotation. The pivoting type is removed by unlocking the footrest,

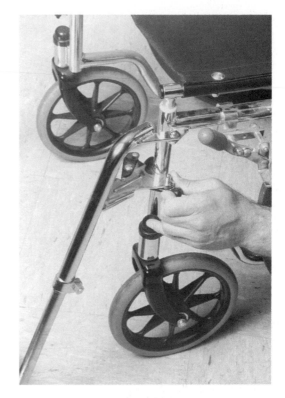

Figure 7.6–5. Unlocking pivoting footrest.

pivoting the footrest to the side, and then lifting the footrest from the pivot pins.

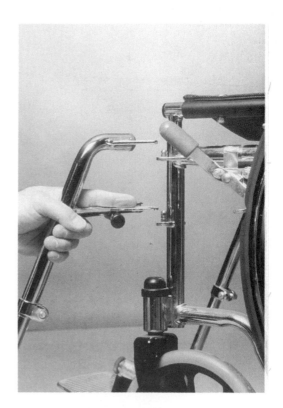

Figure 7.6–6. Removing pivoting footrest.

Elevating Legrests

LO-2

An elevating legrest is necessary when a patient is unable to flex the knee, when a dependent position of the leg contributes to swelling, or with a reclining back wheelchair. A pad provides support for the calf.

LO-3

Legrest position is maintained by a locking mechanism. The lock is released and activated by a lever. The legrest position is adjusted by releasing the lock with one hand, while positioning the legrest with the other hand.

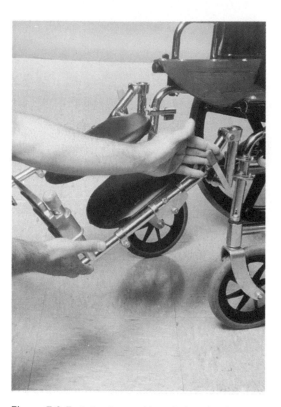

Figure 7.6–7. Adjusting position of elevating legrest.

LO-3

There are two types of removable elevating legrests. One type is removable but does not pivot. The second type is both pivoting and removable. The two types of removable legrests are removed in different ways. The nonpivoting type is removed by unlocking the legrest and sliding the legrest from the frame.

LO-3   To remove an elevating legrest, the calf support is pivoted out of the way. The calf support must be pivoted to the side before the footplate is raised. Failure to use this sequence will not allow the calf support to be moved completely out of the way.

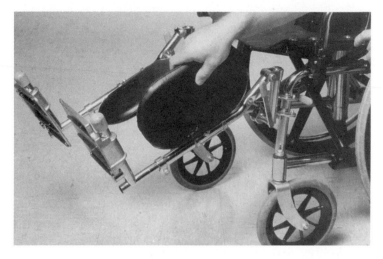

Figure 7.6–8. Raising calf support.

The footplate is raised.

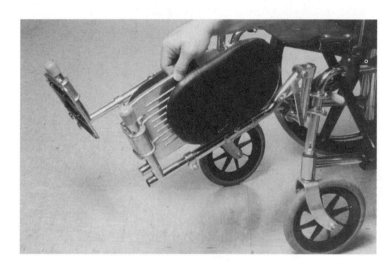

Figure 7.6–9. Raising footplate.

The pivoting and removable elevating legrest is removed in the same manner as a pivoting and removable footrest is removed.

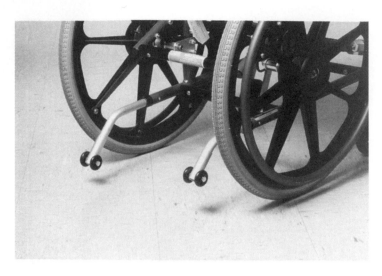

Figure 7.7–1. Antitipping device on rear of wheelchair.

7.7   ANTITIPPING DEVICES

LO-1

LO-2

Small extensions, with or without wheels, attached to the lower horizontal support bar are used to prevent accidental backward tipping of the wheelchair. Adjustment of antitipping devices must permit some tipping of the wheelchair in order to allow front casters to roll over door sills or other low obstructions.

7.8   FOLDING WHEELCHAIRS

LO-3

Wheelchairs can be folded, or collapsed, for storage or transport. A standard wheelchair is folded by raising the footplates and pulling up on the handles located on either side of the seat. The wheelchair should not be folded by pulling up on the middle of the seat upholstery because this may tear the upholstery.

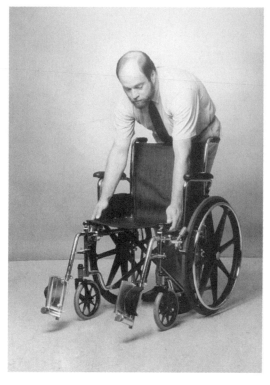

Figure 7.8–1. Starting position for folding standard wheelchair.

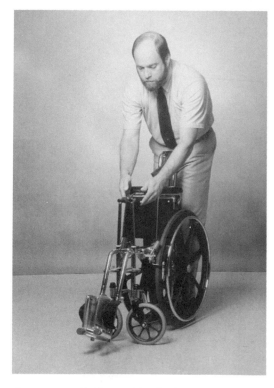

Figure 7.8–2. Ending position for folding standard wheelchair.

7.9   SPECIALIZED WHEELCHAIRS

Different styles of wheelchairs have been developed to meet specific needs. Some styles are minimal modifications of standard wheelchairs. Other styles have required extensive re-engineering of the basic wheelchair. Several, but not all, types of specialized wheelchairs are discussed in this section. In addition to manual wheelchairs, motorized wheelchairs and scooters are available. Motorized devices are not included in this text.

Reclining-Back

LO-1

LO-2

Reclining-back wheelchairs are indicated when a patient is unable to sit erect or to sit erect for long periods of time. There are two types of reclining-back wheelchairs, those that recline completely, and those that recline only partially. An extended back is standard with both types of reclining-back wheelchairs. An extended back provides support for the upper body when the wheelchair back is reclined. Head support is also required for reclining-back wheelchairs, but is not automatically included with the extended back. Reclining-back wheelchairs generally have elevating legrests.

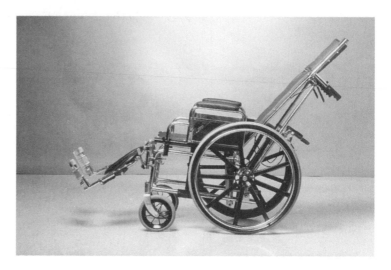

Figure 7.9–1. Reclining-back wheelchair with elevating legrests.

LO-3

There are several mechanisms for unlocking and adjusting the angle of the back. To change the angle of the back, the locking mechanism is released, the angle of the back is adjusted, and the locking mechanism is activated.

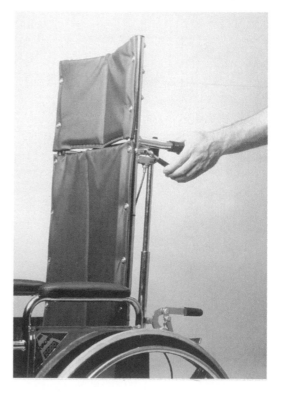

Figure 7.9–2. Lock for back angle adjustment on reclining-back wheelchair.

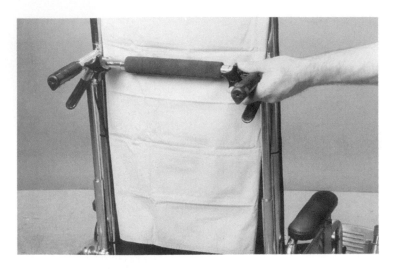

A bar across the back of a reclining-back wheelchair provides support and stability.

LO-2

Figure 7.9–3. Support bar across back of reclining-back wheelchair.

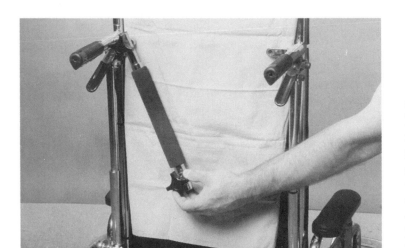

To fold a reclining-back wheelchair, the back support bar must be removed. Several different methods of securing the support bar are available. In the method illustrated, the bar is released by unscrewing a handle on the support bar. A second method uses the push handle as the securing screw. A third method of releasing the support bar is by sliding an outer metal tube to one side, revealing a hinge inside the tube. Pushing down on the hinge once the outer tube is properly positioned releases the hinge so that the wheelchair can be folded in the standard manner.

LO-3

Figure 7.9–4. Releasing support bar in preparation for folding reclining-back wheelchair.

The reclining-back wheelchair can then be folded following the same steps used when folding a standard wheelchair.

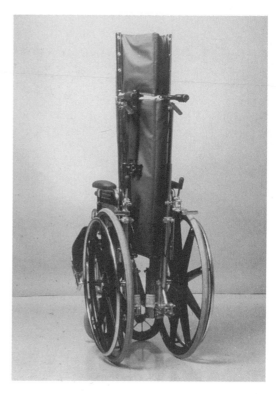

Figure 7.9–5. Reclining-back wheelchair in folded position.

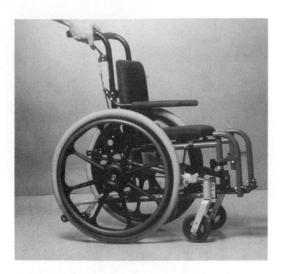

Figure 7.9–6. Starting position to recline tilt-in-space wheelchair.

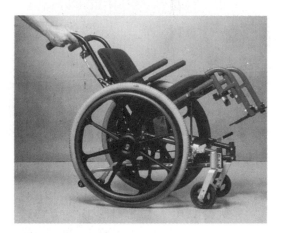

Figure 7.9–7. Tilt-in-space wheelchair in tilted position.

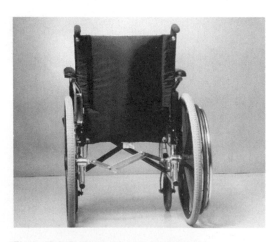

Figure 7.9–8. One-arm drive wheelchair.

Tilt-in-Space

LO-2

A variation of the reclining-back wheelchair is a tilt-in-space frame. The tilt-in-space wheelchair has a fixed seat-to-back angle, even when reclined. This is useful for patients who require customized seating systems to be used in the wheelchair. The tilt-in-space frame permits changes of orientation for pressure relief, or for different activities, while maintaining the postural control of the customized seating system.

One-Arm Drive

LO-1

LO-2

LO-3

A patient with only one functional arm and hand may achieve self-propulsion using a one-arm drive wheelchair. There are two types of one-arm drive mechanisms. One mechanism has two outer rims. These wheelchairs have two handrims on one wheel, and a linking mechanism between the drive wheels. With both rims on one wheel, both rims can be used simultaneously to achieve forward or backward propulsion. Applying force to one rim at a time turns the wheelchair.

A second mechanism uses a lever that is pumped to provide propulsion, and rotated to provide steering. Propulsion is achieved by pumping the lever forward and backward. The direction of travel, forward or reverse, is determined by the position of a shift lever.

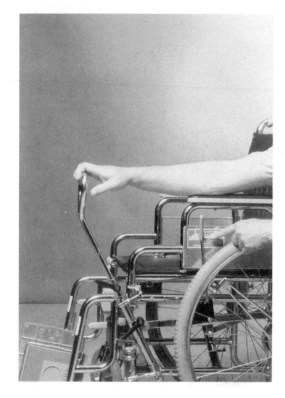

Figure 7.9–9. Pump lever and shift lever on one-arm drive wheelchair.

Rotating the handle of the pump lever turns the caster wheel in the direction the handle is turned.

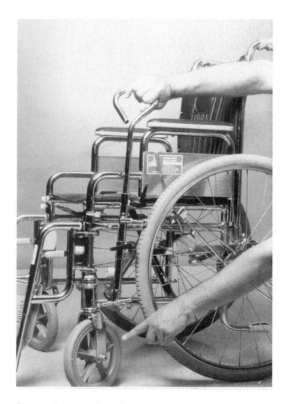

Figure 7.9–10. Pump lever rotating caster wheel on one-arm drive wheelchair.

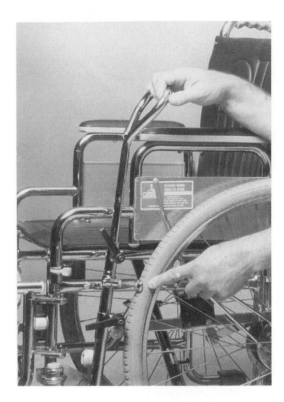

Figure 7.9–11. Engaging the brake on one-arm drive wheelchair.

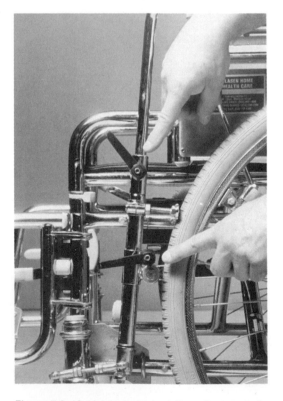

Figure 7.9–12. Height and orientation adjustments for pump lever handle on one-arm drive wheelchair.

Braking is achieved by pulling the handle of the pump lever backward to engage the brake securely against the tire.

The height and orientation of the pump lever handle is adjusted to achieve the most effective position for the patient.

When an attendant is pushing the wheelchair, the pumping mechanism is disengaged at the caster wheel, and the shift lever is in neutral. This is necessary to provide the attendant with full control of the wheelchair.

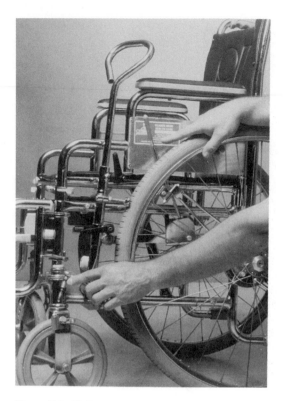

Figure 7.9–13. Pumping mechanism is to be disengaged at caster wheel when propelled by attendant.

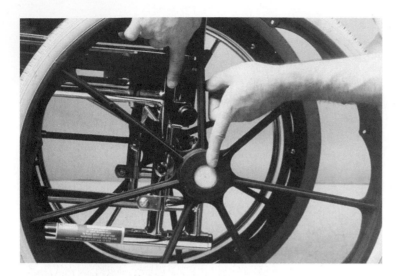

Figure 7.9–14. Offset between drive wheel axle and rear upright on amputee frame wheelchair (chair facing to left).

Amputee Frame

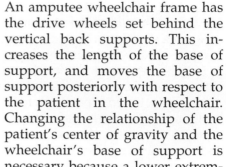

LO-1

LO-2

An amputee wheelchair frame has the drive wheels set behind the vertical back supports. This increases the length of the base of support, and moves the base of support posteriorly with respect to the patient in the wheelchair. Changing the relationship of the patient's center of gravity and the wheelchair's base of support is necessary because a lower extremity amputation moves the patient's center of gravity posteriorly when seated in a wheelchair. If the wheelchair's base of support is not moved posteriorly with respect to the patient, the wheelchair will be less stable, and more likely to tip backward.

7.10 MEASURING TO DETERMINE WHEELCHAIR SIZE

LO-4 Selection of the size and type of wheelchair for an individual depends on such information as the results of patient evaluations, the needs of caregivers, and the environment in which the chair will be used. The size of the wheelchair is determined by selected measurements of patient size. Care must be taken to use measuring equipment properly, and to read the tape measure or ruler accurately. Accurate measurement requires the therapist to assume a position that places the tape measure at the therapist's eye level. In some of the accompanying photographs, the therapist's position is altered to allow the tape measure to be seen.

The best method of obtaining accurate measurements is to have the patient sit on a solid flat surface and lean against a solid flat back. Wood inserts can be used in a wheelchair or straight-back chair to ensure accuracy when measuring a patient.

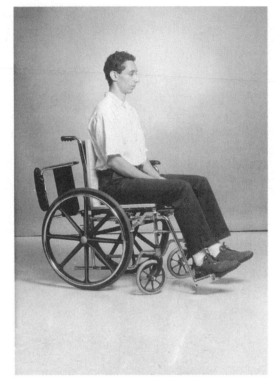

Figure 7.10–1. Flat surfaces used for measuring patient for wheelchair size.

Seat Depth

LO-4 Seat depth is one of the two most important measurements for determining wheelchair size. Proper seat depth provides support for the pelvis and thigh. The front edge of the seat should end 2 to 3 inches from the lower leg or knee. When seat depth is too short, the thighs are not supported properly, which affects weight distribution and comfort adversely. Seat depth that is longer than appropriate may affect circulation or lead to "sacral sitting" by the patient. Sacral sitting occurs when a patient slouches in a chair and the buttocks slide forward. When a patient slouches and the buttocks slide forward on the seat, the pelvis rotates posteriorly, placing the posterior aspect of the sacrum on the seat of the chair. Sacral sitting may result in improper postural alignment, sitting pressure placed on the posterior aspect of the sacrum, excessive pressure leading to skin breakdown, and less efficient propulsion.

The patient must sit with proper alignment, and in contact with both the flat back and the seat. One measurement and one calculation are necessary to determine seat depth. The distance from the flat back surface to the posterior aspect of the lower leg is measured along the solid seat surface. Two or three inches is subtracted from this measurement. The result is the seat depth measurement.

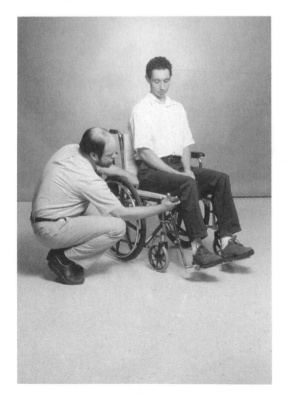

Figure 7.10–2. Measuring for seat depth.

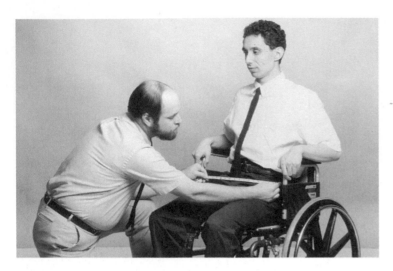

Figure 7.10–3. Measuring for seat width.

Seat Width

LO-4

Seat width is the second of the two most important measurements for determining wheelchair size. Proper seat width results in properly locating the drive wheels and armrests for easy and efficient use by the patient. When a wheelchair is too wide, a patient may have difficulty reaching the drive wheels for effective propulsion, and may lean to one side or the other to rest on the armrests. When a wheelchair is too narrow, excessive pressure on the lateral aspects of the pelvis and thighs may occur, causing discomfort or skin breakdown. In addition to body width, space for clothing, such as winter coats, prosthetic devices when necessary, and ease of movement must be provided.

With the patient sitting in proper alignment on the solid flat seat, the widest aspect of the patient's hips or thighs is measured. Two inches is added to this measurement. The result is the seat width measurement.

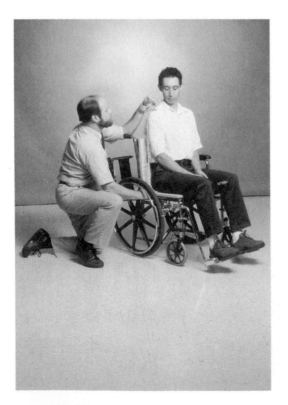

Figure 7.10–4. Measuring for back height.

Back Height

LO-4

Back height is measured with the patient sitting on the solid flat seat in proper alignment. The measurement points depend on how much back support is needed by the patient. In most cases, the distance measured is from the top of the seat to the inferior angle of the scapula. When a seat cushion is to be used, the height of the cushion must be added to this measurement. The result is the back height measurement.

Armrest Height

Proper armrest height permits a patient to rest his forearms comfortably on the armrest when sitting in proper alignment. When armrests are at an improper height, the patient will be unable to sit in proper alignment, and may be subject to unequal pressure on the forearms and ischia.

Armrest height is measured with the patient sitting on the solid flat seat in proper alignment, the upper arm held against the chest wall, and the elbow flexed to 90 degrees. The vertical distance between the solid seat surface and the patient's forearm is measured. When a seat cushion is to be used, the height of the cushion must be added to this measurement. The result is the armrest height.

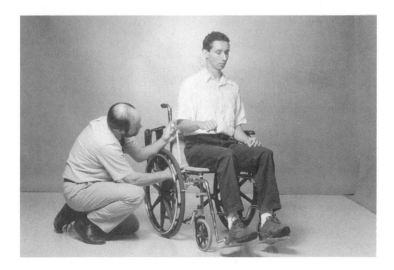

Figure 7.10–5. Measuring for armrest height.

Seat-to-Footplate Length

Seat-to-footplate length significantly affects sitting posture. When the length is too great, the patient may sacral sit in order to rest his feet on the footplate. When the length is too short, weight distribution along the thigh is uneven, forcing excessive weight bearing on the ischia and coccyx. Excessive pressure on the ischia or coccyx may result in skin breakdown.

The length of the patient's lower leg and height of the foot are measured from the posterior aspect of the thigh at the popliteal fossa to the sole of the foot.

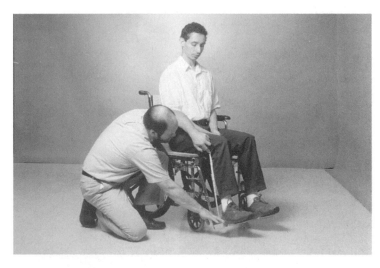

Figure 7.10–6. Measuring for seat-to-footplate length.

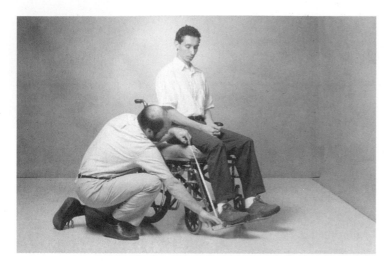

Figure 7.10–7. Measuring for seat-to-footplate length with seat cushion in place.

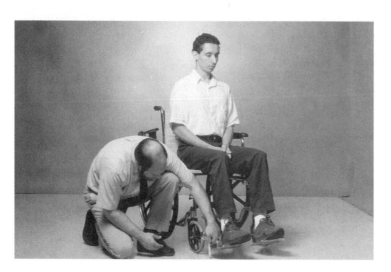

Figure 7.10–8. Measuring floor-to-footplate distance.

When a seat cushion is to be used, the height of the cushion must be subtracted from this measurement. The result is the seat-to-footplate length. This length is used to determine which legrest or footrest will be selected for the wheelchair, as well as to adjust the seat-to-footplate length. This measurement is also a factor when considering the seat-to-floor height of a wheelchair.

A minimum of 2 inches between the floor and the under surface of the footplate is necessary to provide clearance over thresholds and other small obstacles. The distance to be measured is from the lowest point of the footplate to the floor. Seat-to-footplate distance and footplate clearance height must be determined in combination with the type of front rigging and wheel size to be chosen.

Footplate Size

LO-4

Footplate size is determined by the size of the patient's foot. The portion of the foot that must be supported by a footplate extends from the calcaneus to the heads of the metatarsals. Supporting this portion of the foot provides proper support of the lower extremity, and helps to prevent the development of deformities of the foot and ankle. While a specific portion of the foot must be supported, the length of the footrest should be kept to a minimum to avoid interference with wheelchair maneuverability.

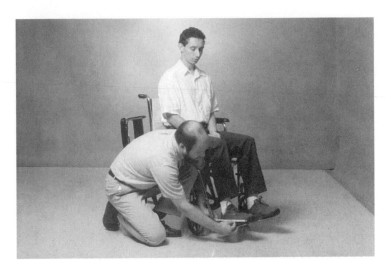

Figure 7.10–9. Measuring footplate size.

7.11   STANDARD WHEELCHAIR MEASUREMENTS

LO-4

Table 7–1 provides standard measurements for wheelchairs of different sizes. Wheelchair dimensions for a particular patient should be appropriately matched to these sizes. Custom fabrication is possible, but costly in comparison to choosing from among standard sizes.

TABLE 7–1. Standard Wheelchair Sizes

	Seat Width (in)	Seat Depth (in)	Seat Height (in)
Adult	18	16	20
Narrow adult	16	16	20
Slim adult	14	16	20
Tall adult	18	17	20
Hemi or low seat			17½
Preschool	10	8	19½
Tiny tot	12	11½	19½
Child	14	11½	18¾
Junior	16	16	18½

7.12 REVIEW QUESTIONS

1. When are wheelchair brakes used?

2. What are the indications for the following variations of wheelchair components?

    Desk-length armrests

    Full-length armrests

    Adjustable-height armrests

    Elevating legrests

    Footrests

3. How does a tilt-in-space wheelchair differ from a reclining-back wheelchair?

4. Describe two styles of one-arm drive wheelchairs.

5. How is an amputee wheelchair frame different from a standard frame?

6. Describe how to measure a patient for a wheelchair, including seat width, seat depth, seat height, back height, and armrest height.

7. How do wheelchair cushions affect measurements used to determine wheelchair fit?

8. What are the effects of inappropriate seat depth, seat width, or armrest height on sitting posture?

9. What is the effect of inappropriate footplate-to-seat distance on sitting posture?

10. What are the standard wheelchair sizes?

7.13 SUGGESTED ACTIVITIES

1. Provide a variety of wheelchair components and types for students to manipulate and for practice as both therapist and patient.

2. Students remove, adjust, and replace all components on the available wheelchairs.

3. Students measure several classmates to determine the correct wheelchair size.

4. Students practice teaching "patients and family" and other health care providers how to adjust and handle wheelchairs correctly.

5. Students document treatment and wheelchair measurements in SOAP note format.

CASE STUDIES

1. The patient is an 8-year-old boy with a diagnosis of cerebral palsy who presents with athetoid movements in the upper extremities. He is non-ambulatory and has difficulty adjusting position and maintaining head alignment. He is unable to manage a joy stick due to athetoid movements in the upper extremities. Make recommendations for a type of wheelchair and components.

2. The patient is a 17-year-old female 10 weeks post complete T10 spinal cord injury. She has indicated that she will use a wheelchair rather than ambulate with crutches and orthosis. Indicate the measurements necessary to determine wheelchair size. Recommend the type of wheelchair and components that would be appropriate.

3. The patient is a 67-year-old male with right hemiplegia (stage 2) following left CVA, presenting with flaccidity in both right extremities.

Chapter

8

Transfers

 Learner Objectives

The student will be able to:

1 List transfers, indicating those that are dependent, assisted, or independent.

2 Describe and correctly perform dependent, assisted, and independent transfers.

3 Describe types and levels of assistance used when transferring a patient.

INTRODUCTION

The transfer of a patient in or out of a wheelchair, bed, or cart may require the maximum assistance of several people, minimal assistance of one person, or no assistance at all. Each patient should be evaluated, or a person knowledgeable about the patient's functional capabilities interviewed, to determine an appropriate method of transfer prior to performing a transfer. Patient and therapist safety must not be compromised.

Whenever in doubt about the level of assistance necessary to transfer a patient safely, obtain additional assistance. The wheelchair, cart, or bed must always be stabilized by securing the brakes, or by other means, ie, bracing against a wall. Using proper body mechanics will reduce the possibility of injury. Before beginning practice of transfers, review the material on body mechanics in Chapter 2.

Dependent transfers are those transfers requiring minimal, or no active participation by a patient. Dependent transfers include the sliding transfer from cart to treatment table, three-person carry, dependent standing pivot transfer, and hydraulic lift transfer.

Assisted transfers are those transfers requiring some patient participation. Assisted transfers include the two-person lift, sliding board transfer, and assisted standing pivot transfer.

Transfers, which may be assisted or independent, include standing pivot, push-up, sliding board, the wheelchair to floor, and floor to wheelchair transfers. Transfers between wheelchair and floor are necessary should the patient fall out of the wheelchair, or when the patient wants to participate in activities on the floor.

Indicating the level and type of assistance required by a patient during an assisted transfer provides other personnel with information needed to complete a transfer safely. **Levels of assistance** can be stated as stand-by, minimal, moderate, or maximum. **Types of assistance** can be stated as verbal cuing of instructions, balance control, and lifting or supporting. For example, one patient may require moderate assistance for balance control. Another patient may require minimal assistance for support. Yet a third patient may require stand-by assistance for verbal cuing of instructions.

As a patient improves, the type of transfer may progress from dependent to assisted to independent. The amount of assistance may progress from maximum to none as the patient improves. The type of assistance may progress from a therapist doing all the lifting to a therapist using verbal cues only as the patient improves. The goal is for the patient to achieve a maximum level of independence that can be performed safely. The transfer chosen is based upon evaluation of a patient, including strength, range of motion, pain, cognitive ability, and movement dysfunction.

It is important for the therapist to have direct contact with a patient during transfers for two major reasons. First, direct contact permits the therapist to maintain the best possible biomechanical posture while working with the patient. The patient can be maintained close to the therapist's base of support, placing less stress on the therapist's back and upper extremities. The therapist's hands can be placed on the appropriate aspect of the patient's anatomy to provide support, such as under the buttocks for lifting or behind the hips for moving the patient into the therapist's base of support. Second, direct contact with a patient permits the therapist's manual contacts to provide input to the patient concerning the direction of movement. Such input assists the patient in determining the proper direction of movement, and provides a learning tool for being an active participant during transfers.

Transfer belts may be used to provide an alternative method of providing control of the patient during transfers when used properly. In situations when direct manual contacts cannot be safely maintained because of the size of a patient, a transfer belt provides a method of controlling a patient securely. When a transfer belt is used, the patient should be maintained close to the therapist, and not at arm's length.

Improper use of transfer belts decreases the safety for both the patient and therapist by moving the patient away from the therapist's base of support. When held at arm's length the patient is not fully supported, and the therapist is at greater risk for back and upper extremity injury. Care must be taken that transfer belts do not become only a handle for maneuvering patients during transfers. Simply pushing, pulling, or lifting on transfer belts alone does not provide the specific support needed by patients during transfers. When used improperly, transfer belts also do not provide the necessary input of manual contacts that help the patient understand the direction of movement required.

In some settings or jurisdictions, transfer belts may be required equipment. Each individual therapist must be responsible for determining the administrative and legal requirements of practicing in a specific setting or jurisdiction. An administrative or legal requirement for specific equipment may exist in an effort to limit injury or liability, but may fail to do so because of incorrect purpose or use. When specific equipment is required to be used, the user must adhere to proper application and use of the equipment.

There is generalizability of transfer techniques. For example, the procedure for transferring from a wheelchair to a treatment table may also be used in transferring from a wheelchair to a bed. With modifications, transfers into bathtubs, cars, or onto toilets, can also be achieved.

A purpose of transfers is to permit patients to function in different environments, or use different pieces of equipment. The goal of clinical treatment, with respect to transfers, is to increase the level of independence of a patient. This entails decreasing physical assistance and verbal reminders. The result is for a patient to progress, whenever possible, from dependent to assisted to independent transfers.

> **CLINICAL NOTE**
> Commands and Cues

A patient should always be informed about the transfer to be performed, and what he is expected to do. The explanation must be understandable to the patient. Commands and counts are used to synchronize the actions of all participants in the transfer. When the assistance of more than one person is required for a transfer, the therapist at the head of the patient explains how the command will be given and gives the commands. For example, the sequence followed by the therapist might be

1. "I will count to three and then give the command to lift."
2. "When I say 'lift,' we will lift."
3. The therapist checks visually and verbally to ensure that all assistants and the patient are ready before the transfer is initiated.
4. "One, two, three, lift."

A transfer is not considered complete until the patient is safe in the new position. The therapist and assistants must not release their control of the patient until he or she is secure in the new place. Appropriate positioning and draping must be completed and necessary equipment must be placed within usable reach of the patient. The patient must feel secure in his or her new position. Only then is a transfer considered complete.

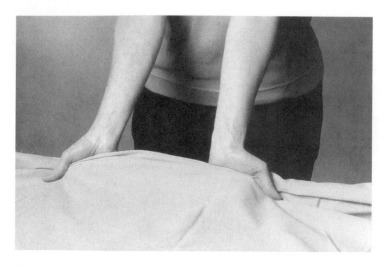

Figure 8.1–1. Grasping draw sheet.

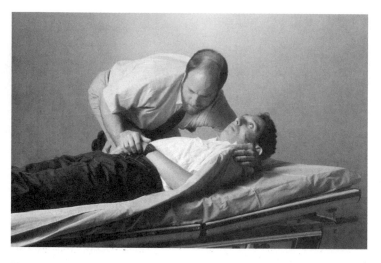

Figure 8.1–2. Supporting patient's head.

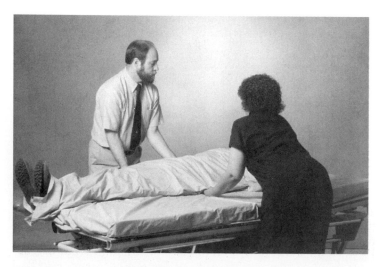

Figure 8.1–3. Wrapping draw sheet around patient.

8.1 SLIDING TRANSFER— CART TO TREATMENT TABLE

LO-2

The cart should be positioned parallel to, and against, the treatment table or bed and secured. The cart should be positioned so the patient moves toward his unaffected side, and so the patient's head will be at the head of the treatment table or bed.

When a patient can transfer predominantly under his own power, one person may assist by stabilizing the cart, and when necessary, providing minimal physical or verbal assistance.

When a patient does not have the functional ability to perform this transfer, the assistance of three people is required. The three people may use a "draw" sheet to move ("draw") the patient from the cart to the treatment table. The draw sheet is placed under the patient, and is rolled and grasped close to the patient. A stronger grip is obtained when grasping with the forearm supinated.

The person at the head should be on the side to which the patient is moving. This person is responsible for coordinating the transfer by instructing the patient, determining when everyone is ready, and issuing the commands.

When a patient is unable to control his head and neck, the person at the head will support the patient's head by placing one arm under the patient's shoulders while cradling the patient's head.

When a patient cannot assist or remain calm during a transfer, a sheet may be wrapped around the patient.

Two people stand on the side to which the patient is to be moved, and one stands on the other side. When the two people on the side to which the patient is to be moved are not able to reach across the treatment table to lift the patient, they may kneel on the treatment table to lift the patient,

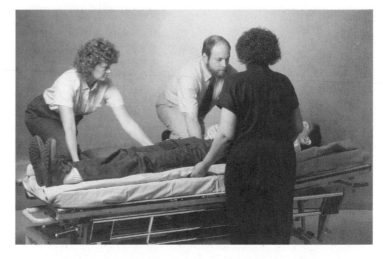

Figure 8.1–4. Starting positions for sliding transfer.

and perform the first part of the transfer movement.

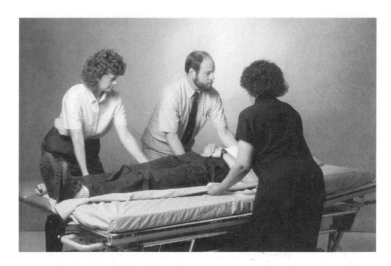

Figure 8.1–5. Mid-point of sliding transfer.

Once the patient has been moved part way onto the treatment table, the therapist must move completely off the treatment table, and complete the transfer.

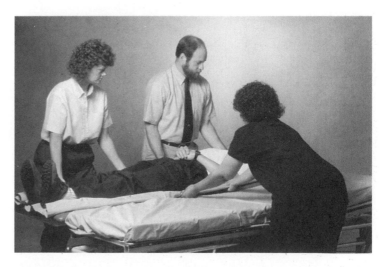

Figure 8.1–6. Completing sliding transfer.

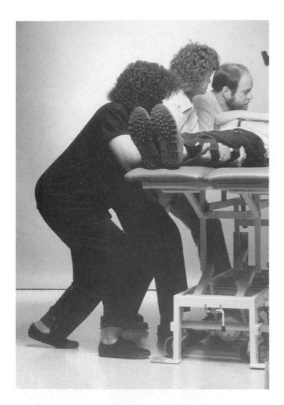

Figure 8.2–1. Starting positions for three-person carry.

8.2   THREE-PERSON CARRY

LO-2

When the cart and treatment table cannot be arranged parallel to each other, or the sliding transfer is deemed unsafe, the three-person carry is used. As the name of the transfer implies, three people are required to carry an adult of average size.

The cart is positioned and secured at right angles to the treatment table, with the head of the cart at the foot of the table, or the foot of the cart at the head of the table. The therapists must remove jewelry before sliding their arms under the patient to avoid scratching the patient. All three therapists stand on the same side of the treatment table, and are positioned in such a manner that one can support the head and upper trunk, one can support the midsection, and one can support the lower extremities. The strongest therapist is usually in the middle or at the head. The tallest therapist is usually at the head. The therapist at the head of the patient is responsible for instructing the patient, determining when everyone is ready, and issuing commands.

The therapists stand in stride with their feet slightly apart and knees bent. The therapists slide their arms under the patient so their elbows are on the treatment table, and the patient is cradled from head to foot. In this figure the cart has been removed to permit a full view of the therapists to illustrate their initial position.

Upon command, the patient is moved to the edge of the treatment table. In the remaining figures for this transfer, the cart has been placed properly, with the head of the cart at the foot of the treatment table.

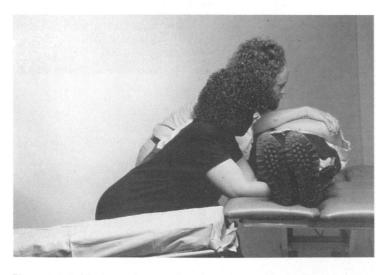

Figure 8.2–2. Moving patient to edge of treatment table.

By flexing their elbows, the therapists roll the patient onto his side in a log roll. The patient is now cradled in the bend of the therapists' elbows, bringing the weight of the patient closer to the center of the therapists' base of support.

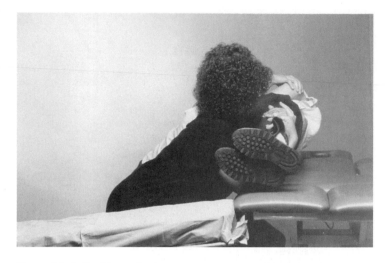

Figure 8.2–3. Cradling patient.

The therapists stand on command, lifting the patient.

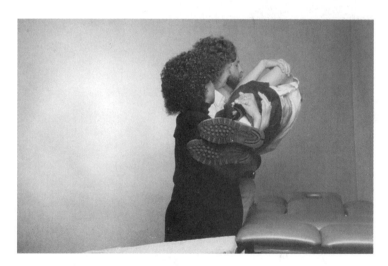

Figure 8.2–4. Lifting patient from treatment table.

On command, the therapists pivot and line up parallel to the cart.

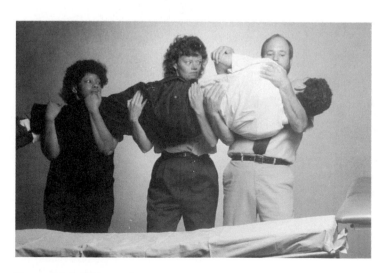

Figure 8.2–5. Facing cart.

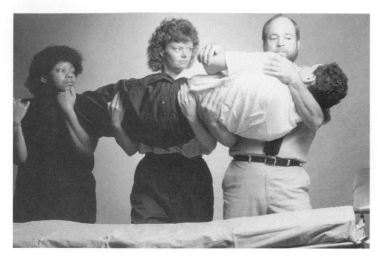

Figure 8.2–6. Advancing to cart.

The therapists then move forward in a straight line until they are next to the cart to which they are moving.

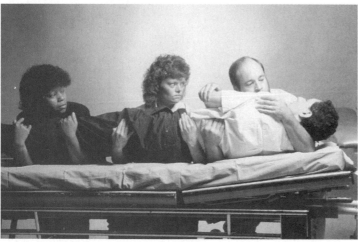

Figure 8.2–7. Lowering patient to cart.

The therapists stand in stride. Upon command, the therapists bend their legs until their elbows rest on the edge of the cart, to lower the patient to the cart.

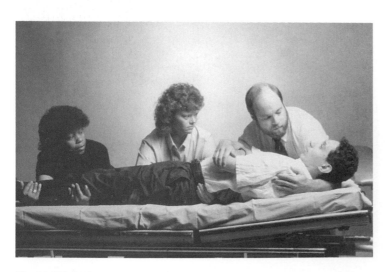

Figure 8.2–8. Uncradling patient onto cart.

The patient is uncradled onto the cart and then moved to the center of the cart and positioned in proper alignment. The therapists then remove their arms carefully.

8.3   HYDRAULIC LIFT

Introduction

Hydraulic lifts are mechanical devices that provide a method for one person to transfer a dependent patient. The hydraulic lift has caster wheels for positioning and maneuvering.

LO-2

The base of the hydraulic lift can be widened to fit around a wheelchair or other equipment. The base is placed in the narrow position when the patient is being moved to make maneuvering easier. To change the width of the base, the long lever attached to the base is moved from one side to the other. This lever is locked by either a slotted mechanism at the bottom of the lever, or by a cam locking mechanism that is activated and deactivated by twisting the lever.

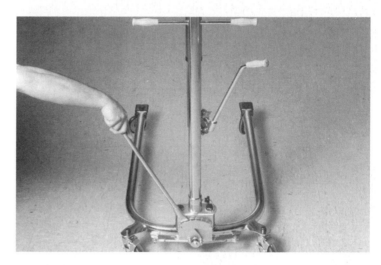

Figure 8.3–1. Narrowing base of hydraulic lift.

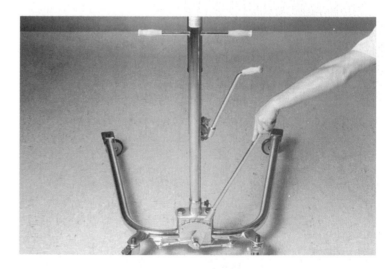

Figure 8.3–2. Widening base of hydraulic lift.

The hydraulic release valve on the front of the upright is closed to allow the arm of the hydraulic lift to be raised and opened slowly to lower the patient.

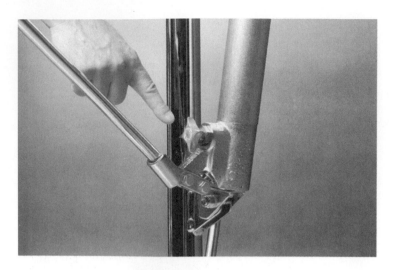

Figure 8.3–3. Hydraulic release valve.

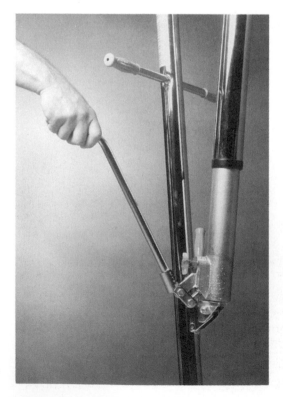

After checking that the hydraulic release valve is closed, the therapist pumps the handle to raise the arm of the hydraulic lift.

Figure 8.3–4. Hydraulic pump handle.

The sling on which the patient rests is attached to a spreader bar on the lift by two chains with hooks. The lengths of the chains are adjusted to accommodate the height of the patient. The chains are attached to each side of the spreader bar such that each chain is divided into two unequal segments. The spreader bar hooks are the dividing points of the two segments of each chain. The shorter segment of each chain is the segment that will be attached to the upper part of the sling, the part that will be supporting the patient's back. The longer segment of each chain is the segment that will be attached to the lower part of the sling, the part that will be supporting the patient's lower extremities. In this way, the patient can be lifted in a sitting position.

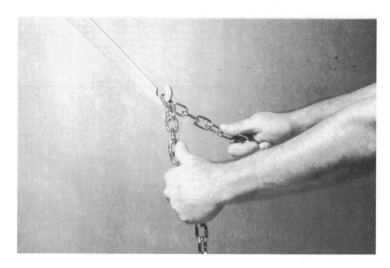

Figure 8.3–5. Setting sling chains on spreader bar.

Slings are made of a variety of fabrics. Some are one piece, and others are two pieces.

The sling is positioned so the seams are on the outside, away from the patient, to avoid pressure areas.

The chain hooks are attached from inside the sling to the outside. This reduces the likelihood of the patient being injured by the hook.

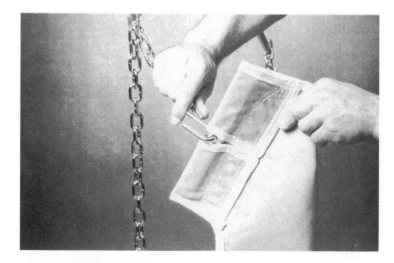

Figure 8.3–6. Attaching chain hooks to sling.

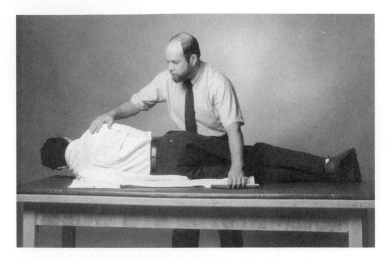

Figure 8.3–7. Turning patient to position sling.

Transfer

LO-2

When the patient is on a treatment table, the sling can be placed under the patient by rolling the patient onto one side and properly positioning the rolled sling on the table. The patient is then rolled to the other side and the sling is unrolled.

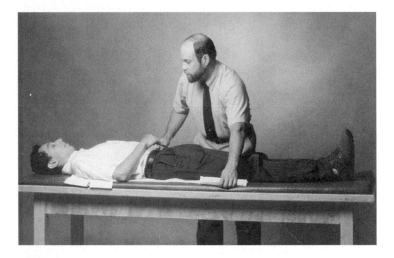

Figure 8.3–8. Final positioning of sling under patient.

Once the patient is positioned on the sling, the hydraulic lift is moved into position so the spreader bar is across the patient. Both ends of each chain are attached to their respective sides of the sling.

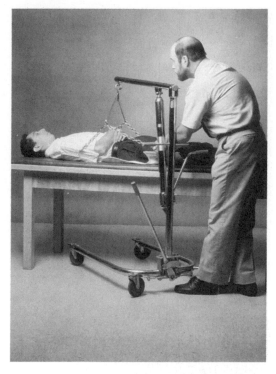

Figure 8.3–9. Attaching chains to sling.

With the valve closed, the therapist pumps the handle to lift the patient. Care should be taken to ensure that a safe sitting position is attained as the patient is raised.

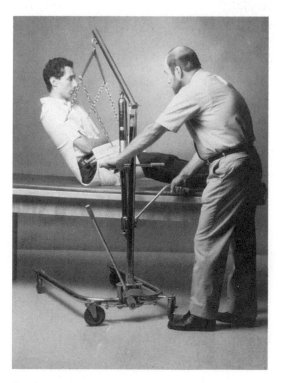

Figure 8.3–10. Lifting patient.

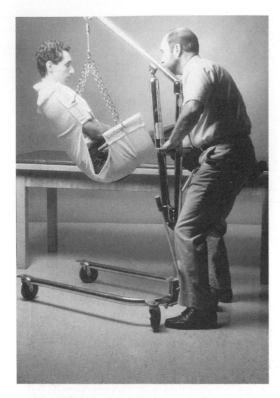

Figure 8.3–11. Assisting patient's lower extremities off of table.

Placing an arm under the patient's lower extremities, the therapist assists the patient's lower extremities off the treatment table.

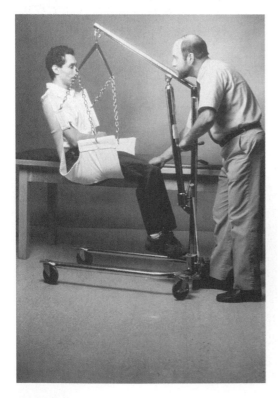

Figure 8.3–12. Steadying patient.

After lowering the lower extremities from the table, the therapist steadies the patient to prevent excessive sway during moving.

The patient is moved to a locked wheel-chair and the base is placed in the wide position.

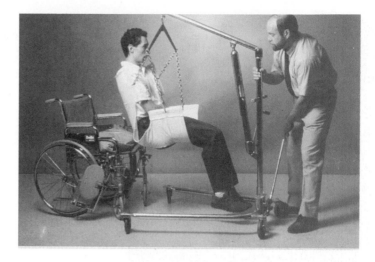

Figure 8.3–13. Widening base to fit around wheelchair.

The lift is maneuvered so that the patient is over the seat of the locked wheelchair.

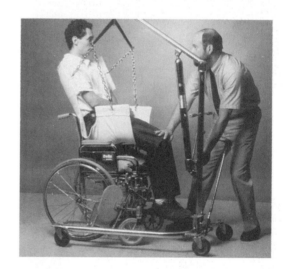

Figure 8.3–14. Maneuvering patient over wheelchair seat.

The hydraulic release valve is opened slowly to lower the patient into the wheelchair. Properly seating the patient in the wheelchair requires a slight pressure in the horizontal plane applied at the knees or thighs. This places the patient into the wheelchair completely, with the patient's back resting firmly against the back of the wheelchair.

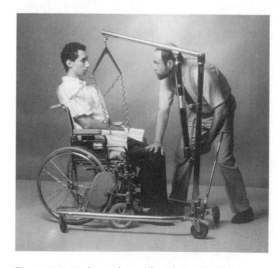

Figure 8.3–15. Lowering patient into wheelchair seat.

Once the patient is seated in the wheelchair, the hydraulic release valve is closed to avoid the potential of the arm striking the patient. The chains are then removed from the sling.

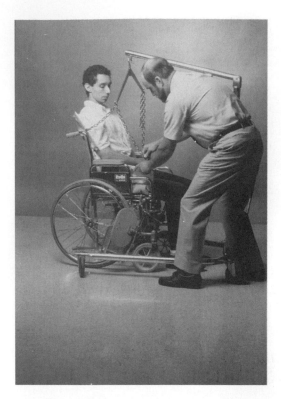

Figure 8.3–16. Removing chains from sling.

The therapist must ensure that the patient is secure when sitting without assistance before moving the hydraulic lift. While moving the hydraulic lift away from the patient, the therapist must ensure that the spreader bar and chains do not swing and strike the patient.

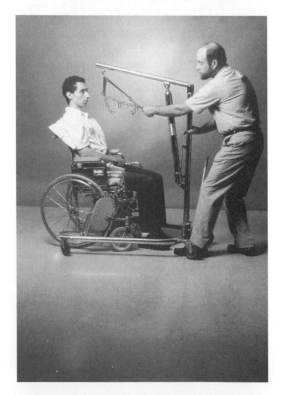

Figure 8.3–17. Moving hydraulic lift away from patient.

The seat belt is secured and the patient's feet are placed properly on the footrests. A one-piece sling is left in place under the patient. When a two-piece sling has been used, the portion behind the patient's back may be removed, thus the need to position the sling appropriately to avoid pressure from the seams.

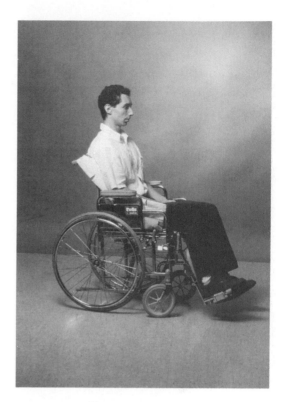

Figure 8.3–18. Sling remains under patient in wheelchair.

8.4   TWO-PERSON LIFT

Wheelchair to Floor

LO-2

When a patient has some upper extremity strength and trunk control, the two-person lift can be used. This transfer is often used to move the patient between the wheelchair and the floor.

To prepare for the two-person lift transfer, the wheelchair is locked and the patient's feet are removed from the footrests. The footplates are raised. The footrests are removed from the wheelchair when possible, or swung out of the way. The armrest on the side of the wheelchair to which the patient will be transferred is removed.

The patient crosses his upper extremities in front of his trunk. Standing behind the patient, the therapist reaches under the patient's upper extremities and grasps the opposite wrists of the patient (left on right and right on left). This prevents the patient from abducting his upper extremities during the lift.

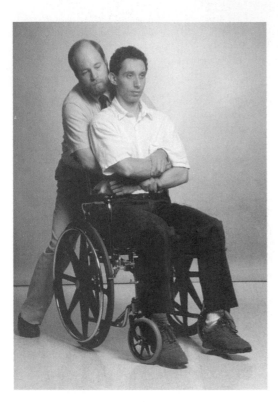

Figure 8.4–1. Hand placement for two-person lift.

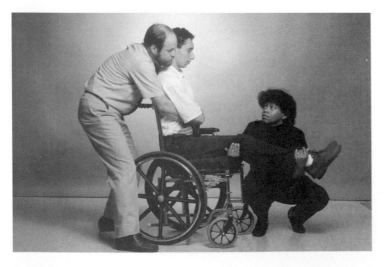

Figure 8.4–2. Starting position for two-person lift from wheelchair.

The therapist at the head of the patient places one foot on either side of the wheel and leans around the handle. The position of the therapist may be modified depending on the size of the therapist and patient, and the configuration of the wheelchair. The second therapist supports the patient's lower extremities by placing one hand under the thighs, well above the knees. The other hand supports the lower legs. The second therapist should face in the direction of the intended transfer, and have her feet in stride with hips and knees flexed.

On command from the therapist at the head of the patient, both therapists straighten, lifting the patient to a height that will ensure that he clears all parts of the wheelchair.

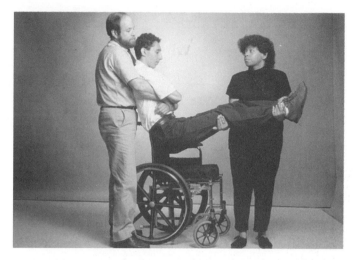

Figure 8.4–3. Lifting patient.

As a unit, the therapists step to the side or forward, as necessary to clear the wheelchair, and then lower the patient to the floor. The patient is not released until he is in a position he can maintain.

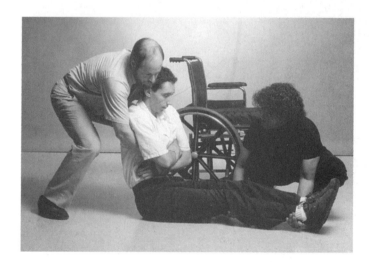

Figure 8.4 4. Placing patient on floor.

Floor to Wheelchair

LO-2

To return the patient to the wheelchair, the maneuver is reversed. The armrests and footrests are removed as described previously.

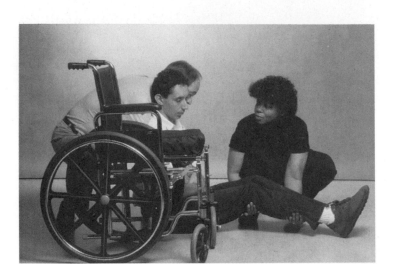

Figure 8.4–5. Starting position for two-person lift from floor.

With the patient in a long sitting position alongside the wheelchair, the therapist at the head of the patient squats behind the patient and grasps the patient's wrists as described previously. The therapist lifting the patient's lower extremities starts in a squatting position, with one arm under the thighs and one arm under the lower legs. Starting in a half-kneeling position would necessitate a movement into the squatting position, increasing the risk of injury to all participants.

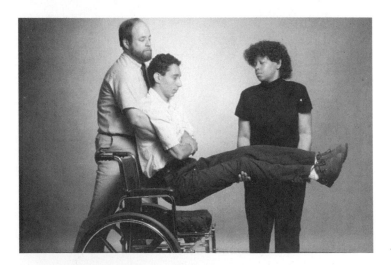

Figure 8.4–6. Lifting patient.

On command from the therapist at the head of the patient, the patient is lifted to a height that will ensure clearing all parts of the wheelchair.

The therapists step sideways or forward, as appropriate, so the patient is centered over the seat of the wheelchair. The therapist supporting the patient's lower extremities should gently pull the patient's lower extremities away from the back of the wheelchair so the patient will clear the upright of the back of the wheelchair seat. Once the wheelchair back upright has been cleared, the patient must be pushed toward the back of the wheelchair for the assumption of proper sitting posture.

When the patient is seated in a position he can maintain, the seatbelt is secured, the armrest and footrests are replaced, and the patient's feet are placed on the footrests.

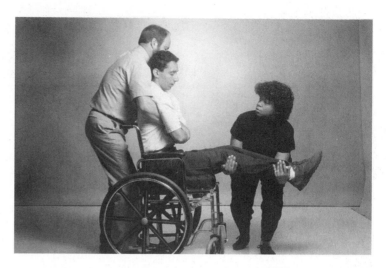

Figure 8.4–7. Placing patient in wheelchair.

8.5   DEPENDENT STANDING PIVOT

LO-2

The dependent standing pivot transfer is used for patients who are unable to stand independently, but who can bear some weight on their lower extremities. This includes patients with weakness, paresis, or paralysis.

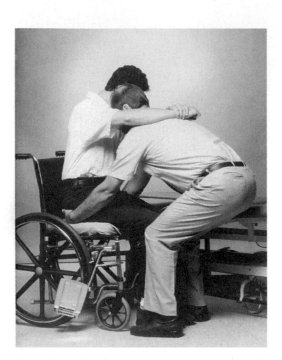

Figure 8.5–1. Starting position for dependent standing pivot transfer.

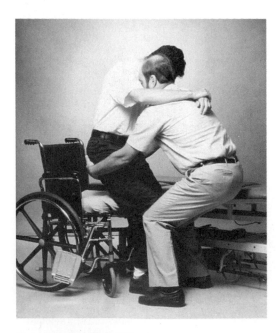

Figure 8.5–2. Lifting patient.

To perform a dependent standing pivot transfer, the wheelchair is placed parallel to the treatment table and locked. The patient's feet are placed on the floor, the footplates are raised, and the footrests are removed from the wheelchair when possible, or swung out of the way. The armrest nearest the treatment table is removed. To facilitate clearing the wheel, the patient is moved forward in the wheelchair.

To provide stability for the patient's lower extremities during the transfer, the therapist must "block" the patient's lower extremities. Blocking the lower extremities is performed in different ways for different transfers. In this transfer, blocking is achieved by placing the therapist's feet and knees outside the patient's feet and knees, with the therapist holding the patient's knees between his knees.

The patient's lower extremities are blocked, and the therapist's hands are placed under the patient's buttocks. The patient places his upper extremities around the therapist's upper back. Care must be taken that the patient's arms are not placed around the therapist's neck, and that the therapist maintains a static spinal posture throughout the transfer. The purpose of the placement of the patient's arms is to provide control for the patient's upper trunk, and not to provide assistance in lifting using the therapist's upper back musculature. Failure to keep the patient's arms from around the neck, or to maintain an erect posture in the upper spine, may lead to injury of the therapist, and subsequent loss of control of the patient during transfer.

In some settings or jurisdictions there may be regulations that limit the placement of a patient's arms around or close to a therapist's neck. Each therapist must be individually responsible for determining the requirements of practicing in a specific setting or jurisdiction.

To synchronize the effort of both the therapist and patient, the therapist counts and gives commands. As the therapist counts, he initiates a rocking motion in time to the counts in order to develop momentum. On the command "up," the therapist straightens his legs and lifts the patient from the wheelchair. The lift is only high enough to clear the wheelchair and any height difference between the wheelchair and the treatment table.

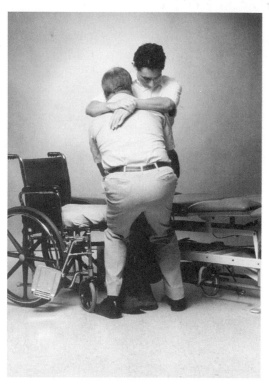

Figure 8.5–3. Pivoting patient.

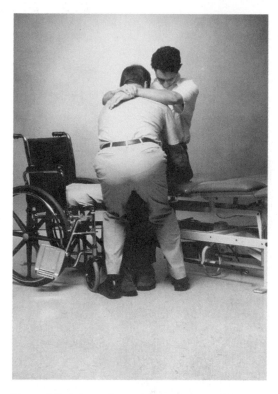

Figure 8.5–4. Lowering patient to sitting position.

The therapist pivots toward the treatment table, rotating the patient to the proper position for sitting on the table.

The patient is lowered to a sitting position on the table by the therapist.

The patient is not released until he is in a position that can be maintained independently.

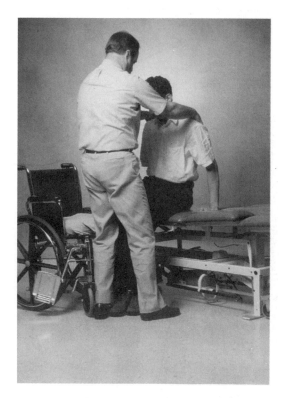

Figure 8.5–5. Guarding patient after transfer.

8.6   SLIDING BOARD

LO-2

The sliding board transfer is used when a patient has enough strength to lift most of the weight off her buttocks and sufficient sitting balance to move in the sitting position, but is not able to perform a push-up transfer.

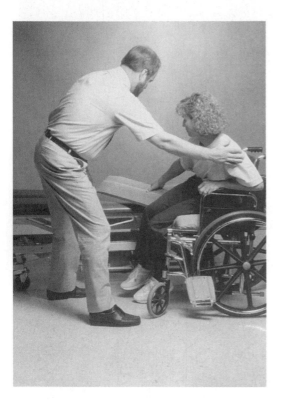

Figure 8.6–1. Positioning sliding board.

To perform a sliding board transfer, the wheelchair is positioned parallel, or at a slight angle, to the treatment table and locked. The patient's feet are removed from the footrests and placed on the floor. The footplates are raised, and the footrests are removed from the wheelchair when possible, or swung out of the way. The patient moves forward on the seat of the wheelchair and the armrest on the side nearest the treatment table is removed.

The therapist guards the patient by standing in front of her, and may block her knees to prevent her from sliding off the sliding board. The therapist can provide assistance for lifting by placing his hands under the patient's buttocks and lifting as the patient performs a sitting push-up.

When the patient needs assistance for balance, the therapist can place his hands on the patient's shoulders. The therapist decreases assistance as the patient improves.

The patient leans away from the treatment table, and the sliding board is placed well under the buttocks. Care must be taken not to pinch the patient between the sliding board and the wheelchair seat.

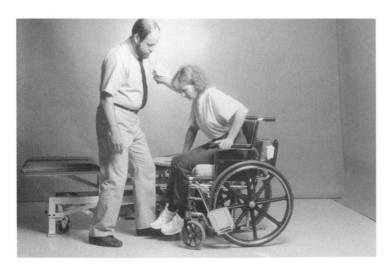

Figure 8.6–2. Patient moves back into upright position.

The patient moves back into an upright sitting position, with the buttock nearest the treatment table resting on the sliding board.

The patient performs the transfer by doing a series of push-ups. By straightening the upper extremities and depressing the shoulders, the patient lifts her body to decrease her weight on the sliding board. While her body weight has been lifted, she slides her buttocks toward the treatment table, and then lowers herself back onto the sliding board again. The patient repositions her hands. This sequence is repeated until she is on the treatment table with only one buttock remaining on the sliding board.

When necessary, the therapist can assist the patient by lifting with his hands under the patient's buttocks.

The patient may place her palms flat on the sliding

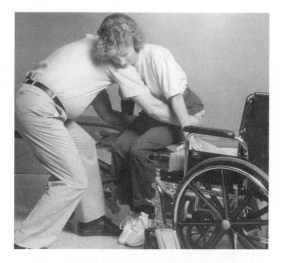

Figure 8.6–3. Therapist assists patient by lifting.

board, or make a fist and place the outside of her fists on the sliding board to achieve higher lift during the push-ups. The armrest can be used for the first few push-ups to gain greater height. The patient must not grasp the edge of the sliding board as her fingers may be pinched as she performs the push-ups.

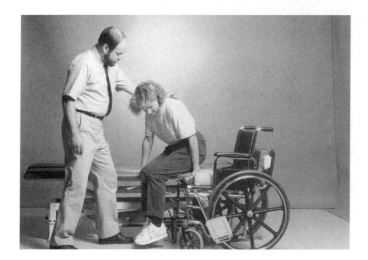

Figure 8.6–4. Patient performs sitting push-ups.

The patient leans away from the wheelchair to remove the sliding board.

The therapist does not release the patient until the patient is in a position that can be maintained independently.

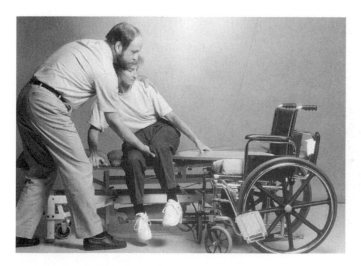

Figure 8.6–5. Removing sliding board.

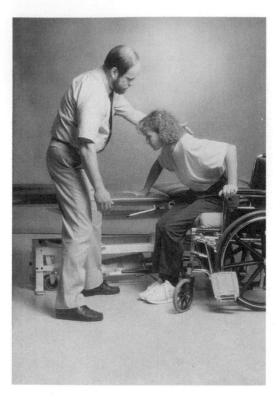

Figure 8.7–1. Starting position for push-up transfer.

8.7   PUSH-UP

LO-2

The push-up transfer is performed in a manner similar to the sliding board transfer, except that the push-up transfer does not use a sliding board for support. When a patient is able to perform the sliding board transfer independently, has developed enough strength to lift her buttocks clear of the supporting surface, and has developed sufficient sitting balance and endurance, the sliding board transfer may be replaced by the push-up transfer. For these patients, the sliding board is eliminated.

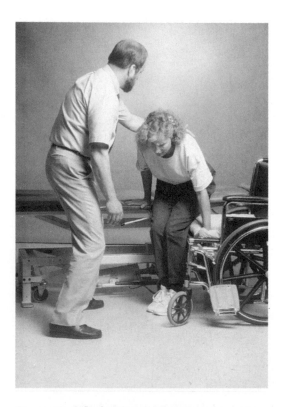

Figure 8.7–2. Performing sitting push-up.

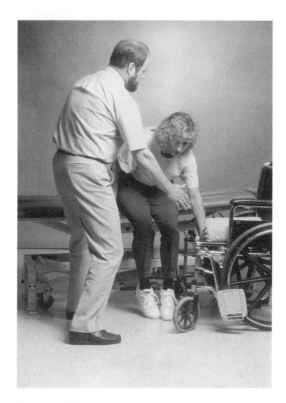

Figure 8.7–3. Lowering onto treatment table.

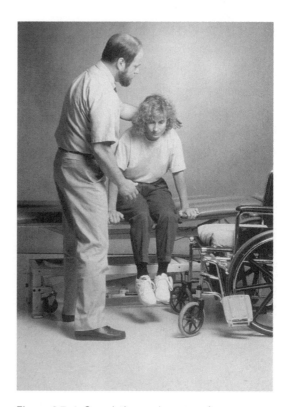

Figure 8.7–4. Completing push-up transfer.

8.8 ASSIST TO FRONT EDGE OF CHAIR

LO-2

A patient must be able to maneuver to the front edge of a wheelchair seat prior to standing or performing many transfers. Sitting on the front edge of the wheelchair seat allows a patient to get his center of gravity over his base of support rapidly and easily as he comes to standing.

When a patient is unable to maneuver forward in a wheelchair independently, assistance must be provided. One of several methods can be used to assist the patient. As a patient's ability improves, assistance is reduced until the patient is performing the task independently.

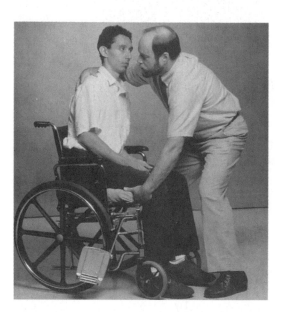

Figure 8.8–1. Shifting patient's weight to one side.

Side-to-Side Weight Shifting

LO-2

In the side-to-side weight shifting method, the therapist assists the patient to the front edge of a seat by placing one arm around the patient's shoulders from one side, and the other arm under the thigh of the opposite lower extremity. In this figure, the therapist's right arm is placed around the patient's left shoulder, and the therapist's left hand is placed under the patient's right thigh.

The patient's weight is shifted to the left to unweight his right buttock. While the right buttock is unweighted, the therapist assists the patient in moving his right thigh forward.

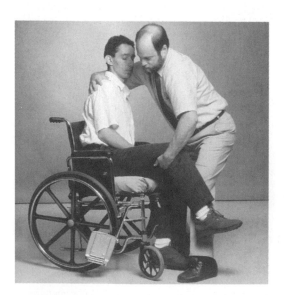

Figure 8.8–2. Assisting lower extremity forward.

The patient's right lower extremity is lowered to the supporting surface, and the patient is returned to an erect sitting position.

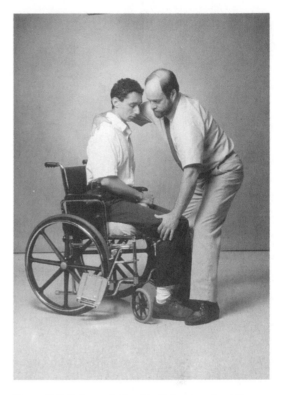

Figure 8.8–3. Lowering patient's lower extremity.

The therapist reverses the position of his arms, and performs the same maneuver to the other side.

This sequence is repeated from side to side until the patient reaches the front edge of the seat.

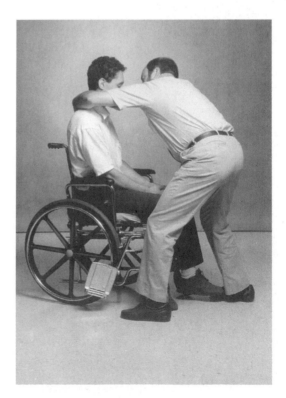

Figure 8.8–4. Shifting patient's weight to opposite side.

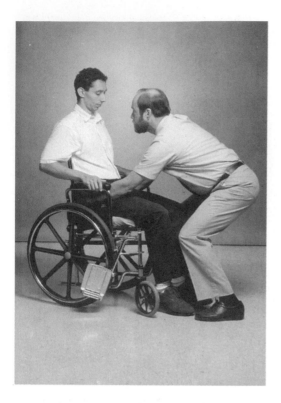

Figure 8.8–5. Starting position to slide patient's pelvis forward.

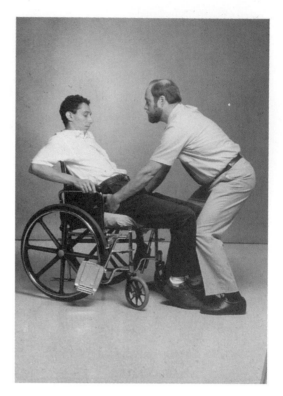

Figure 8.8–6. Buttocks are at front edge of seat.

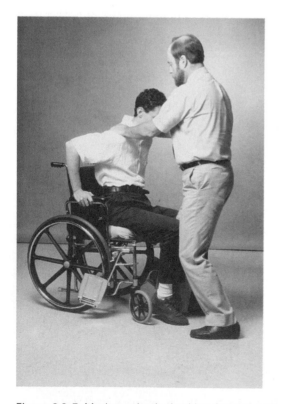

Figure 8.8–7. Moving patient's shoulders forward over pelvis.

Pelvic Slide

LO-2

The pelvic slide method of assisting a patient to the front edge of a seat involves moving the patient's pelvis and upper trunk as separate units. The therapist places both hands under the patient's buttocks, and assists the patient to lift and slide his buttocks to the front edge of the seat.

The therapist then places his hands behind the patient's shoulders and assists the patient in moving his shoulders forward over his pelvis into an erect sitting position.

Sitting Push-Up

LO-2

The sitting push-up method of assisting a patient to the front edge of a seat requires the patient to perform sitting push-ups. The therapist may assist by lifting under the patient's buttocks, or by guarding at the shoulders.

Each time the patient lowers himself back to the wheelchair seat, he lowers himself closer to the front edge of the seat.

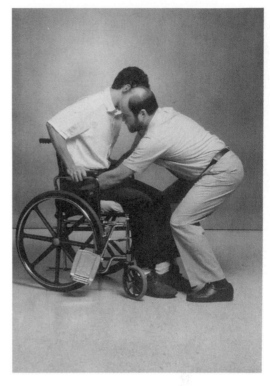

Figure 8.8–8. Starting position to assist sitting push-up.

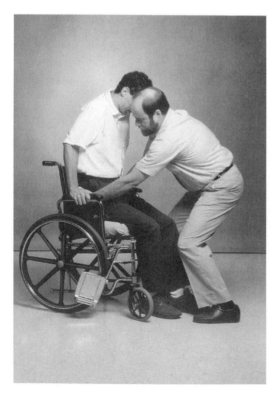

Figure 8.8–9. Assisted sitting push-up.

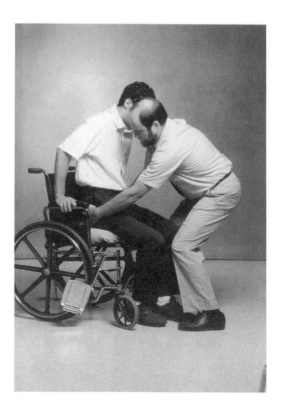

Figure 8.8–10. Lowering at front edge of seat.

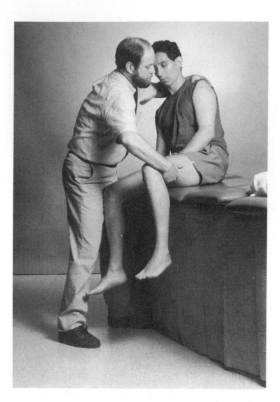

Figure 8.9–1. Weight shifting to assist patient onto treatment table.

8.9   ASSIST TO SITTING ON TREATMENT TABLE

LO-2

When a patient sits on the edge of a treatment table and is unable to move more completely onto the table, the therapist can assist by using a reversal of the maneuver used to move the patient forward in the wheelchair. In this case, the therapist assists the patient in moving the thigh backwards onto the table, rather than moving the thigh forward to the edge of the seat. The therapist must guard against the patient sliding off the front edge of the table as the patient's weight is shifted onto one buttock. This maneuver can also be used to assist a patient in seating himself fully against the back of a wheelchair.

8.10 ASSISTED STANDING PIVOT

Introduction

LO-2 The assisted standing pivot transfer is used when a patient can sit, stand, pivot, and bear some weight on the lower extremities, but has some weakness, paresis, or paralysis that necessitates assistance to transfer safely. This transfer is also used to teach the patient to transfer independently. The therapist reduces the amount of assistance provided to the patient until the highest possible level of independence is achieved.

By varying hand position, the therapist can vary the amount and type of assistance provided to a patient performing this transfer. By placing a hand under the buttocks, the therapist can assist by lifting as the patient rises to standing.

By placing a hand on the side of the pelvis, the therapist can guide the patient as he rises to standing. The therapist is in a position to control excessive lateral shift of the pelvis. From this position, the therapist's hand can be moved quickly to the posterior aspect of the pelvis to support the patient when necessary.

By placing a hand on the anterior aspect of the pelvis, the therapist can guide or resist movement as the patient rises to standing. Resistance may provide facilitation, making the activity easier, and teaches the patient to bring his pelvis forward as he rises.

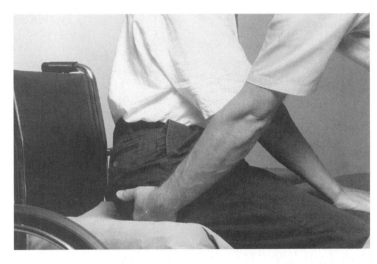

Figure 8.10–1. Hand position under buttock.

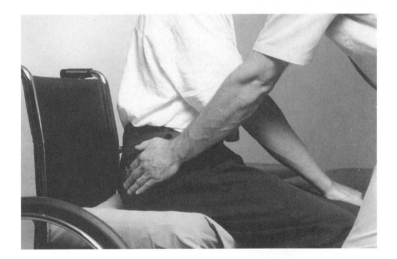

Figure 8.10–2. Hand on lateral aspect of pelvis.

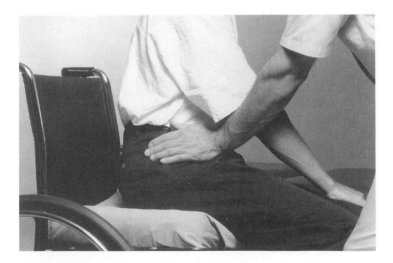

Figure 8.10–3. Hand on anterior aspect of pelvis.

In the following methods of performing the assisted standing pivot transfer, the patient is role-playing greater strength on one side, as might be observed in a patient with hemiplegia. For complete independence, the patient must be able to transfer to both sides. When first teaching the patient to transfer, moving toward the uninvolved side is easier for many patients. Teaching the patient to transfer toward the involved side reinforces the patient's awareness, and use, of the involved side.

Guarding the Uninvolved Lower Extremity

LO-2

In the first method, the patient is positioned so he can move toward his uninvolved side during the transfer. The wheelchair is placed parallel, or at a slight angle, to the treatment table and locked. The patient's feet are placed on the floor, the footplates are raised, and the footrests are removed from the wheelchair when possible, or swung out of the way. The patient moves forward to the front edge of the wheelchair seat (with assistance when necessary), as previously described.

When the therapist is unfamiliar with a patient's capability, he initially guards the patient's uninvolved lower extremity to ensure support on at least one side during the transfer. The therapist always guards the hip and knee on the same side of the patient by having his knee in contact with the anterolateral aspect of the patient's knee, and his hand in contact with the posterior aspect of the patient's hip. In this example the therapist guards the patient's left knee with his left knee, and the patient's left hip with his right hand. This position prevents the patient from collapsing at these joints. The therapist's other hand is on the patient's opposite shoulder to prevent the patient from falling to that side. The therapist stands in stride with his left foot medial to the patient's left foot. This position provides a base of support in the direction of the transfer, and permits both the patient and therapist to move without tangling feet once the patient is standing.

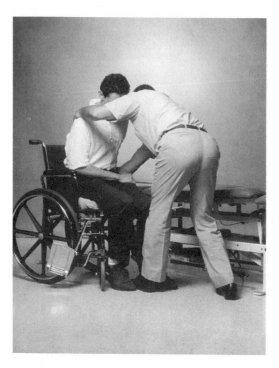

Figure 8.10–4. Starting position when guarding uninvolved lower extremity.

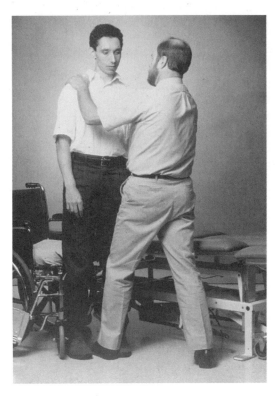

Figure 8.10–5. Standing under control with lower extremity blocked.

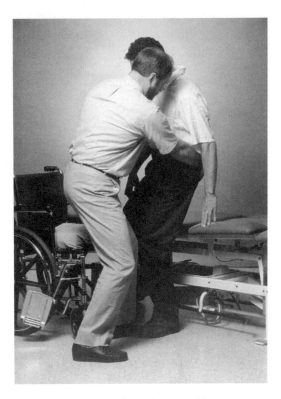

Figure 8.10–6. Lowering to sitting position.

The patient pushes to standing using the armrest of the wheelchair. A full upright position must be attained, and be under control, before the patient pivots or reaches for the treatment table.

The patient pivots and then reaches for the treatment table. The patient lowers himself, with assistance when necessary.

The therapist does not release the patient until the patient is in a position that can be maintained independently.

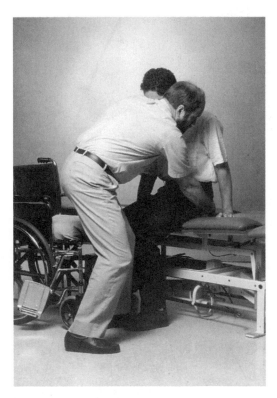

Figure 8.10–7. Adjusting final sitting position.

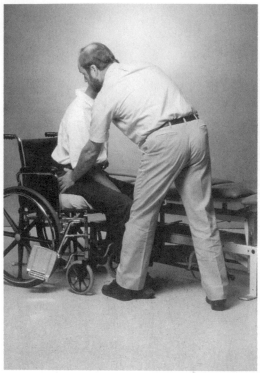

Figure 8.10–8. Starting position when guarding involved lower extremity.

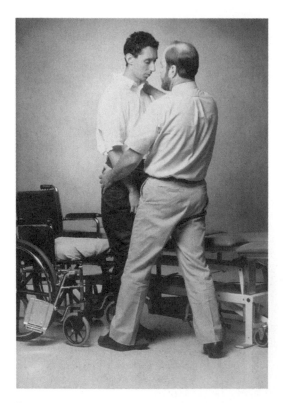

Figure 8.10–9. Standing under control with lower extremity blocked.

Guarding the Involved Lower Extremity

LO-2

A second method of the assisted standing pivot transfer is used once the patient has demonstrated that the uninvolved lower extremity is capable of supporting the patient in a standing position. When this occurs, the therapist can concentrate on guarding the involved lower extremity. This permits the therapist to evaluate the ability of the patient to use the involved lower extremity during transfers, and to assist the patient in using the involved lower extremity in a functional manner. The sequence of the transfer is the same; however, the position of the therapist with respect to the patient changes. The therapist now guards the patient's right knee with his left knee, and the patient's right hip with his left hand. The therapist's left foot is lateral to the patient's right foot. The therapist's right hand is on the patient's left shoulder. The therapist stands in stride to provide a base of support in the direction in which the patient is moving. This permits the therapist to move out of the patient's way as he comes to standing, and to move with him as he completes the transfer.

The patient pushes to standing using the armrest of the wheelchair. A full upright position must be attained, and be under control, before the patient pivots or reaches for the treatment table.

The patient pivots and then reaches for the treatment table. The patient lowers himself, with assistance when necessary, to a seated position.

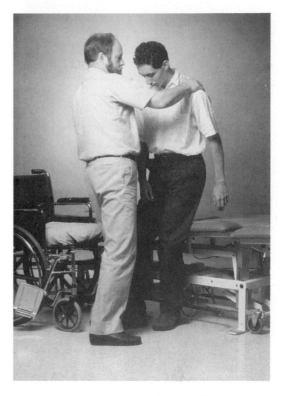

Figure 8.10–10. Lowering to sitting position.

The therapist does not release the patient until the patient is in a position that can be maintained independently.

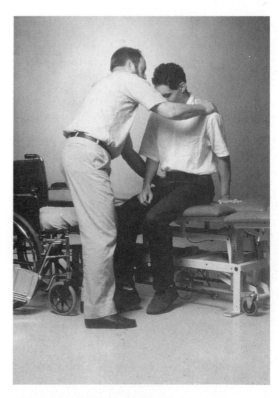

Figure 8.10–11. Adjusting final sitting position.

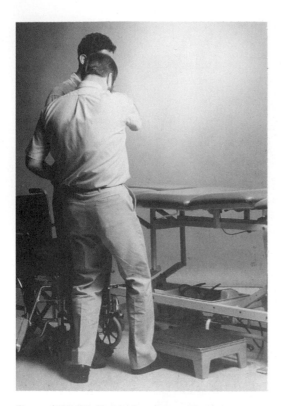

Figure 8.10–12. Positioning step stool.

Wheelchair to Treatment Table—Using a Step Stool

LO-2

Transferring a patient to a high treatment table will require the use of a step stool, especially when a patient is short. The position of the wheelchair, guarding techniques, and the activity of coming to standing are performed as in the assisted standing pivot transfer. In the following sequence, the patient is demonstrating a transfer to the side of his uninvolved lower extremity.

The step stool must be placed close to the therapist so that the therapist can retrieve and position the step stool while guarding the patient, once the patient has attained a standing position.

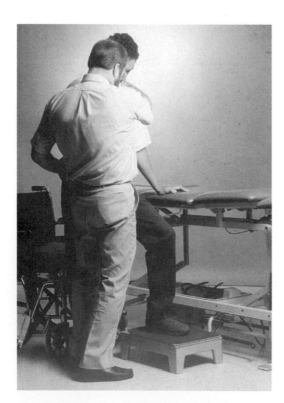

Figure 8.10–13. Uninvolved lower extremity is placed on stool.

The stool is placed alongside the treatment table, and in front of the patient. Having attained a standing position, the patient places his hand on the treatment table. With his hand on the table, the patient places the foot of his uninvolved lower extremity onto the stool. The therapist must guard the involved lower extremity carefully to ensure adequate support as the patient lifts and places his uninvolved foot on the stool.

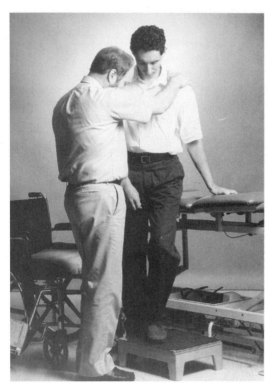

Figure 8.10–14. Stepping up onto stool.

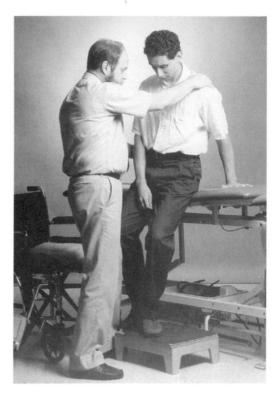

Figure 8.10–15. Pivoting and sitting on edge of treatment table.

The patient steps onto the stool, lifting his body over the stool. This raises the pelvis above the level of the table.

The patient then pivots on his uninvolved lower extremity, and sits on the table.

The patient is moved completely onto the table, and the therapist does not release the patient until the patient is in a position that can be maintained independently.

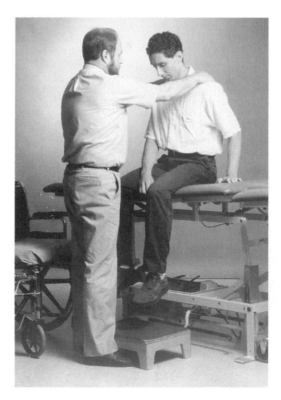

Figure 8.10–16. Adjusting final sitting position.

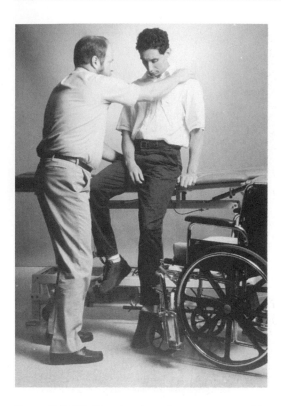

Figure 8.10–17. Stepping down from treatment table.

Treatment Table to Wheelchair

LO-2

To prepare for returning to a wheelchair from a high treatment table, the wheelchair is positioned and locked. In this example, the wheelchair is placed to the patient's uninvolved side. When this position is used, the wheelchair is on the same side of the treatment table as for transferring onto the treatment table, but is facing in the opposite direction. To alight from a high treatment table, a step stool is not necessary. Depending on the status of the patient, either lower extremity may need to be guarded for the patient's safety. In this example, the therapist guards the involved lower extremity as the patient slowly slides off the table onto the uninvolved lower extremity.

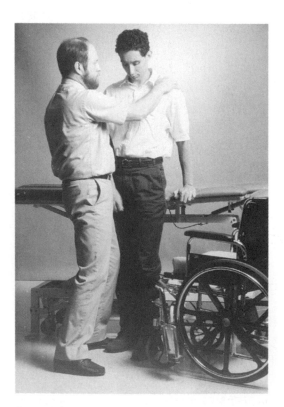

Figure 8.10–18. Standing under control.

The remainder of the steps and instructions for this transfer are the same, whether the patient is transferring from a high or low treatment table to a wheelchair. The therapist guards the patient's right knee with his left knee, and the patient's right hip with his left hand. The therapist's left foot is lateral to the patient's right foot. The therapist's right hand is on the patient's left shoulder. The therapist stands in stride to provide a base of support in the direction in which the patient is moving. This permits the therapist to move out of the patient's way as he comes to standing, and to move with him as he completes the transfer.

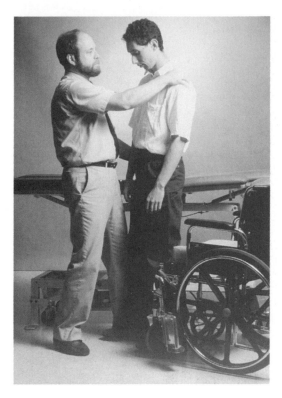

Figure 8.10–19. Therapist in position to move with patient.

The patient pivots and steps backward until he feels the front edge of the wheelchair seat at the back of his knees.

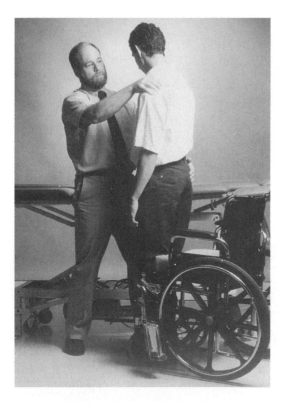

Figure 8.10–20. Pivoting and standing at front edge of seat.

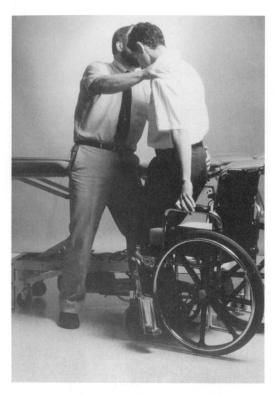

Figure 8.10–21. Grasping armrest and lowering to seat.

Grasping the armrest of the wheelchair, the patient lowers himself, with assistance when necessary, to a sitting position.

The therapist does not release the patient until the patient is in a position that can be maintained independently.

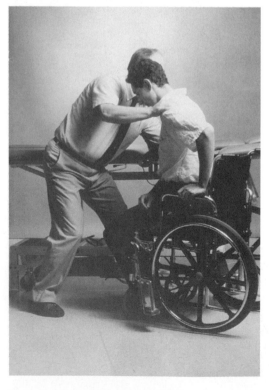

Figure 8.10–22. Sitting on wheelchair seat.

8.11 DEPENDENT ONE-PERSON TRANSFER— FLOOR TO WHEELCHAIR

LO-2

Occasionally a patient may fall out of, or tip over, a wheelchair. When a patient is unable to transfer from the floor to the wheelchair independently, either a one-person or two-person transfer may be used to get the patient back into the wheelchair. While the two-person transfer is desired because it is safer for the patient and those assisting, the one-person transfer may be necessary.

To perform the one-person transfer, the wheelchair is positioned on its back, at the patient's feet. The therapist places one arm under the patient's lower extremities, and the other arm behind the patient's upper back, such that the patient's lower extremities are flexed at the hips and knees. The patient is moved so that the ankles are placed over the front edge of the wheelchair seat.

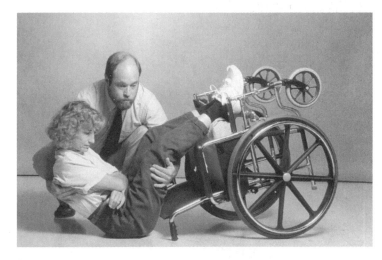

Figure 8.11–1. Initial lift of patient into wheelchair.

The therapist performs a series of short lifting and sliding maneuvers to move the patient into the wheelchair.

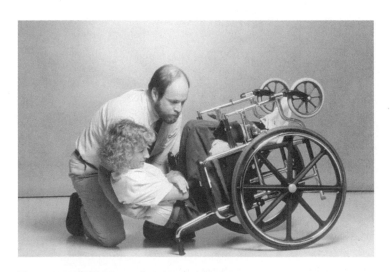

Figure 8.11–2. Placing patient in wheelchair.

At the back of the wheelchair, the therapist squats and grasps both handles of the wheelchair while cradling the patient's upper trunk. The patient and wheelchair are lifted as a unit as the therapist moves to a standing position.

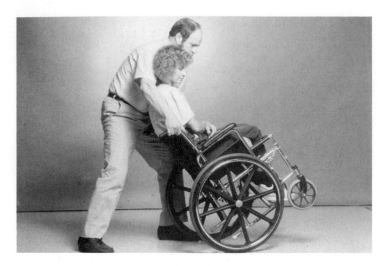

Figure 8.11–3. Lifting patient and wheelchair.

When the patient is tall, or the back of the wheelchair is low, the therapist may grasp one handle of the wheelchair with one hand, and support and lift the patient's trunk with the other hand.

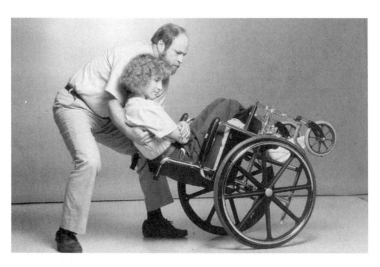

Figure 8.11–4. Alternative arm position for lifting patient and wheelchair.

As the wheelchair approaches the upright position, the therapist shifts one arm to guard the anterior aspect of the patient's upper trunk to prevent her from falling forward.

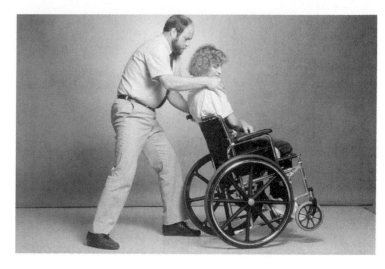

Figure 8.11–5. Guarding patient as wheelchair reaches upright position.

8.12   INDEPENDENT TRANSFER FROM WHEELCHAIR TO FLOOR AND RETURN

Introduction

LO-2

Many patients can, and must, learn to move safely from their wheelchair to the floor and back into the wheelchair. There are several methods for performing this type of transfer. The method of transfer selected depends on the strength, range of motion, agility, and confidence of the patient.

The first steps of each of these procedures are similar. The wheelchair casters are turned forward, as they would be when a patient is wheeling backward in a wheelchair, to increase the base of support of the wheelchair. When the casters are not properly positioned, the wheelchair may tip forward as the patient moves forward on the wheelchair seat. After the casters have been turned forward, the wheelchair is locked. The patient's feet are placed on the floor, the footplates are raised, and the footrests are removed from the wheelchair when possible, or swung out of the way.

During training, the patient must be guarded and assisted to prevent injury or bruising that may result in skin breakdown. A therapist is not pictured in the remaining photographs in this chapter to avoid obstructing the view of the patient, and because eventually these are to be independent transfers.

Forward Lowering—Wheelchair to Floor

LO-2

The forward lowering to the floor and the backward lift into the wheelchair require the most strength and agility of the several methods illustrated.

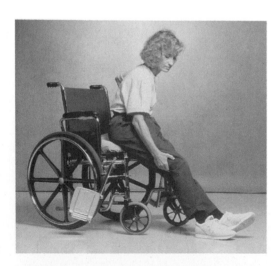

Figure 8.12–1. Positioning lower extremities when at front edge of wheelchair seat.

The wheelchair is positioned and locked with the caster wheels forward. The footrests are removed from the wheelchair when possible, or swung out of the way. The patient moves to the front edge of the wheelchair seat, and the lower extremities are positioned in extension.

One hand is positioned on the side, and toward the front edge, of the wheelchair seat. The other hand is placed on the caster or floor, depending upon the length of the patient's upper extremity, strength, and range of motion.

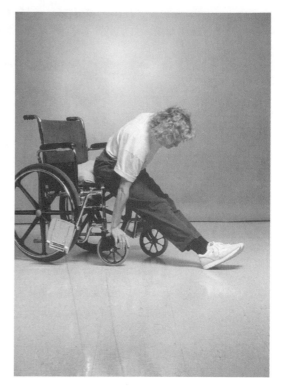

Figure 8.12–2. Using caster for support.

The patient then lowers herself to the floor.

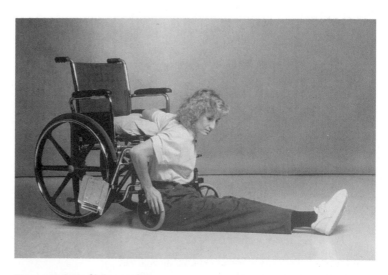

Figure 8.12–3. Sitting on floor.

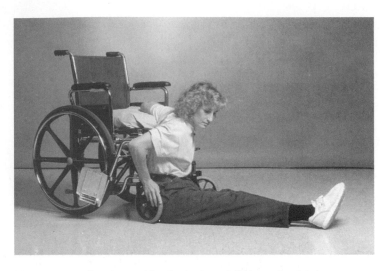

Figure 8.12–4. Starting position for backward lift into wheelchair.

Backward Lift—Floor to Wheelchair

LO-2

The wheelchair is locked with the caster wheels in the forward position. The footrests are removed from the wheelchair when possible, or swung out of the way. The patient assumes the long sitting position with her back against the front edge of the wheelchair. One hand is placed on the side, and toward the front edge, of the wheelchair seat. The other hand is placed on the caster or floor.

The patient pushes up by extending her upper extremities and depressing her shoulder girdles.

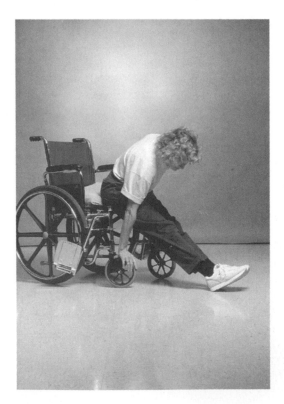

Figure 8.12–5. Lifting to front edge of wheelchair seat.

She balances on the upper extremity that is holding the edge of the seat, and quickly moves the other hand from the caster to the armrest.

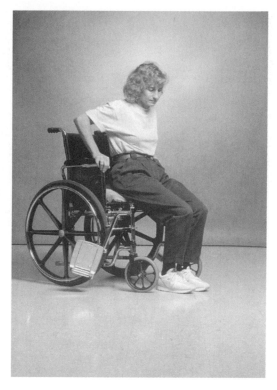

Figure 8.12–6. Balancing while moving upper extremities from caster to armrest.

Using the hand already on the armrest for support, the other hand is then brought from the seat of the wheelchair to the other armrest. Pushing on both armrests, the patient lifts her body over the seat of the wheelchair, and lowers herself onto the seat.

The patient completes the transfer by attaching the footrests, placing her feet on the footplates, and positioning herself properly in a sitting position.

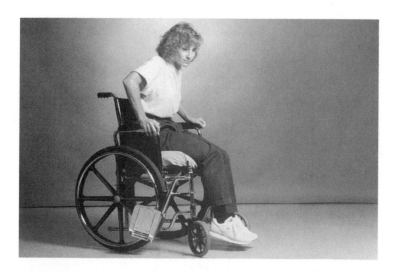

Figure 8.12–7. Lowering onto wheelchair seat.

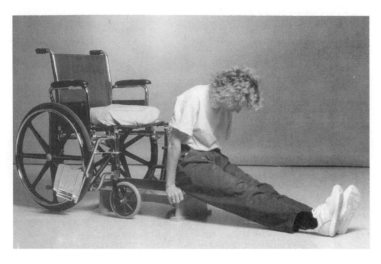

Figure 8.12–8. Pushing up onto stool.

Backward Lift Using a Step Stool— Floor to Wheelchair

LO-2

When a patient is unable to perform a floor to wheelchair transfer directly, a step stool may be used. The reverse of this sequence may be used initially to teach a patient to move from the wheelchair to the floor.

The wheelchair is positioned and locked with the casters forward. A step stool is placed in front of the wheelchair. The patient assumes a long sitting position on the floor in front of the step. With both hands on the step, the patient does a sitting push-up to raise herself onto the step.

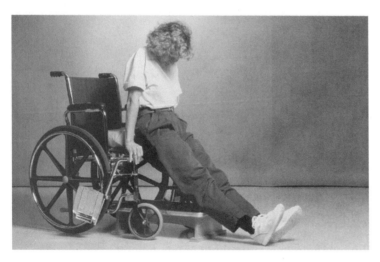

Figure 8.12–9. Pushing up onto front edge of wheelchair seat.

While sitting on the step, the patient places both hands on the front edge of the wheelchair seat, or the lower portion of wheelchair desk armrest. Performing a sitting push-up, the patient lifts herself onto the front edge of the wheelchair seat.

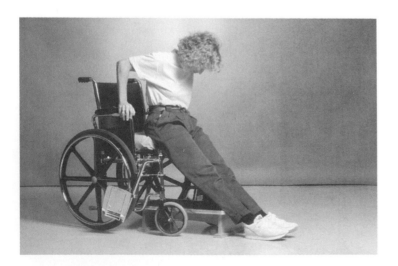

Figure 8.12–10. Moving upper extremities to armrests.

The patient moves her hands to the highest part of the armrest. Using the armrest, the patient performs a sitting push-up to lift herself further onto the seat.

Supporting herself with one hand, the patient uses the other hand to position one lower extremity with the foot resting on the step. This maneuver is repeated for the other lower extremity.

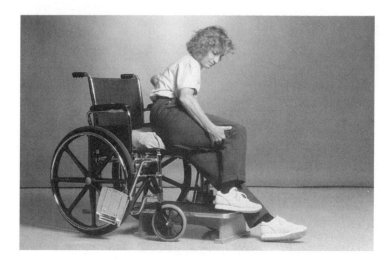

Figure 8.12–11. Positioning lower extremities.

The patient adjusts her position in the wheelchair until she is sitting erect, well back in the wheelchair.

The footrests can then be properly positioned, and the patient's feet placed on the footplates. When necessary, the wheelchair can be unlocked and wheeled backward to clear the step prior to positioning the footrests and the feet.

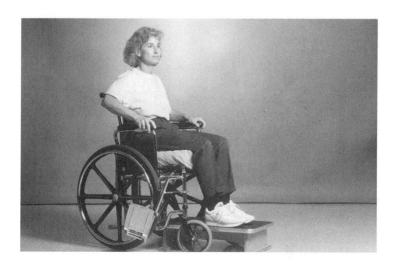

Figure 8.12–12. Moving back onto wheelchair seat.

Turn Around—Wheelchair to Floor

LO-2 The wheelchair is positioned and locked with the casters forward. The footrests are removed from the wheelchair when possible, or swung out of the way. The patient moves to the front edge of the wheelchair seat. She then turns partially onto one hip. In this example the patient is turning to her right.

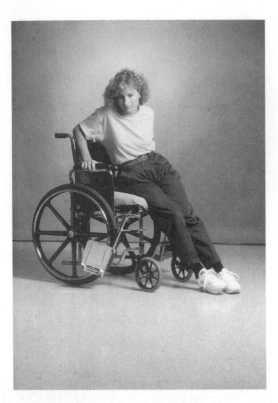

Figure 8.12–13. Turning onto one hip.

The patient moves her right hand behind her, grasping the left side of the seat. Her left hand is moved across the front of her body to grasp the right side of the seat.

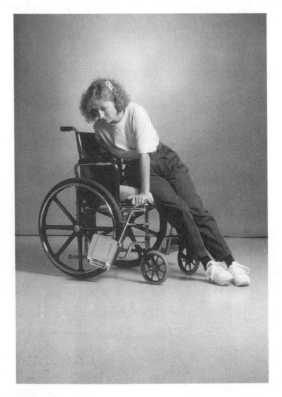

Figure 8.12–14. Positioning upper extremities.

As the patient extends her upper extremities and depresses her shoulder girdles, she lifts herself and completes the turn, facing the back of the wheelchair.

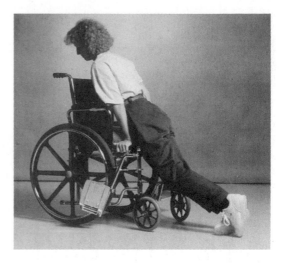

Figure 8.12–15. Supporting on arms and completing turn.

Once the turn has been completed, the patient lowers herself to a kneeling position.

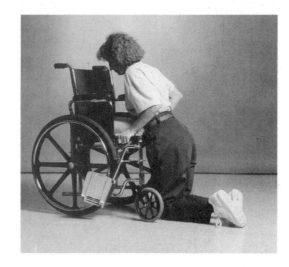

Figure 8.12–16. Lowering to kneeling position.

From the kneeling position, the patient can move directly to either a side-sitting or hands–knees position.

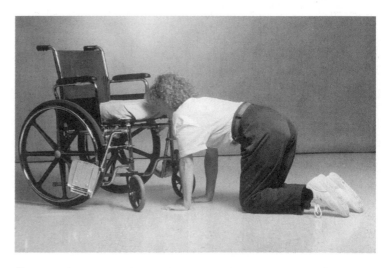

Figure 8.12–17. Assuming hands–knees position.

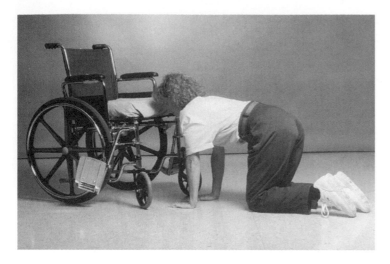

Figure 8.12–18. Starting position to move into wheelchair.

Turn Around—Floor to Wheelchair

LO-2

The wheelchair is positioned and locked with the casters forward. The footrests are removed from the wheelchair when possible, or swung out of the way. The patient assumes a hands–knees position in front of the wheelchair.

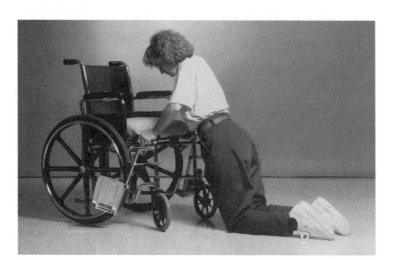

Figure 8.12–19. Moving upper extremities to wheelchair seat and attaining kneeling position.

The patient places one hand on the side of the seat toward the front edge, or on the lower part of a desk armrest when available. She places the other hand in the same position on the opposite side of the wheelchair seat. By extending her upper extremities, she achieves a kneeling position.

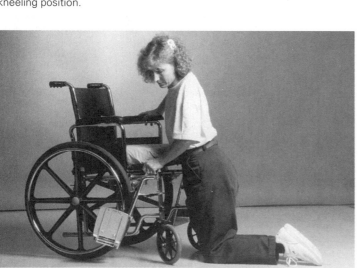

Figure 8.12–20. Positioning upper extremities for lifting.

One hand is moved from the seat or lower part of the armrest to the top of the armrest. Some patients may keep both hands on the lower part of the armrest as they push up.

By extending her upper extremities and depressing her shoulder girdles, the patient lifts herself and starts to turn.

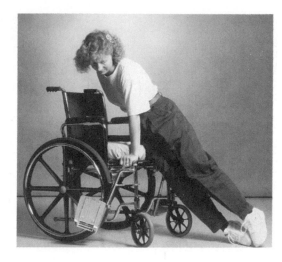

Figure 8.12–21. Lifting and turning.

The patient continues to turn as she lowers herself onto the seat of the wheelchair.

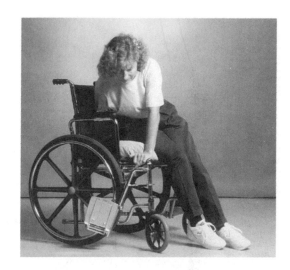

Figure 8.12–22. Lowering to wheelchair seat.

The patient repositions her hands onto the appropriate armrests, and completes the turn.

The patient can then position herself properly in the wheelchair.

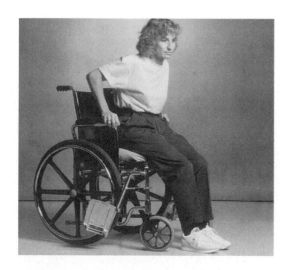

Figure 8.12–23. Positioning upper extremities on armrests.

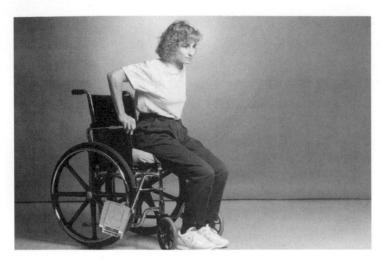

Figure 8.12–24. Sitting at front edge of wheelchair seat.

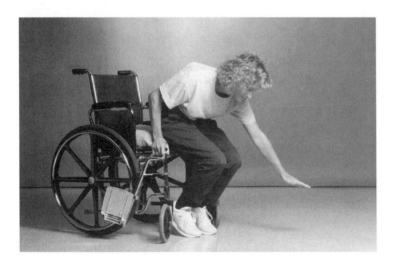

Figure 8.12–25. Reaching for floor with one upper extremity.

Forward to Hands–Knees—Wheelchair to Floor

LO-2 The wheelchair is positioned and locked with the casters forward. The footrests are removed from the wheelchair when possible, or swung out of the way. The patient moves forward to the front edge of the wheelchair seat and places her feet on the floor under the front edge of the wheelchair.

Grasping the seat, or the lower portion of the armrests when available, with one hand, the patient reaches for the floor with the other hand as she moves off of the wheelchair seat.

When the patient's upper extremity that reaches for the floor is able to support her, the other hand is moved from the wheelchair seat or armrest to the floor.

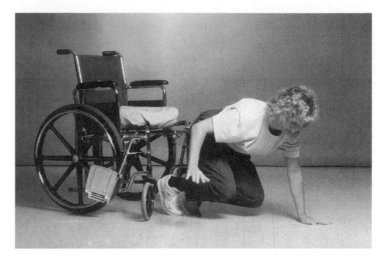

Figure 8.12–26. Reaching for floor with other upper extremity.

The patient completes the movement, ending in a hands–knees position.

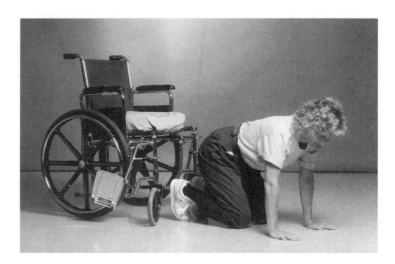

Figure 8.12–27. Assuming hands–knees position.

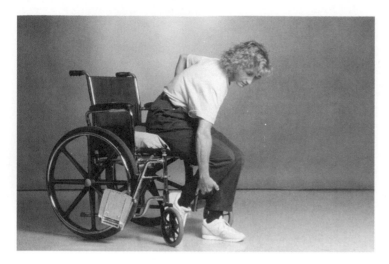

Figure 8.12–28. Positioning lower legs.

Forward to Kneeling—Wheelchair to Floor

LO-2

The wheelchair is positioned and locked with the casters forward. The footrests are removed from the wheelchair when possible, or swung out of the way. The patient moves forward to the front edge of the wheelchair seat, and places her feet on the floor under the front edge of the wheelchair seat.

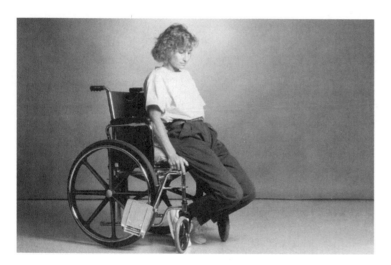

Figure 8.12–29. Lowering to floor.

Grasping both sides of the seat, or the lower portion of the armrests when available, the patient lowers herself to a kneeling position.

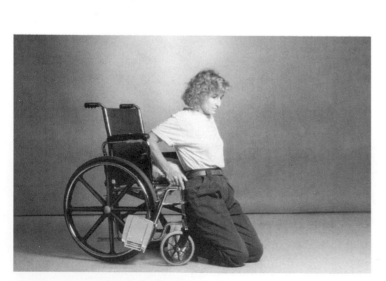

Figure 8.12–30. Assuming kneeling position.

One hand remains on the wheelchair as the other hand is placed on the floor.

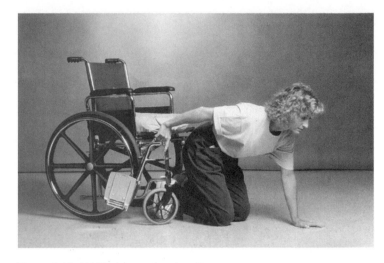

Figure 8.12–31. Placing one hand on floor.

The other hand is moved from the wheelchair to the floor. The patient is now in a hands–knees position.

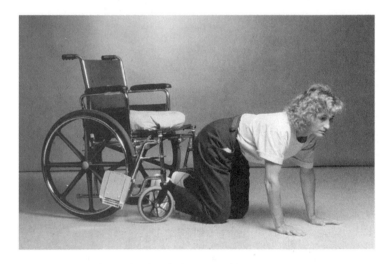

Figure 8.12–32. Assuming hands–knees position.

From the hands–knees position the patient may assume a side-sitting position.

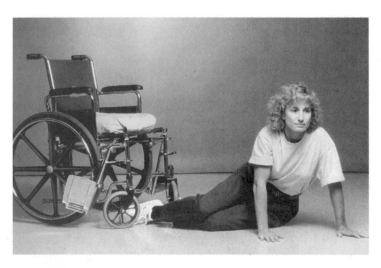

Figure 8.12–33. Assuming side-sitting position.

8.13 REVIEW QUESTIONS

1. Differentiate between dependent, assisted, and independent transfers.

2. What are the purposes of verbal commands during transfers?

3. Describe the sequences for performing the following transfers:

    Sliding transfer

    Three-person carry

    Hydraulic lift

    Two-person lift

    Dependent standing pivot

    Sliding board

    Push-up

    Assist to front edge of chair—three methods

    Assist onto treatment table

    Assisted standing pivot—three methods

    Independent one-person transfer from floor to wheelchair

    Independent transfer from wheelchair to floor and return—seven methods

8.14 SUGGESTED ACTIVITIES

1. Demonstrate the transfer procedures to students.

2. Students practice transfers working in groups of 2 to 4 people, with each student participating as a patient, lead therapist, and assistant.

3. Students practice transfers with partners role-playing the patient. The student should role-play patients with different diagnoses such as CVA (right or left hemiplegia), spinal cord injury (quadriplegia or paraplegia), multiple sclerosis, cerebral palsy, or Parkinson's disease. The student role-playing the patient can add "character" to enhance the activity by being cooperative, noncooperative, in pain, hard of hearing, apprehensive, faint, flaccid, or spastic. The patient must role-play the diagnosis and character consistently.

4. Students practice teaching transfers to "patients and family" and other health care providers.

5. Students document treatment using the SOAP note format.

CASE STUDIES

For the following case studies, students are to develop a progression of transfers appropriate for progressing a patient from dependent to independent (as much as feasible) transfer status. Students should progress the transfer method and the type and amount of assistance.

1. The patient is a 23-year-old female with a diagnosis of multiple sclerosis. She was independent in all activities of daily living (ADLs) and ambulated with a cane for balance until 2 weeks ago. At that time, she experienced an exacerbation that has left her totally dependent in all transfers and unable to ambulate. She becomes faint when moved from supine to sitting, or sitting to standing, too quickly. She is expected to recover most of her prior level of independence.

2. The patient is a 63-year-old male with left CVA onset 20 hours ago, presenting with right hemiplegia and global aphasia (both receptive and expressive aphasia). The cause was a blood clot. Because he received immediate medical treatment, recovery is anticipated to be nearly complete. At present, he is dependent in all ADLs, including transfers and ambulation.

3. The patient is a 18-year-old male who sustained a complete T12-L1 spinal cord lesion in a motorcycle accident 2 weeks ago. Following surgery, he is wearing a thoraco-lumbar-sacral orthosis (TLSO). He has medical clearance to begin transfer training while wearing his TLSO.

4. The patient is a 23-year-old female with cerebral palsy, presenting with spastic quadriplegia. While living with her parents, her father lifted her for all her transfers. Following her recent college graduation, she is

living in a group home for the first time. She ambulates by using a power wheelchair. The staff of the group home requests assistance in selecting appropriate transfers. The staff would like a program to assist her in becoming an active participant in her transfers. Would the transfer method selected be different if she was 5 feet tall weighing 250 pounds versus 5 feet tall weighing 96 pounds?

5. The patient is a 49-year-old female with severe rheumatoid arthritis. She is 5 feet 3 inches tall, and weighs 175 pounds. Transfers are currently accomplished using a pneumatic lift. She ambulates by using a power wheelchair. Because her arthritis is in remission at this time, she would like to learn to transfer without the pneumatic lift so she can get out in the community more.

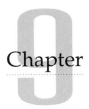

Chapter

9

Ambulation
With Assistive Devices

Learner Objectives

The student will be able to:

1 State indications for use of assistive devices to ambulate.
2 State the uses of parallel bars during gait training.
3 List the causes of fatigue during gait training, and methods to reduce the effects of fatigue.
4 Discuss the effect of patient concentration on gait training.
5 Describe the use of a scale to teach weight-bearing limits.
6 Describe methods of instruction appropriate for gait training.
7 List the activities that a patient must master to be independent in ambulation with an assistive device.
8 List assistive devices in order from those providing most stability to least stability.
9 List assistive devices in order from those requiring the most coordination to least coordination.
10 List the evaluations used to determine appropriate assistive devices for different patients and pathologies.
11 Adjust the height of assistive devices properly.
12 Describe the variety of styles of walkers, crutches, and canes.
13 Describe and demonstrate common gait patterns used with assistive devices.
14 Guard a patient properly when using assistive devices during ambulation on level surfaces, stairs and curbs, the assumption of sitting from standing and standing from sitting, moving through doorways, falling without injury, and resumption of ambulation after falling.
15 Instruct a patient in the proper method of using various assistive devices to perform different gait patterns on level surfaces, stairs and curbs, moving through doorways, the assumption of sitting from standing and standing from sitting, falling without injury, and resumption of ambulation after falling.
16 Discuss the use of the tilt table during gait training.

INTRODUCTION

LO-1

Assistive devices permit some patients who cannot ambulate without assistance to ambulate safely. Three major indications for using assistive devices are

1. Structural deformity or loss, injury, or disease, which decreases the ability to bear weight on the lower extremities
2. Muscle weakness or paralysis of the trunk or lower extremities
3. Inadequate balance

Assistive devices increase a patient's base of support and provide additional means of support. Thus, assistive devices provide a larger area within which the patient's center of gravity can shift without loss of balance, and a redistribution of support within the wider base of support.

9.1   TEACHING TIPS

Parallel Bars

LO-2

CLINICAL NOTE

Patients should feel secure

Instruction in a gait pattern often begins in a set of parallel bars. Parallel bars provide maximum stability, and require the least amount of coordination by a patient. A patient can become accustomed to the upright posture and learn a gait pattern in the relative safety of parallel bars. Assistive devices can be fitted while a patient stands in parallel bars. When appropriate, a patient can practice standing or a gait pattern while waiting for the therapist to adjust assistive devices, providing efficient use of treatment time.

Initial use of assistive devices can be in, or alongside, parallel bars. Patients have reassurance that the stable parallel bars are readily available. A patient may, however, become too dependent on the parallel bars. The therapist must progress a patient to ambulation away from the parallel bars as rapidly as possible.

Fatigue

LO-3

CLINICAL NOTE

Fatigue can interfere with learning

Fatigue may occur during gait training as a result of

1. Performing an activity that has not been performed for a while
2. Using assistive devices during ambulation
3. Greater concentration levels while learning a new gait pattern with additional equipment
4. Physiological responses to the stresses of injury or illness

These factors can cause a patient to fatigue rapidly. Frequent rest periods may be necessary during initial gait training sessions. Several short sessions of gait training, rather than one long session, may be more effective.

Patient Concentration

LO-4

When first using assistive devices, the need to concentrate can be very high. During initial training sessions, a patient will require greater concentration to learn a gait pattern properly. Often patients will look at their feet and assistive devices as they learn to walk. Patients do so because they need input as to where their feet and assistive devices are with respect to their body. Looking at feet and assistive devices also reduces distractions of other objects and activities in the immediate area.

High levels of concentration by patients on their feet and assistive devices makes ambulation an activity requiring active thought, interfering with a patient's ability to respond to other inputs, such as conversation. A patient may stop walking to answer questions. Conversation with, and around, a patient not directly related to ambulation should be avoided during initial gait training. Later in training, however, such additional inputs can be used to test the degree to which a patient has mastered use of an assistive device and a new gait pattern. When ambulation has become an automatic activity again, patients will be able to respond to questions and other activity in the environment without losing concentration or coordination during ambulation. At this time, patients will usually start to look up and around as they ambulate. When this occurs, patients can take over the responsibility of monitoring the environment for themselves, and more complex environments can be used for gait training.

Initial gait training should occur in an environment that is as free of distractions as possible. The therapist should monitor the environment for the patient. Patient rooms or therapy departments are usually less distracting than public corridors. When more complex environments are needed to challenge a patient, public corridors can be used for gait training.

CLINICAL NOTE

Walk and talk test

Weight Bearing

LO-5

When teaching a patient with a restriction of weight bearing, a bathroom scale can be useful. By placing one lower extremity on the scale, different levels of weight bearing, and the attendant feeling, can be demonstrated. When using this method, the lower extremity not placed on the scale must be placed on a solid surface at the same level as the scale to avoid an uneven supporting surface. In some cases, two scales may be used, with one lower extremity placed on each scale.

Instruction

LO-6

Before a patient begins ambulating, the therapist describes and demonstrates the proper use of the assistive device and the appropriate gait pattern. A demonstration is the primary method of instruction, with verbal descriptions reinforcing the demonstration. Verbal descriptions should be kept simple. Observing other patients who are using assistive devices correctly can also be a useful method of instruction.

Once a patient is proficient in the use of an assistive device and gait pattern on level surfaces, instruction in the use of stairs, curbs, ramps, elevators, doors, and falling safely, is provided. The patient should be taught to ascend and descend stairs on the side appropriate for the country in which they live. In the United States this is the patient's right side facing the stairs.

INSTRUCT BY

Demonstration
Verbal description
Observing other patients

LO-7

Instruction in sitting down and standing up when using chairs with and without arms, low or soft sofas and chairs, toilets, and car seats is also necessary. Patients must be taught to sit in a controlled manner, rather than collapsing into a sitting position.

Uneven surfaces may present specific problems to patients. Gravel, grass, broken sidewalks and paving, and curb cuts may require additional instruction and practice. Patients should be cautioned to avoid small throw rugs that may slip or become entangled with their feet or assistive devices. Wet or highly polished floors should also be avoided whenever possible. When ambulating on icy, wet, or highly polished surfaces, smaller movements of assistive devices and smaller steps should be used. Forces placed on assistive devices should be directed downward as much as possible to prevent assistive devices from slipping on wet or unstable surfaces.

Patients must be instructed to check that assistive devices are in safe working condition. Rubber tips on assistive devices will not grip the floor properly if they become worn excessively or dirt fills the grooves. Wing nuts on crutches often loosen with use.

A therapist will not always be available to instruct a patient in how to perform a task outside of a rehabilitation setting. Therefore patients are assisted in solving problems on their own when using assistive devices.

9.2   CHOOSING AN ASSISTIVE DEVICE

Introduction

CLINICAL NOTE

Stability and support

A variety of assistive devices for ambulation are available. Some devices provide more stability and support than others. Some devices require more coordination to use. As a patient's abilities increase, the patient may change from a device that provides relatively greater stability and support to one that provides relatively less stability and support. Other patients continue to use the same device throughout the entire time an assistive device is required. Patients with progressive disorders change from devices that provide relatively less stability and support to devices that provide relatively greater stability and support.

The following list of assistive devices is ordered from those providing the most stability and support to those providing the least stability and support.

LO-8

1. Parallel bars
2. Walker
3. Axillary crutches
4. Forearm (Lofstrand) crutches
5. Two canes
6. One cane

The following list of assistive devices is ordered from those requiring the least patient coordination to those requiring the most patient coordination.

LO-9

1. Parallel bars
2. Walker
3. One cane
4. Two canes
5. Axillary crutches
6. Forearm (Lofstrand) crutches

Some patients may use one crutch as an intermediate step between two crutches and one cane, or instead of one cane.

When selecting an assistive device, the therapist must choose one that will provide the necessary support, and that the patient can manipulate. The choice of an assistive device is based on an assessment of a patient's strength, range of motion, balance, stability, coordination, and general condition. For example, a patient with a fractured lower extremity who must be non-weight bearing may use either crutches or a walker, based on the results of an evaluation. Crutches may be used when the necessary strength, stability, and coordination are present. Another patient with the same fracture may require the use of a walker because of poor stability, coordination, or a medically debilitating condition.

LO-10

A platform for the forearm can be attached to walkers or crutches for patients who are unable to bear weight through their hand, wrist, or forearm, or who have poor grasp.

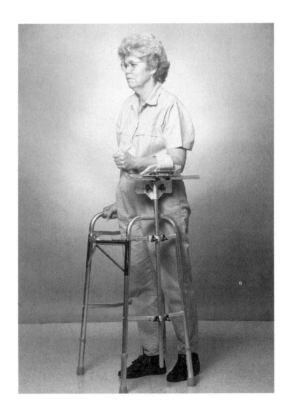

Figure 9.2–1. Platform attached to walker.

Assistive devices come in several sizes—tall, standard, junior, and child. Most assistive devices are adjustable within a given range, and there is usually some overlap of adjustment between sizes. Some assistive devices have ranges of height marked on them by the manufacturer. These markings are estimates only. Accurate measurement must be performed and confirmed by the therapist for each individual patient.

Walkers

LO-12

Walkers provide a relatively greater degree of stability, and are generally easy to use. Walkers are chosen for patients with generalized weakness, debilitating conditions, a need to reduce weight bearing on one or both lower extremities, relatively poor balance and coordination, or an injury to one lower extremity coupled with the inability to use crutches. This may mean that walkers are used more often with elderly patients.

When ambulating with a walker, lifting of the body to decrease weight bearing is achieved by shoulder depression and elbow extension.

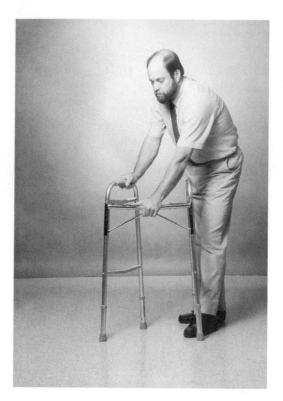

Figure 9.2–2. Folding a collapsible walker.

Walkers may, however, be cumbersome. A collapsible walker should be used with patients who will ambulate in the community. A collapsible walker is easier to transport in a car, and place out of the way in public places, such as movies and restaurants, than is a noncollapsible walker.

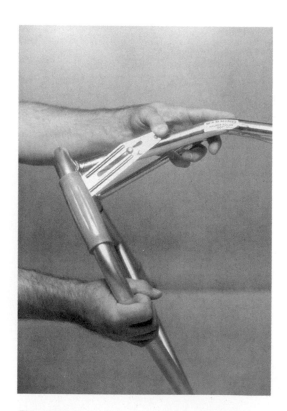

Figure 9.2–3. Locking mechanism on collapsible walker.

LO-11

Walkers are usually made of aluminum, and are adjustable in height. To adjust the height of a walker, the walker is inverted.

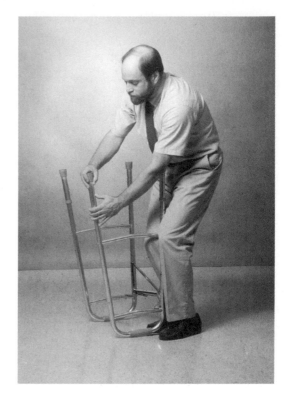

Figure 9.2–4. Adjusting height of walker.

Each leg has a push button lock with a telescoping leg. All legs are adjusted to the same height.

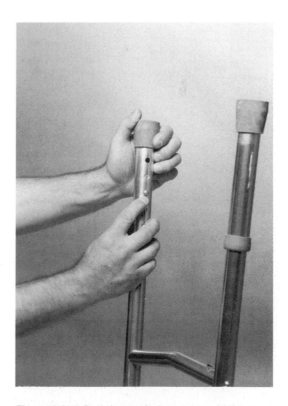

Figure 9.2–5. Push button lock on telescoping leg.

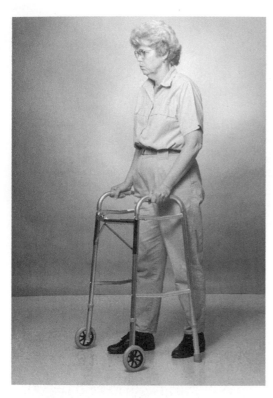

Figure 9.2–6. Wheeled walker.

LO-12   Wheeled walkers are available with either two or four wheels. Walkers with four wheels should have a brake that is activated during weight bearing on the walker to ensure stability.

A stair climbing walker is available for patients who must use stairs frequently. This walker has an additional pair of handgrips on the rear legs that are used when the patient is on the stairs. These handgrips make the walker larger, increasing the difficulty of maneuvering in small areas.

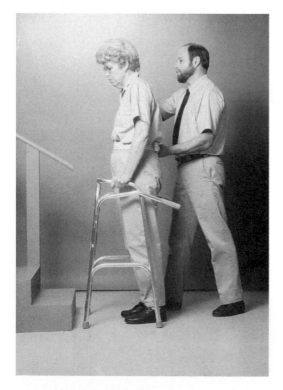

Figure 9.2–7. Stair climbing walker.

Other special walkers are available. A walker with a trunk support is used for patients who have adequate reciprocal lower extremity movements but lack adequate trunk support. These walkers are called ring walkers. Ring walkers are larger than standard walkers and are not collapsible. An adduction board may be added to a ring walker. The adduction board is suspended from the frame of the walker to prevent the patient's lower extremities from adducting during the swing phase of gait. Although cumbersome, for some patients an adduction board may be the difference between walking and not walking.

A reciprocal walker is designed with joints that permit one side of the walker to be advanced at a time. A reciprocal walker is used when a patient lacks the strength or balance to lift a walker completely to advance the walker.

A reverse walker, with or without wheels, is used frequently with children. The patient stands in the walker with her back to the cross bar. The reverse walker is designed to encourage erect posture.

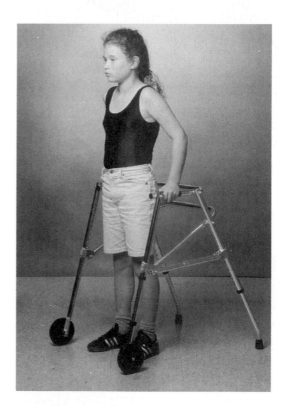

Figure 9.2–8. Reverse walker.

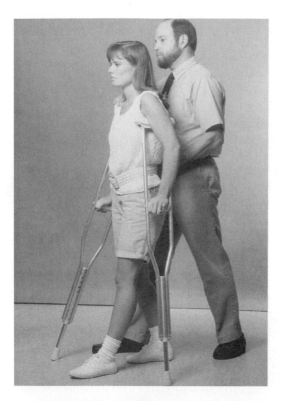

Figure 9.2–9. Axillary crutches.

Axillary Crutches

LO-12   Axillary crutches provide a moderate degree of stability, and are slightly harder to use than walkers. Axillary crutches are generally chosen for patients with weakness of one or both lower extremities, a need to reduce weight bearing on one or both lower extremities, or who need some support of the trunk.

When ambulating with crutches, lifting of the body to decrease weight bearing is achieved by shoulder depression and elbow extension. Patients must also adduct their upper extremities to keep the crutches in place under the axillae.

Axillary crutches were traditionally made of wood, but now may be made of wood or aluminum. Wing nuts and bolts are used to adjust the crutch length and handgrip height of axillary crutches. Push button locks and telescoping legs may be used on some aluminum crutches.

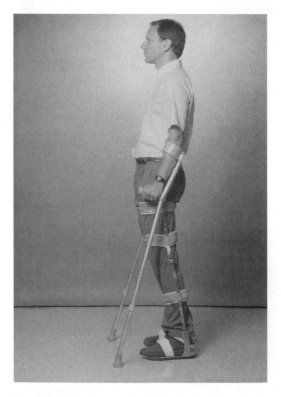

Figure 9.2–10. Forearm (Lofstrand) crutches.

Forearm (Lofstrand) Crutches

LO-12   Forearm (Lofstrand) crutches are slightly harder to use than axillary crutches, but provide more ease of movement. When ambulating with forearm crutches, lifting of the body to decrease weight bearing is achieved by shoulder depression and elbow extension. The cuff on forearm crutches permits a patient to use his hand for manipulating the environment without dropping the crutch. Forearm crutches are recommended for patients with the same problems as with axillary crutches, with the exception of decreased trunk stability. Patients who will need crutches permanently, or for long periods of time, may find forearm crutches more desirable because they are lighter and more maneuverable than axillary crutches.

Canes

LO-12

Canes provide limited stability and weight bearing capability. They are made of either aluminum or wood. Aluminum canes are adjustable using push button locks and telescoping legs. Wooden canes are adjusted by cutting them to length, which limits their adjustability. Canes are generally chosen for patients with slight weakness of muscles of the lower extremities, pain in the lower extremities, or for patients who need assistance with balance while ambulating.

When using one cane to limit weight bearing on one lower extremity, the cane is initially used in the hand on the side opposite the involved lower extremity. This placement provides a second point of support on the uninvolved side. Increasing the base of support toward the uninvolved side permits a patient to shift weight to the uninvolved side during stance on the involved lower extremity. When weight bearing on the involved lower extremity is permitted, the cane is used on the involved side to increase the base of support toward the involved side. This encourages weight shifting onto the involved lower extremity during stance on the involved lower extremity. Depending upon the severity of a patient's problem, either one or two canes may be required. Two canes are used primarily for bilateral involvement, or for assistance with balance.

Several styles of canes are available. The standard cane has a handgrip, shaft, and a single tip. The most common shape of a standard cane is a J-line cane, named by its shape.

A variation of the cane is the quad cane, named because it has four feet. The quad cane is available with two base sizes, large and small. The design of a quad cane makes it stable. The patient can let go of the cane without concern that it will fall or slide to the floor as standard canes do. A disadvantage of the large base quad cane is that because of the size of the base, it will not fit on a standard stair unless turned sideways.

Another variation for canes is an offset shaft. An offset shaft is available for both the standard and quad cane. The purpose of the offset shaft is to have weight bearing occur directly over the tip of a cane or center of the base of a quad cane. The handgrip is available in varied shapes and textures to make grasp easier.

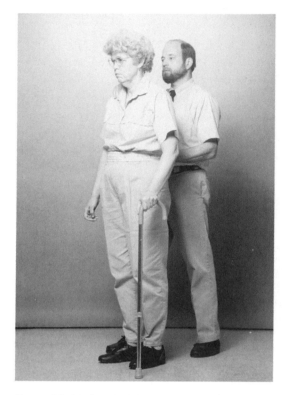

Figure 9.2–11. Standard J-line cane.

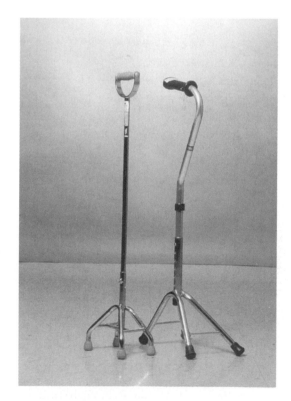

Figure 9.2–12. Small base (left) and large base (right) quad canes. Large base quad cane with offset handle.

LO-13

9.3   CHOOSING A GAIT PATTERN

Gait patterns define the sequence of moving the assistive device(s) and lower extremities. Five gait patterns are commonly used. The gait patterns described in this section are described for forward progression. These patterns, however, are also used for turning and backward progression. A change in the direction of placement of the assistive devices and lower extremities is necessary when turning or performing backward progression.

Weight Bearing

Weight bearing is the amount of weight that can be borne on a lower extremity during standing or ambulation. The amount of weight bearing permitted is dependent on the patient's condition and the medical management of the condition.

The amount of weight bearing on a lower extremity can vary from full weight bearing to non-weight bearing. The amount of weight bearing is controlled by the extent to which assistive devices are used for weight bearing. Commonly used phrases that describe degrees of weight bearing are defined as follows.

Non-weight bearing: The involved lower extremity is not to be weight bearing, and is usually not permitted to touch the ground.

Toe touch: The patient can rest the toes of the involved lower extremity on the ground for balance, but not for weight bearing.

Partial weight bearing: A limited amount of weight bearing, such as 5 pounds, is permitted for the involved lower extremity. When a specific weight is not provided, minimal weight bearing should be permitted on the involved lower extremity until a specific weight is confirmed by the treating physician.

Weight bearing as tolerated: The patient determines the amount of weight bearing that will occur on the involved lower extremity. The amount of weight bearing may vary from minimal to full, depending upon the tolerance of the patient.

Full weight bearing: The patient is permitted full weight bearing on the involved lower extremity. Assistive devices should not be used to decrease weight bearing on the involved lower extremity, but may be used for balance.

Two-Point Gait

A two-point gait pattern is used when two assistive devices, such as two canes or two crutches, are required. This gait pattern is used with patients who have muscle weakness, pain, or problems with balance.

One assistive device and the opposite lower extremity are lifted and moved forward simultaneously. When the assistive device and lower extremity have been placed on the ground, the patient's weight is shifted to these supports. The other assistive device and its opposite lower extremity are then moved forward. This two-part sequence is repeated. Each combination of one assistive device and the opposite lower extremity is considered "one point." A complete cycle includes "two points," providing the name two-point gait pattern.

Four-Point Gait

A four-point gait pattern is often described as a deliberate two-point gait pattern. This gait pattern is used when two assistive devices, such as two canes or two crutches, are required. A four-point gait pattern is used with the same type of patients who use a two-point gait pattern, but for which the problems are more severe. A four-point gait pattern may also be used as a starting point to teach a patient coordination on crutches or canes before they graduate to using a two-point gait pattern.

One assistive device is moved forward and placed on the floor, followed by the opposite lower extremity. The other assistive device is moved forward and placed on the floor, followed by its opposite lower extremity. Each time an assistive device or lower extremity is lifted to be moved forward, weight bearing is shifted to the three supports remaining in contact with the floor. This four-part sequence is repeated. Each movement of an assistive device or lower extremity is considered a "point." A complete cycle includes "four points," providing the name four-point gait pattern.

Three-Point Gait

A three-point gait pattern is used by patients who have one involved lower extremity. This lower extremity may be weak, painful, injured, or require decreased weight bearing. The levels of weight bearing described above may be used by patients ambulating with a three-point gait pattern. This gait pattern requires two crutches or canes, or a walker. The example that follows assumes the use of two crutches. The use of two canes follows the same pattern. The use of a walker requires that both sides of the walker be advanced as a unit, mimicking the simultaneous advancement of two crutches or canes.

As patients initially learn this gait pattern, both crutches are moved forward and placed on the floor. The involved lower extremity is then moved forward between the two crutches. After the involved lower extremity is moved, weight bearing is shifted to the upper extremities and involved lower extremity as permitted. The uninvolved lower extremity is then moved forward. Weight bearing is then shifted to the uninvolved lower extremity in preparation for the next forward movement of the crutches and involved lower extremity. This three-part sequence is repeated. The assistive devices are considered "one point," and each lower extremity is considered a "point." Thus, a complete cycle includes "three points," providing the name three-point gait pattern.

As patients become more confident, the crutches and involved lower extremity are moved forward simultaneously. The shifting of weight bearing and movement of the uninvolved lower extremity follow as before.

Initially, patients may advance the uninvolved lower extremity forward only to the involved lower extremity and crutches. Patients should be encouraged to step beyond the placement of the involved lower extremity and crutches for a faster and more normal gait pattern.

Swing-To Gait

A swing-to gait pattern requires the use of two crutches or a walker. This gait pattern is used for patients who have lower extremity muscle weakness, paresis, paralysis, or require decreased weight bearing on one lower extremity. The levels of weight bearing described above may be used by patients ambulating with a swing-to gait pattern. The example that follows assumes the use of two crutches.

The patient moves both crutches forward simultaneously, and places the tips on the floor. Weight bearing is shifted onto the assistive devices. Both lower extremities are moved forward simultaneously to the same point as the assistive devices were advanced, and are placed on the floor. Weight bearing is shifted to the lower extremities for support so the assistive devices can be advanced again. This two-part sequence is repeated. Each cycle requires that the lower extremities be "swung to" the same point as the assistive devices were advanced, providing the name swing-to gait pattern.

Swing-Through Gait

A swing-through gait pattern requires the use of two crutches or a walker. This gait pattern is used for patients who have lower extremity muscle weakness, paresis, paralysis, or require decreased weight bearing on one lower extremity, but who have greater confidence and ability using assistive devices. The levels of weight bearing described previously may be used by patients ambulating with a swing-through gait pattern. The example that follows assumes the use of two crutches.

The patient moves both crutches forward simultaneously, and places the tips on the floor. Weight bearing is shifted onto the assistive devices. Both lower extremities swing forward simultaneously beyond the point to which the assistive devices were advanced, and are placed on the floor. Weight bearing is shifted to the lower extremity(ies) for support so the assistive devices can be advanced again. This two-part sequence is repeated. Each cycle requires that the lower extremities be "swung through" the point to which the assistive devices were advanced, providing the name swing-through gait pattern.

9.4   GUARDING

LO-14

Guarding is the process of protecting a patient from falling. Proper guarding requires use of a gait belt. Guarding by holding onto a patient's belt may be uncomfortable for the patient because the narrow belt or belt buckle can bind or pinch the patient. Clothing may tear, and does not fit snugly enough to provide control during guarding. A gait belt should fit snugly around the patient's waist. Handles for the therapist to grasp may or may not be present on gait belts.

When a patient arises from, or sits down in, a chair, the therapist stands in stride, to one side and slightly behind the patient. In some situations the therapist may stand in front of the patient, as for an assisted standing pivot transfer. Standing in front of the patient permits the therapist to provide more physical assistance, and to have the patient move into the therapist's base of support.

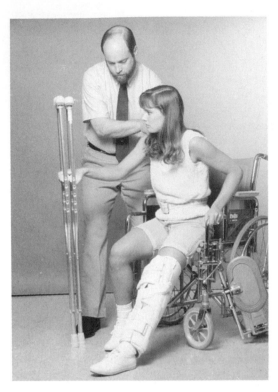

Figure 9.4–1. Therapist's position to guard assumption of standing.

When a patient ambulates, the therapist stands in stride, behind and slightly to one side of the patient. The therapist grasps the gait belt with a supinated forearm because this provides a stronger grasp. The therapist's other hand is placed over the patient's shoulder, not on the upper extremity where it may interfere with free motion needed to control an assistive device.

In all situations, the therapist must be positioned in a way that permits the therapist to move as the patient moves. This is extremely important because the therapist's position must not interfere with the patient's movement. This also requires that the therapist be alert to the patient's position and movements, and to obstacles in the environment.

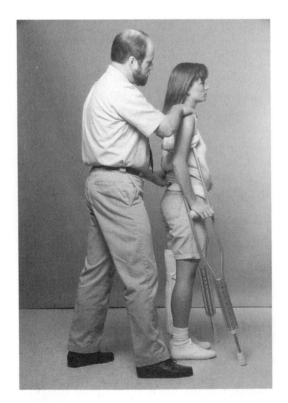

Figure 9.4–2. Therapist's position to guard during ambulation.

During initial gait training, the therapist stands close to the patient to provide increased support and control. As the patient walks, the therapist moves with the patient. The therapist's "outside" foot moves when the assistive device on that side is moved. The therapist's "outside" foot is the foot that is most lateral to the patient. The therapist's "inside" foot is moved when the patient's foot on the side the therapist is guarding is moved. The therapist's "inside" foot is the foot that is behind the patient. The "outside" and "inside" foot may be either the therapist's left or right foot, depending on the side of the patient on which the therapist stands. This allows the therapist to move smoothly without kicking or tripping the patient, and without interfering with the assistive device.

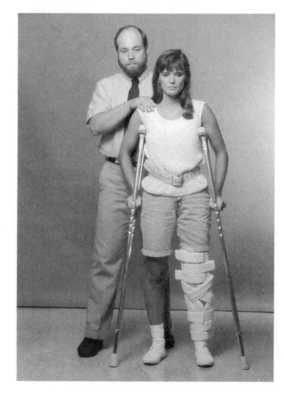

Figure 9.4–3. Therapist's position for close guarding.

As the patient's capabilities improve, the therapist can remove the hand from the shoulder, and stand farther away. Eventually the therapist walks near the patient without holding the gait belt.

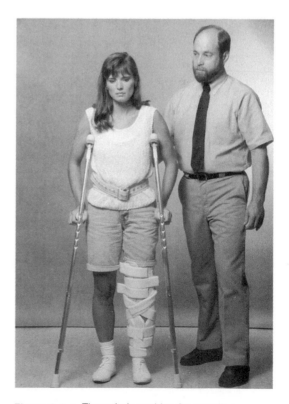

Figure 9.4–4. Therapist's position for guarding as patient improves.

When a patient starts to fall, the therapist must decide whether to prevent the fall, or to permit a controlled fall in a manner that will prevent injury to the patient or himself. The therapist must be alert to a patient's movements at all times, and be able to react quickly to prevent or control a fall. Proper guarding and attention focused on the patient are required at all times.

Pulling a patient toward the therapist is the safer and stronger method of preventing a fall. A therapist is able to exert more control on a patient's weight when the patient is pulled into the therapist's base of support, rather than being pushed away from the therapist. When a patient starts to fall, the therapist is able to provide support, and protect the involved lower extremity by shifting weight onto the uninvolved lower extremity. This combination of measures is best achieved by guarding a patient on the uninvolved side.

Initially, the therapist may stand on the patient's uninvolved side. During early stages of gait training, patients usually lean away from the involved lower extremity because they fear pain or further injury if they put too much weight on the involved lower extremity. Guarding on the patient's uninvolved side permits shifting the patient's weight onto the uninvolved lower extremity, and into the therapist, should the patient start to fall.

Later, the therapist may guard on the patient's involved side to encourage a more upright posture during gait, and weight bearing on the involved lower extremity when appropriate.

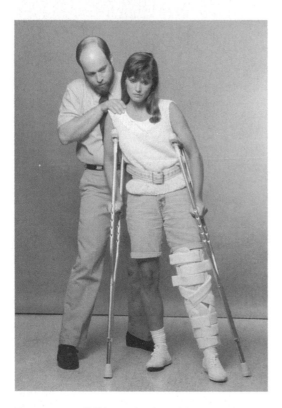

Figure 9.4–5. Shifting patient's weight onto uninvolved lower extremity, and into therapist.

When guarding a patient on stairs, the therapist positions himself below the patient, whether the patient is moving up or down the stairs. One of the therapist's hands grasps the gait belt, and the other hand holds the handrail. Holding the handrail provides the therapist with a point of stability. The therapist stands in stride. As the patient and therapist move on the stairs, the therapist places his feet on different stair treads and avoids placing his feet on the same stair tread simultaneously. The stride position enables the therapist to shift his weight as the patient moves, and permits the therapist to shift the patient's weight into his base of support should the patient begin to fall.

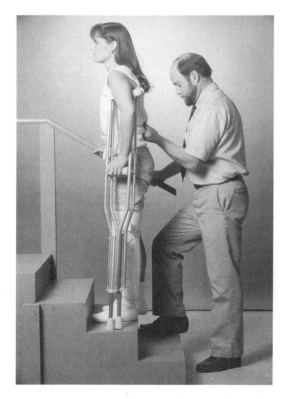

Figure 9.4–6. Therapist's position to guard on stairs.

Occasionally a second therapist is needed to guard a patient on stairs. The second therapist stands in stride on the stairs above the patient, and also holds the gait belt and handrail.

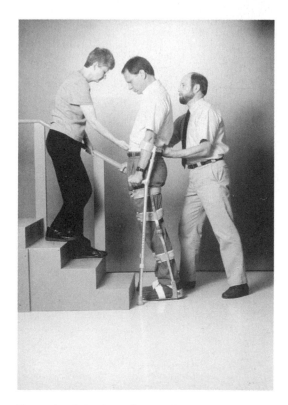

Figure 9.4–7. Positions for two therapists to guard on stairs.

9.5 ASSUMPTION OF STANDING AND SITTING

LO-15

When assuming standing from a wheelchair, or sitting in a wheelchair from standing, the wheelchair wheels are always locked, and positioned against a wall if possible. The footplates are raised and the footrests are removed when possible, or swung out of the way. When footrests are removed, they must be put in a place that will not interfere with the patient or therapist.

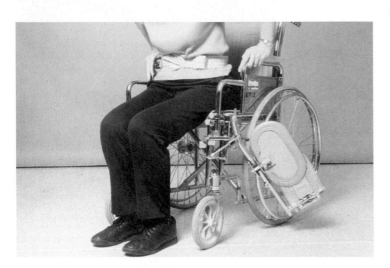

Figure 9.5–1. Patient's feet side by side.

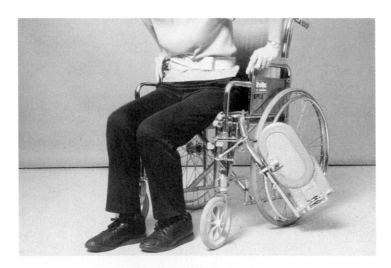

Figure 9.5–2. Patient's feet in stride.

To assume a standing position, the patient must be sitting at the front edge of the seat. This can be achieved using procedures presented in Chapter 8. Once the patient has moved to the front edge of the seat, the feet are placed flat on the floor below the front edge of the seat. In this position the patient's center of gravity can be brought over the base of support quickly as standing is assumed. The feet may be placed side by side, or they may be placed in a short stride position. Using a stride position increases the patient's base of support. When moving to standing with the feet in stride, the foot of the uninvolved lower extremity is placed slightly farther forward than the foot of the involved lower extremity. Having the patient place her hands on the armrests will also increase the base of support, and will provide initial assistance to push to a standing position.

Assistive devices to be used for ambulation must be accessible to the patient when sitting in the chair, and after the assumption of standing. Initially, assistive devices may not be used for the assumption of standing. Both hands are then used on the armrests of the chair to assist with pushing to standing. In such cases, the assistive devices must be accessible to the therapist, who hands them to the patient once standing has been achieved. When using assistive devices to assume standing, one of the patient's hands may be placed on the assistive devices, and the other hand may be placed on the armrest. Whichever hand position is used, the movement to assume standing should be a controlled continuous motion.

To assume a sitting position, patients must approach the front edge of the chair, and turn to face away from the chair. When performing this maneuver, patients may initially feel more confident turning toward their uninvolved side. This occurs because they are turning into their strength. They must, however, be able to turn in both directions, toward both their involved and uninvolved sides. As patients approach the wheelchair, they must check to ensure that the wheelchair is locked and the footrests are out of the way.

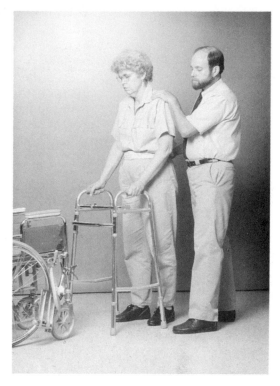

Figure 9.5–3. Approaching wheelchair to assume sitting.

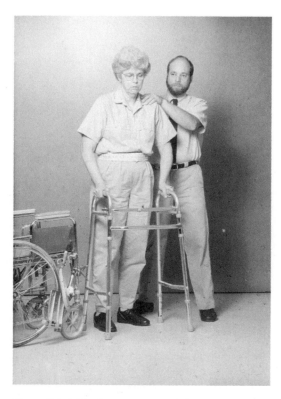

Figure 9.5–4. Turning to assume sitting.

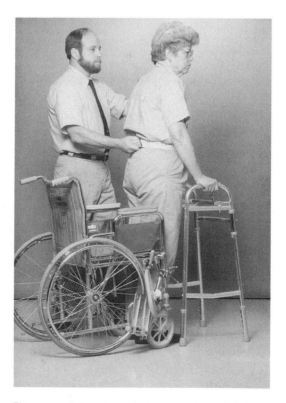

Figure 9.5–5. Positioned facing away from chair to assume sitting.

With the patient standing at the front edge of the seat, and facing away from the chair, the patient's center of gravity can be maintained over the base of support as sitting is assumed. The feet may be placed side by side, or they may be placed in a short stride position. Using a stride position increases the patient's base of support. When moving to sitting with the feet in stride, the foot of the uninvolved lower extremity is slightly farther back than the foot of the involved lower extremity. Having the patient reach for, and use, the armrests as she lowers herself to sitting will also increase the patient's base of support, and will provide assistance to control the latter stages of lowering.

Initially, assistive devices may not be used for the assumption of sitting. In such cases, the assistive devices are handed to the therapist before the patient begins to sit. Both hands are then used on the armrests of the chair to assist with controlled lowering. When using assistive devices during assumption of sitting, one of the patient's hands, usually the hand on the side of the involved lower extremity, is placed on the assistive devices. The other hand is placed on the armrest. The patient should lower herself in a controlled manner onto the front edge of the seat.

During the assumption of standing and sitting, the relative placement of the feet of the involved and uninvolved lower extremities permits patients to move into their strength during the movement. As a patient assumes standing, she shifts her weight forward within her base of support, and onto her uninvolved lower extremity. As a patient assumes sitting, she shifts her weight backward within her base of support, and onto her uninvolved lower extremity.

When assuming a standing position, the patient must lean forward to shift her center of gravity over her feet, extend her knees and hips, and initially push directly downward with her upper extremities. Pushing at an angle creates a horizontal component of the pushing force vector that does not assist the patient to rise. The horizontal component of the pushing force may also propel the patient horizontally, and thus off balance.

9.6   ASCENDING AND DESCENDING STAIRS

LO-15

When ascending or descending stairs, the patient places the tips of the assistive device one half to two thirds of the way forward, with respect to the direction in which the patient is facing, on the stair tread. When two assistive devices are used, the assistive devices are placed far enough apart to allow room for the patient to move between the assistive devices. When ascending stairs, the uninvolved lower extremity is moved to the next higher stair first because it must lift the body. The involved lower extremity and assistive devices follow as the body is lifted. When descending stairs, the assistive devices are moved to the next lower stair first, to provide support for the involved lower extremity. The uninvolved lower extremity is used to lower the body until the assistive devices are on the next lower stair. The involved lower extremity may be moved with the assistive devices or may follow. Weight is shifted to the assistive devices and involved lower extremity when appropriate. The uninvolved lower extremity is then moved down to the same stair.

Some patients may progress to a step-over-step pattern on the stairs.

9.7 CURBS

The sequence for ascending and descending curbs is the same as the sequence for ascending and descending stairs. When ascending or descending curbs, only the assistive devices are available for support because of the absence of handrails.

LO-15

9.8 MOVING THROUGH DOORWAYS

There are many combinations of extremity involvement and doorway conditions that may arise. A patient may have one or two functional upper extremities, and the involvement of the patient's lower extremities may vary. The door may open toward or away from the patient, the door may be hinged on the left or right, the room around the door available for maneuvering may be ample or quite limited, and doors may or may not have automatic door openers or closers. Each combination of factors will require modifications to the general method of ambulating through doorways. The most important fact to remember is that the patient's safety must not be endangered. Key guidelines are that the patient's balance must not be compromised, and the door should not be permitted to strike the patient.

LO-15

The therapist's position for guarding during these maneuvers is the same position as for guarding during ambulation with walkers, crutches, and canes. Realizing that shorter steps and abrupt turns may be required, the therapist must be prepared to move with the patient, avoiding interference with the patient's freedom of movement, or the arc of movement of the door. During initial gait training through doorways, the therapist may need to control opening and closing of the door to protect the patient.

Less force and rapidity of movement is necessary when moving through a doorway without an automatic door closer. When a door does not have an automatic closer, the door does not have to be opened greater than the width of the patient to prevent the door from closing forcefully on the patient. The rapid movement of assistive devices to block the door is not necessary.

In the sections on ambulation through doorways presented later in this chapter, text and photographs depict independent ambulation. This method was used so a therapist does not obscure the desired photographic views of the patient.

9.9   TILT TABLE

LO-16

Some patients must be reacclimated to upright posture in a safe manner before sitting, standing, or ambulation can be initiated. This is usually necessitated by the existence of orthostatic hypotension in patients who have been in bed for extended periods. Readjustment of the cardiovascular system may be necessary to avoid dizziness or fainting as these patients assume an upright posture. A tilt table is a safe method to provide maximum support for such patients. Support is provided while a patient is raised slowly to an upright position by the tilt table, leaving the therapist free to control the tilt table and monitor the patient.

Vital signs are measured, as presented in Chapter 3, before and during the process of raising the patient to an upright posture. The patient should be lowered when he reports feeling faint. A patient who is lowered after feeling faint must be monitored until his vital signs return to normal, and the patient no longer reports feeling faint. Medical assistance should be obtained when necessary.

Figure 9.9–1. Monitoring vital signs on tilt table.

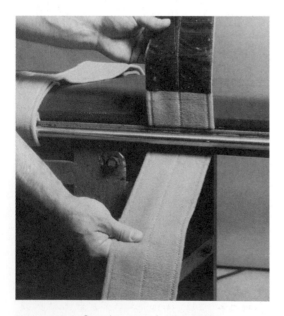

Straps are used to secure a patient to a tilt table. A variety of styles of straps are available. A bar extends along each side of the tilt table surface and the straps used to secure a patient on the tilt table are attached to the bar on one side of the table.

Figure 9.9–2. Securing strap on tilt table bar.

The straps are passed over the patient and secured to the bar on the other side. The location of the straps across the patient depends on the patient's condition. If upper trunk stability is required, a chest strap, with the upper extremities free, is used. A strap over the pelvis stabilizes the lower trunk. A strap at knee level is used if the patient cannot maintain knee extension.

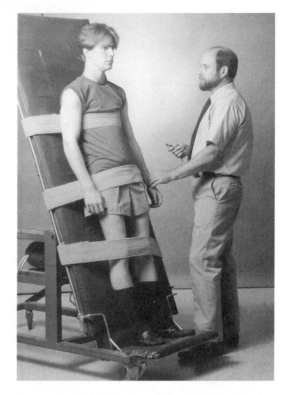

Figure 9.9–3. Patient secured on upright tilt table.

The angle of table tilt is adjusted to a position the patient can tolerate safely. Changes in the position of the table should be performed slowly and steadily. Greater degrees of tilt may be assumed as the patient's cardiovascular system adjusts to the demands of upright posture. For many patients the full upright position provides a sensation of falling forward; therefore, this position is usually avoided.

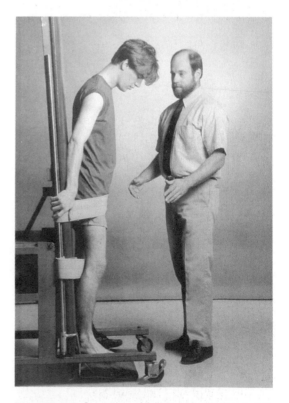

Figure 9.9–4. Sensation of falling with tilt table in full upright position.

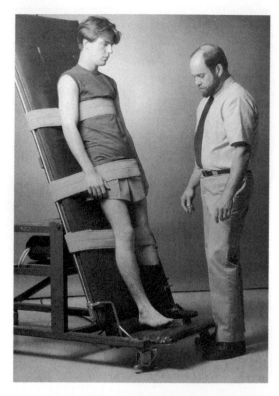

Figure 9.9–5. Involved lower extremity non-weight-bearing and free from strap for exercise.

When weight bearing is not permitted on one lower extremity, a lift can be placed under the uninvolved lower extremity. This prevents the involved lower extremity from reaching the supporting surface. Thus, the involved lower extremity is not weight bearing.

When an exercise program for one of the lower extremities is to be implemented, the strap across the knees can be loosened, or placed only around the opposite lower extremity. This permits the therapist to implement the patient's lower extremity exercise program.

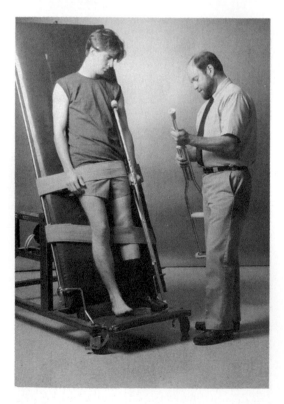

Figure 9.9–6. Adjusting assistive devices with patient on tilt table.

Gait training can begin on the tilt table with the fitting of assistive devices. Patients who cannot sit may find it easier to be brought to an upright posture on a tilt table, and then to walk off the tilt table.

9.10   WALKERS

Fitting

 To measure a walker for the proper height, the patient stands upright, with shoulders relaxed, within the walker with the crossbar in front. The

LO-11 top of the handgrip should be approximately at the level of the patient's ulnar styloid process when her upper extremity is relaxed at her side. When the patient grasps the handgrip, the shoulders should be level and relaxed, and the elbows flexed to 20 to 30 degrees.

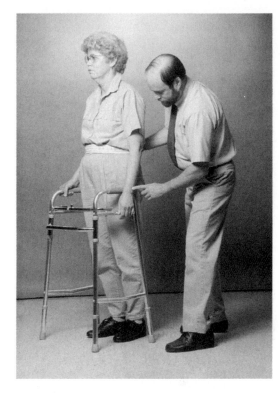

Figure 9.10–1. Fitting height of walker.

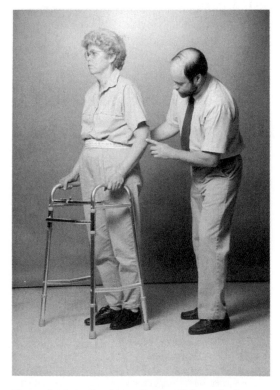

Figure 9.10–2. Checking amount of elbow flexion.

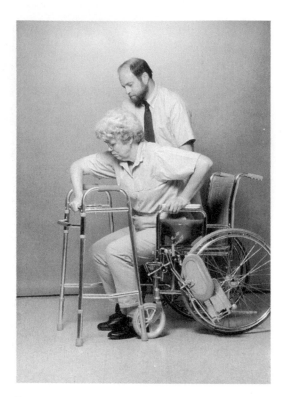

Figure 9.10–3. Starting position to assume standing using crossbar of walker.

In and Out of a Wheelchair

LO-15 Two methods of getting in and out of a wheelchair will be described. In both methods, the wheelchair is prepared and the patient positioned in the manner described earlier in this chapter under "Assumption of Standing and Sitting." Reversing wheelchair desk armrests so the higher portion is at the front of the wheelchair will assist patients in pushing to standing and lowering to sitting. The therapist is positioned in the manner described earlier in this chapter under "Guarding."

Assuming Standing Using a Walker

The wheelchair is locked and the footrests moved out of the way. The patient is positioned at the front edge of the seat, with her feet in stride or side by side. Positioned in stride, and behind and to one side of the patient, the therapist grasps the patient's gait belt and shoulder.

The patient's hand on the uninvolved side grasps and pushes down on the crossbar of the walker, and the hand on the involved side is placed on the armrest of the wheelchair. This ensures that the patient is moving into her strength.

The patient pushes to standing.

Figure 9.10–4. Patient pushes to standing.

The patient's hand on the involved side is moved from the armrest of the wheelchair and placed on the proper handgrip of the walker.

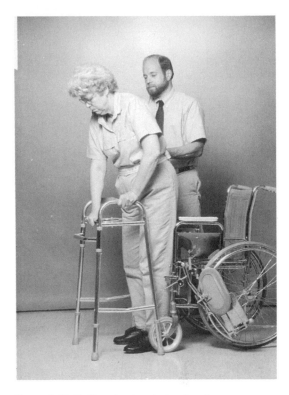

Figure 9.10–5. Grasping handgrip of walker.

The patient's hand on the uninvolved side is moved from the crossbar to the proper handgrip.

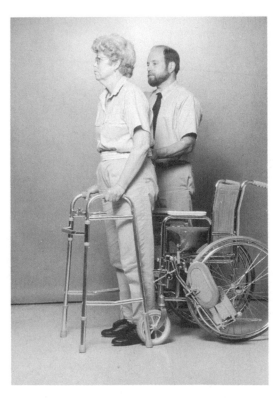

Figure 9.10–6. Grasping both handgrips of walker.

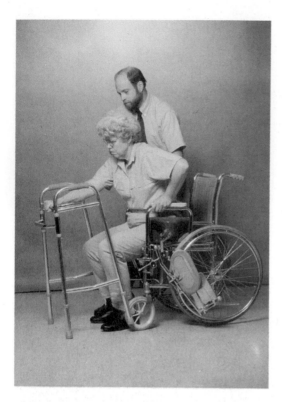

The force exerted on the crossbar of the walker must be exerted directly downward to avoid tipping the walker.

Figure 9.10–7. Incorrect direction of force causing walker to tip forward.

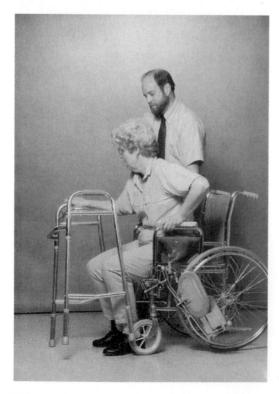

The patient's hand on the uninvolved side may be placed on a handgrip instead of the crossbar. There are two disadvantages of this method. First, the handgrip is at the very outside of the walker's base of support and a slight deviation from pushing directly downward will cause the walker to tip. Second, the handgrip is located higher on the walker than the crossbar. This location of the handgrip may make pushing directly downward more difficult for a patient.

Figure 9.10–8. Incorrect direction of force causing walker to tip sideways.

Assuming Sitting Using a Walker

LO-15   The wheelchair is locked and the footrests moved out of the way. To sit, the patient positions herself at the front edge of the wheelchair seat, facing away from the wheelchair. The front edge of the wheelchair seat is felt against the back of the lower extremities. The patient's feet are positioned in stride or side by side. Positioned in stride, and behind and to one side of the patient, the therapist grasps the patient's gait belt and shoulder.

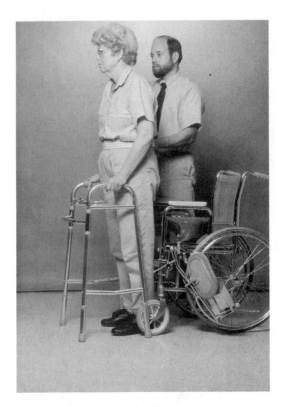

Figure 9.10–9. Starting position to assume sitting.

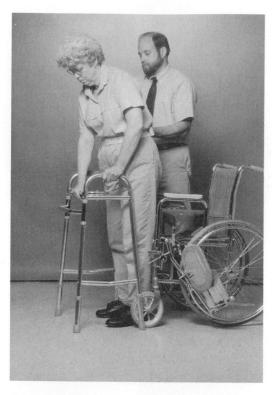

Figure 9.10–10. Grasping crossbar of walker.

The patient grasps the middle of the crossbar with the hand on the involved side,

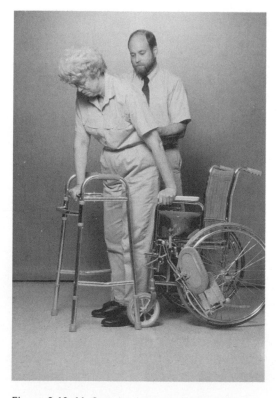

Figure 9.10–11. Grasping armrest of wheelchair.

and then reaches backward and grasps the armrest with the hand on the uninvolved side.

The patient lowers herself in a controlled manner to sitting onto the front edge of the seat.

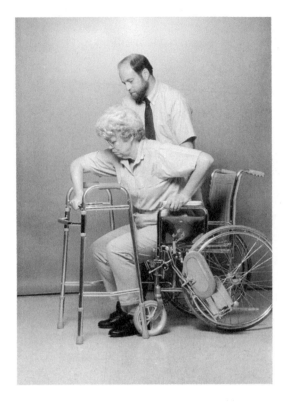

Figure 9.10–12. Lowering to sitting.

The hand on the involved side is moved to the armrest. The patient moves back into the seat, and adjusts her sitting position.

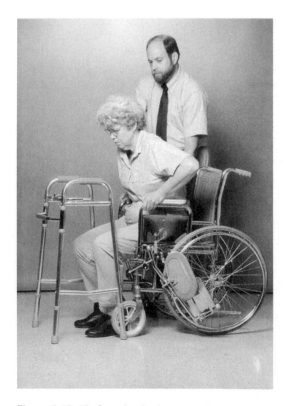

Figure 9.10–13. Grasping both armrests.

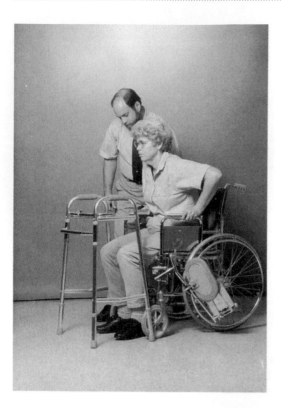

Figure 9.10–14. Starting position to assume standing using both armrests.

Assuming Standing Using Both Armrests

LO-15

The wheelchair is locked and the footrests moved out of the way. The patient is positioned at the front edge of the seat, with her feet in stride or side by side. Positioned in stride, and behind and to one side of the patient, the therapist grasps the patient's gait belt and shoulder.

Sitting on the front edge of the seat, the patient places both hands on the armrests.

Using the armrests, the patient pushes to standing.

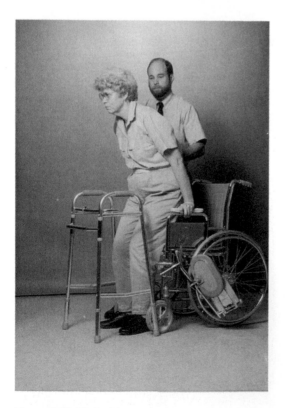

Figure 9.10–15. Pushing on both armrests to standing.

The patient's weight must be completely shifted over her feet.

She then moves one hand at a time from an armrest to the proper handgrip of the walker.

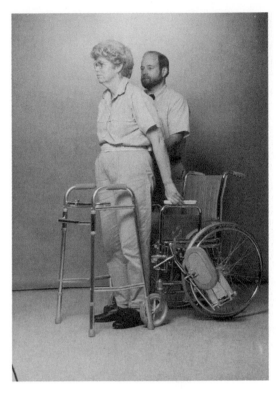

Figure 9.10–16. Shifting weight over feet.

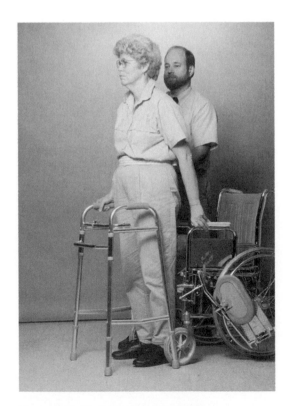

Figure 9.10–17. Grasping one handgrip.

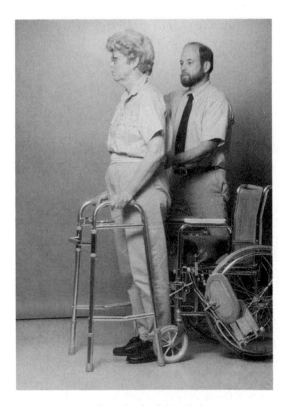

Figure 9.10–18. Grasping both handgrips.

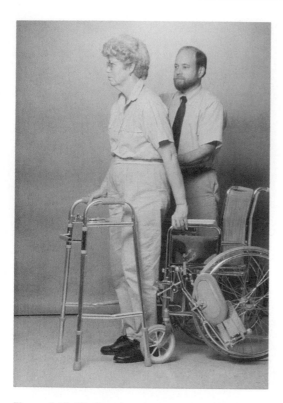

Figure 9.10–19. Grasping one armrest.

Assuming Sitting Using Both Armrests

LO-15 The wheelchair is locked and the footrests moved out of the way. To sit, the patient positions herself at the front edge of the wheelchair seat, facing away from the wheelchair. The front edge of the wheelchair seat is felt against the back of the lower extremities. The patient's feet are positioned in stride or side by side. Positioned in stride, and behind and to one side of the patient, the therapist grasps the patient's gait belt and shoulder.

The patient retains her grasp on one handgrip of the walker while reaching back with the other hand to grasp the armrest.

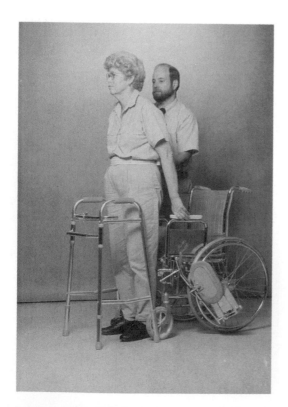

Figure 9.10–20. Grasping both armrests.

After grasping one armrest, the other hand moves from the handgrip of the walker and grasps the other armrest.

The patient lowers herself to sitting in a controlled manner onto the front edge of the seat.

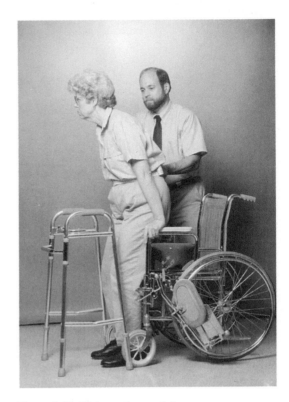

Figure 9.10–21. Lowering to sitting.

Once seated, she moves back into the seat and adjusts her sitting position.

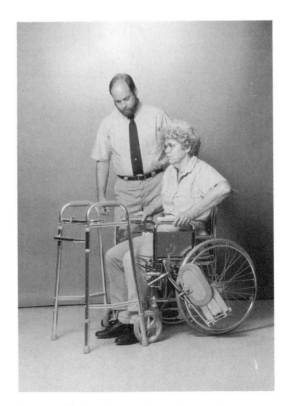

Figure 9.10–22. Adjusting final sitting position.

Moving a Walker

LO-15 The walker is moved by picking it up, moving it a stride length forward, and placing it on the floor. The walker should be lifted and set down so that all four legs clear, or contact, the floor simultaneously.

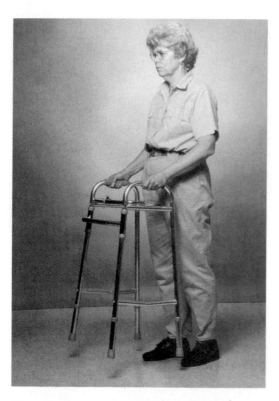

Figure 9.10–23. Correct method of using walker.

Some patients will "rock" the walker, lifting and setting down two legs and rocking onto the other two legs. Rocking the walker reduces the base of support and stability a walker provides when used properly. Rocking the walker should be discouraged.

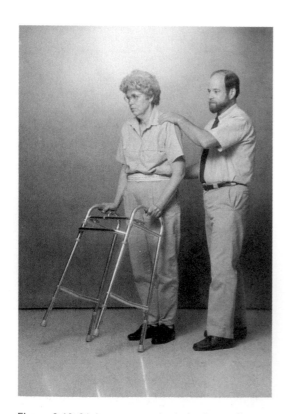

Figure 9.10–24. Incorrect method of using walker.

The patient's lower extremity should not be placed beyond the crossbar. Doing so prevents weight shifting over this lower extremity. When stepping beyond the crossbar occurs, the base of support and stability provided by a walker are reduced.

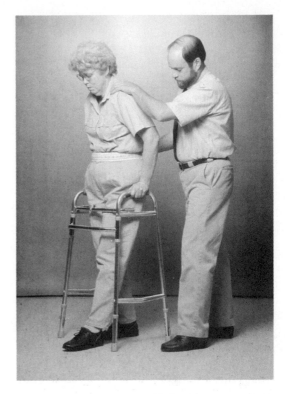

Figure 9.10–25. Improper stride length.

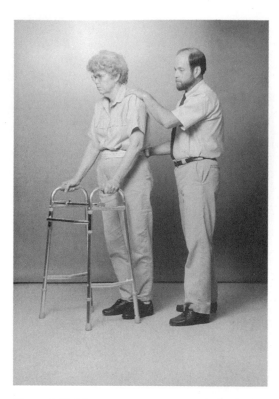

Figure 9.10–26. Walker moved forward.

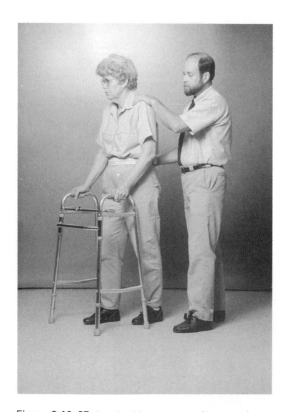

Figure 9.10–27. Involved lower extremity moved forward.

Ambulating Using a Three-Point Gait Pattern

Partial to Full Weight Bearing

Positioned in stride, behind and to one side of the patient, the therapist grasps the patient's gait belt and shoulder.

LO-15   To ambulate using the three-point gait pattern, the patient stands centered within the walker. The walker is lifted and advanced forward. All four legs of the walker must be lifted from, or lowered to, the floor simultaneously.

As the patient moves the walker, the therapist advances his left, or outside, foot.

The patient advances her involved lower extremity, moving into the strength and stability of the walker.

The patient bears weight through her upper extremities as she advances her uninvolved lower extremity. She may step to, or slightly beyond, her other foot. Equal step lengths should be encouraged. The therapist advances his right, or inside, foot to move with the patient.

The total sequence is repeated for continued progression.

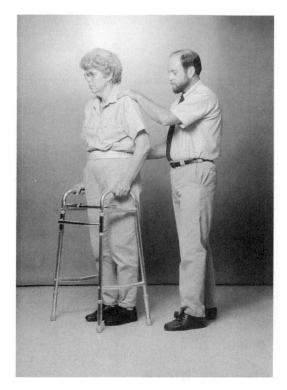

Figure 9.10–28. Uninvolved lower extremity moved forward.

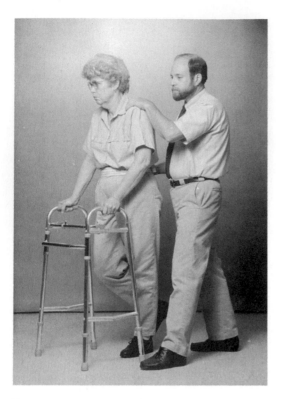

Figure 9.10–29. Walker moved forward.

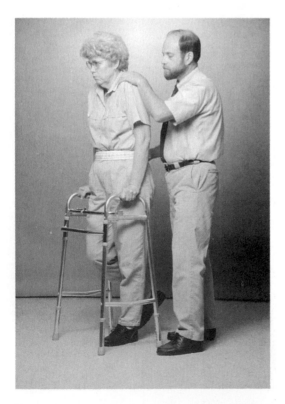

Figure 9.10–30. Uninvolved lower extremity moved forward.

Non-Weight Bearing

 Positioned in stride, behind and to one side of the patient, the therapist grasps the patient's gait belt and shoulder.

LO-15   To ambulate using the three-point gait pattern non-weight bearing on the involved lower extremity, the patient stands centered in the walker. The involved lower extremity is not rested on the floor. It may be held with the knee in extension, putting the foot in front of the patient, or it may be held with knee flexion, putting the foot behind the patient. The uninvolved lower extremity and both upper extremities provide support.

The walker is lifted and advanced forward. All four legs of the walker must be lifted from, or lowered to, the floor simultaneously.

As the patient moves the walker, the therapist advances his left, or outside, foot.

Bearing weight through her upper extremities, the patient steps into the walker with the uninvolved lower extremity. The therapist advances his right, or inside, foot to move with the patient.

The total sequence is repeated for continued progression.

Ambulating Using a Swing-To Gait Pattern

LO-15

Positioned in stride, behind and to one side of the patient, the therapist grasps the patient's gait belt and shoulder.

To ambulate using a swing-to gait pattern, the patient stands centered in the walker. The walker is advanced, and the therapist advances his left, or outside, foot.

Bearing weight through her upper extremities, and depressing her shoulders while pushing down on the handgrips of the walker, the patient lifts her body. The patient can then let her body swing forward ("swing-to") into the walker. The therapist moves his right, or inside, foot as the patient swings forward.

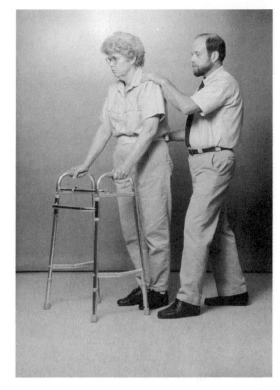

Figure 9.10–31. Walker moved forward.

The patient lowers herself at the end of the swing and bears weight on her lower extremities.

The sequence is repeated for continued progression.

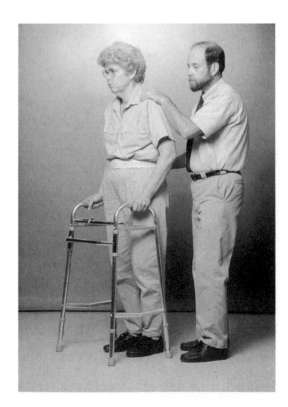

Figure 9.10–32. Patient's body swings to walker.

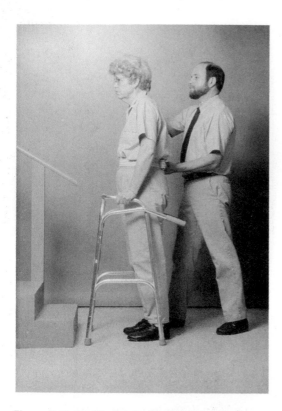

Figure 9.10–33. Starting position to ascend stairs.

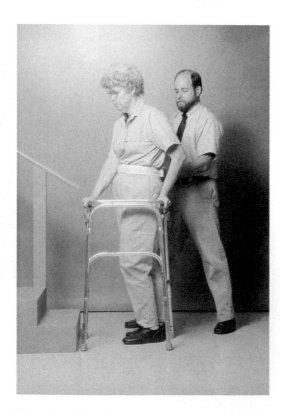

Figure 9.10–34. Walker turned with crossbar to side of patient.

Stairs

Ascending Using a Stair Climbing Walker

LO-15

Ambulation on the stairs using a walker can be accomplished with a standard walker or with a stair climbing walker. When a patient will negotiate stairs frequently a stair climbing walker should be used.

Positioned in stride behind the patient, the therapist grasps the patient's gait belt and shoulder. The patient stands facing up the stairs, with the walker in the usual position for ambulation.

The stair climbing walker is first turned so the crossbar is to the side of the patient.

The stair climbing walker is then turned so the crossbar is behind the patient.

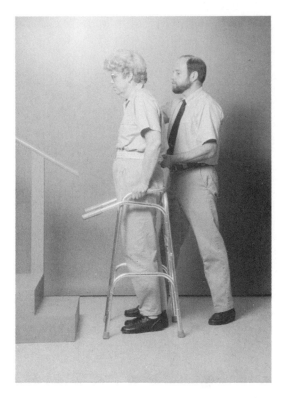

Figure 9.10–35. Walker turned with crossbar behind patient.

The two legs of the walker closest to the stairs are placed on the first stair.

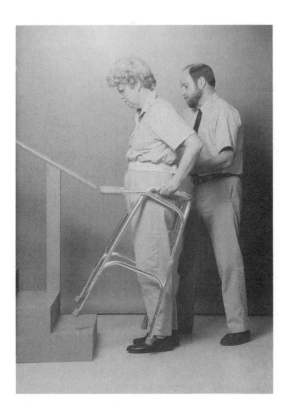

Figure 9.10–36. Lifting walker onto first stair.

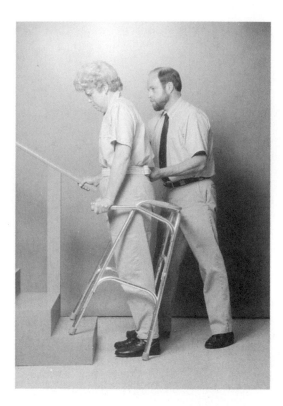

Figure 9.10–37. Grasping stair climbing handgrips.

Grasping the stair climbing handgrips, the patient supports her weight on her upper extremities. Continuing to stand in stride behind the patient, the therapist keeps one hand on the gait belt and moves the other hand from the patient's shoulder to the handrail.

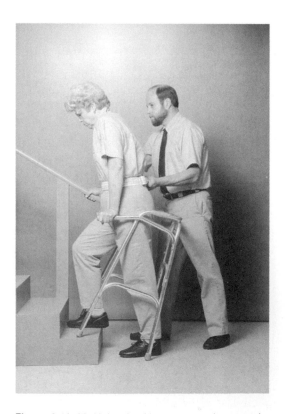

Figure 9.10–38. Uninvolved lower extremity moved to next stair.

The patient steps onto the same stair as the forward-most legs of the walker with her uninvolved lower extremity.

Extending her uninvolved lower extremity, the patient lifts her body. The involved lower extremity is placed on the same stair as the uninvolved lower extremity. Guarding becomes more difficult for the therapist at this point because the placement of the walker prevents the therapist from maintaining a close position behind the patient.

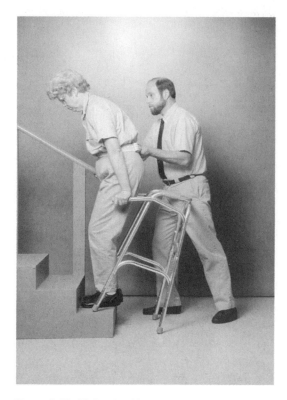

Figure 9.10–39. Involved lower extremity lifted to same stair.

The walker is lifted and advanced to the next stair. At this time the therapist can move closer behind the patient again.

The sequence is repeated to ascend the remaining stairs.

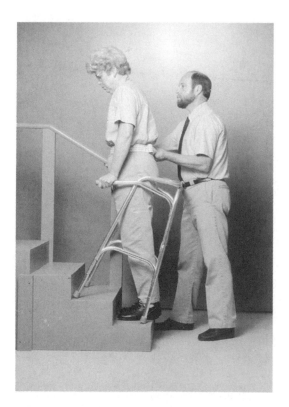

Figure 9.10–40. Walker lifted to next stair.

Descending Using a Stair Climbing Walker

LO-15 To descend stairs using a stair climbing walker, the patient stands facing down the stairs. The walker is positioned with the crossbar of the walker in front of the patient. The patient grasps the stair climbing handgrips and positions the walker so the forwardmost legs are on the lower stair.

Positioned in stride in front of the patient, the therapist grasps the patient's gait belt and handrail.

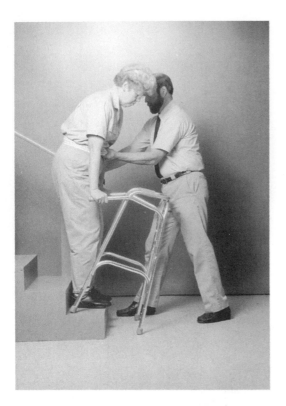

Figure 9.10–41. Walker lowered to next stair.

The patient lowers her involved lower extremity to the same stair as the forwardmost legs of the walker by flexing her uninvolved lower extremity.

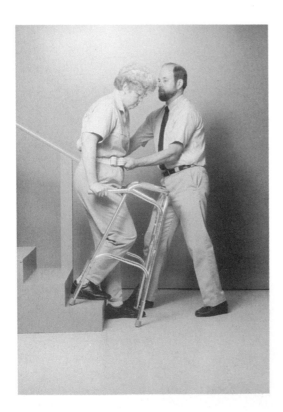

Figure 9.10–42. Involved lower extremity lowered to next stair.

Supporting herself with her upper extremities on the walker, the patient lowers her uninvolved lower extremity to the same stair.

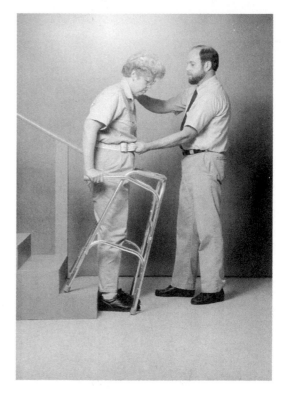

Figure 9.10–43. Uninvolved lower extremity lowered to same stair.

The sequence is repeated until the patient finishes descending the stairs. When the patient has finished descending the stairs and reaches the landing or floor level, she grasps the handgrips of the walker and positions the walker for ambulation.

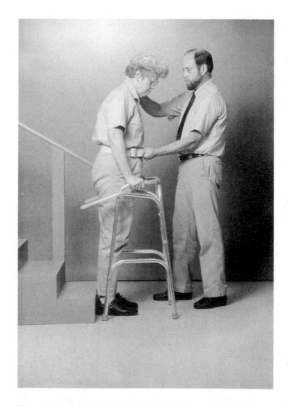

Figure 9.10–44. Walker positioned for ambulation.

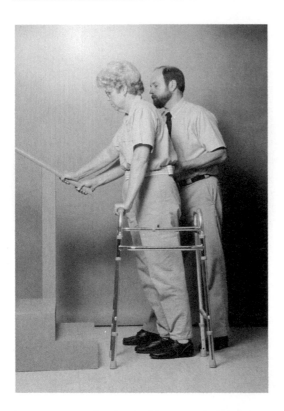

Figure 9.10–45. Starting position to ascend stairs.

Ascending Using a Standard Walker

  Although not the most stable device on stairs, a standard walker can be used when ambulating on the stairs.

LO-15   To ascend stairs using a standard walker, the patient stands facing up the stairs with the walker in the usual position for ambulation. The patient turns the walker sideways so the crossbar is away from the patient. The patient's hand closest to the walker is placed on the forwardmost handgrip of the walker. The patient's other hand grasps the handrail. Positioned in stride behind the patient, the therapist grasps the patient's gait belt and handrail.

The patient places the two forwardmost legs of the walker on the first stair.

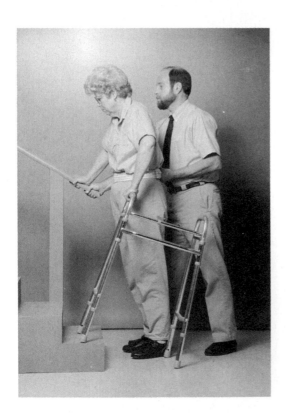

Figure 9.10–46. Walker lifted to next stair.

The patient advances her uninvolved lower extremity onto the same stair as the forwardmost legs of the walker.

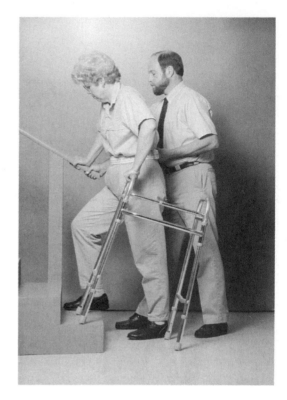

Figure 9.10–47. Uninvolved lower extremity lifted to next stair.

Extending her uninvolved lower extremity, the patient lifts her body. The patient places her involved lower extremity on the same stair as the uninvolved lower extremity.

The sequence is repeated to ascend the remaining stairs.

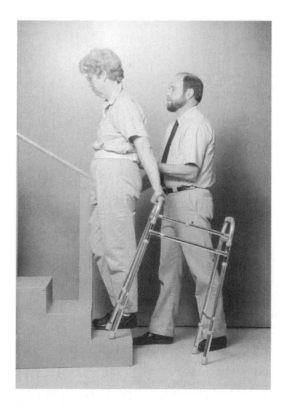

Figure 9.10–48. Involved lower extremity lifted to same stair.

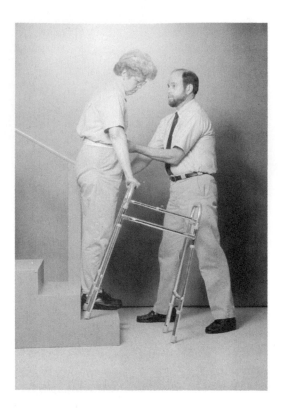

Figure 9.10–49. Walker lowered to next stair.

Descending Using a Standard Walker

LO-15 To descend stairs using a standard walker the patient stands facing down the stairs. The walker is turned sideways as for ascending the stairs. The two forwardmost legs of the walker are placed on the lower stair. With the hand closest to the walker, the patient grasps the rear handgrip of the walker. The patient's other hand grasps the handrail.

Positioned in stride in front of the patient, the therapist grasps the patient's gait belt and handrail.

The patient lowers her involved lower extremity to the same stair as the forwardmost legs of the walker by flexing her uninvolved lower extremity.

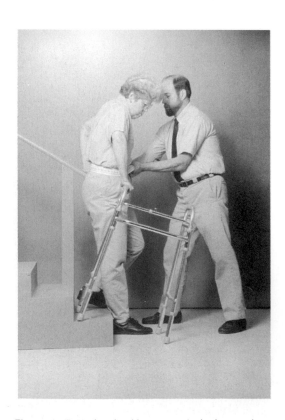

Figure 9.10–50. Involved lower extremity lowered to next stair.

Supporting her weight and balancing using her upper extremities, the uninvolved lower extremity is brought to the same stair as the involved lower extremity.

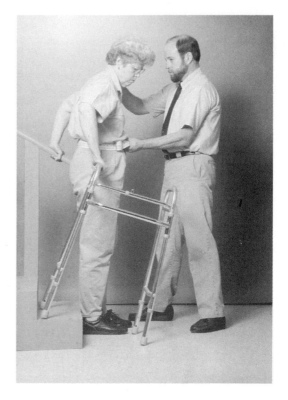

Figure 9.10–51. Uninvolved lower extremity lowered to same stair.

The sequence is repeated until the patient finishes descending the stairs. When the patient has reached the landing or floor level, she grasps both handgrips and positions the walker for ambulation.

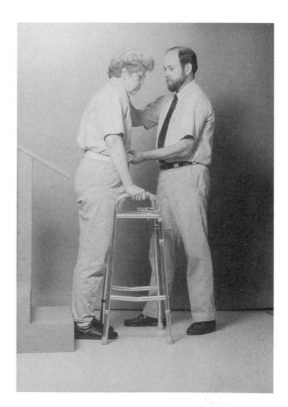

Figure 9.10–52. Walker positioned for ambulation.

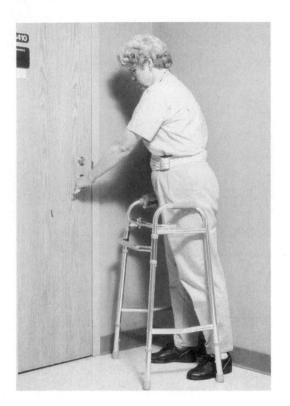

Figure 9.10–53. Positioned beyond door's arc of motion.

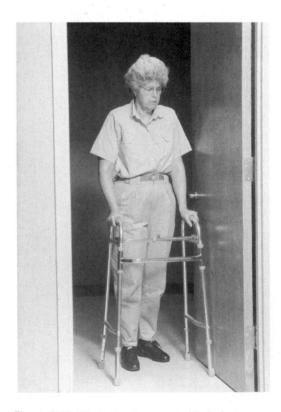

Figure 9.10–54. Walker tips used to block door closing.

Doorways With Automatic Door Closers

Door Opens Toward the Patient

LO-15

The patient approaches the latch edge of the door, standing outside the arc through which the opening door will move. The patient shifts her weight to the side of the walker away from the hand that will be placed on the door handle. The unweighted hand is then placed on the door handle. Preferably, weight is shifted to the side closest to the door handle, and the hand farthest from the door handle is used to pull open the door.

Using a pulling motion, the door is opened wider than the width of the patient. This is necessary because the door will start to close automatically before the patient can progress through the doorway. The automatic closing of the door must be blocked by the tips of the walker's legs to allow the patient time to progress through the doorway.

The hand used to open the door is quickly returned to the walker. The walker is lifted and moved forward into the doorway. All four legs of the walker are placed on the floor, and the tips of the two legs closest to the door serve as door stops. Using this method, the closing door hits the tips of the walker's legs, and not the patient.

Using the tips of the walker's legs as a doorstop, the patient progresses through the doorway.

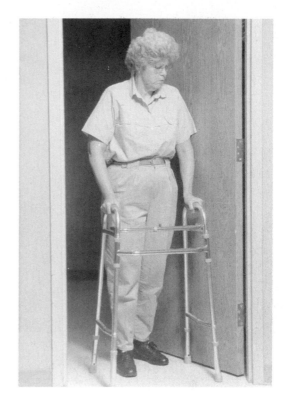

Figure 9.10–55. Moving through doorway.

Once the patient has moved completely through the doorway, the door closes behind the patient.

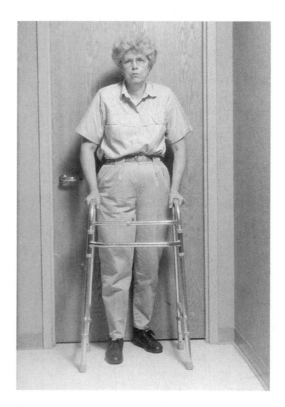

Figure 9.10–56. Door closes behind patient.

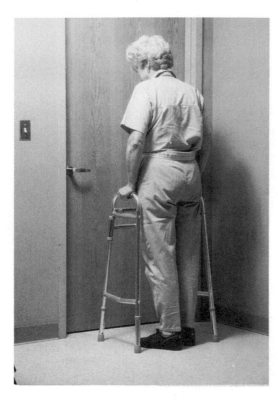

Figure 9.10–57. Approaching door.

Door Opens Away from the Patient

The patient approaches the door.

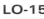
LO-15

The patient shifts her weight to the side of the walker away from the hand that is closest to the door handle. The unweighted hand is then placed on the door handle.

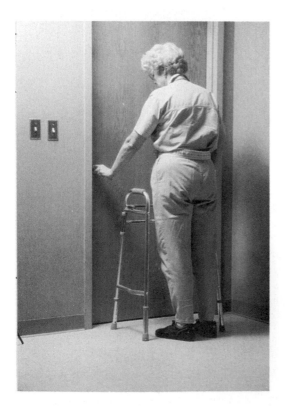

Figure 9.10–58. Grasping door handle.

Using a pushing motion, the door is opened wider than the width of the patient. Opening the door wider than the width of the patient is necessary because the door will start to close automatically before the patient can progress through the doorway. The automatic closing of the door must be blocked by the tips of the walker's legs to allow the patient time to progress through the doorway.

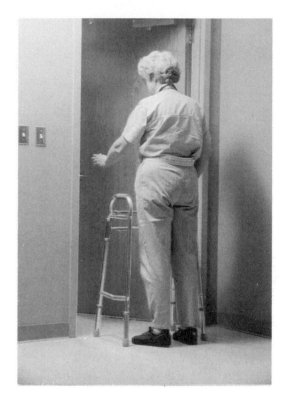

Figure 9.10–59. Opening door.

The hand used to open the door is quickly returned to the walker. The walker is lifted and moved forward into the doorway. All four legs of the walker are placed on the floor, and the tips of the two legs closest to the door serve as door stops. Using this method, the closing door hits the tips of the walker's legs, and not the patient.

Once the patient has moved completely through the doorway, the door closes behind the patient.

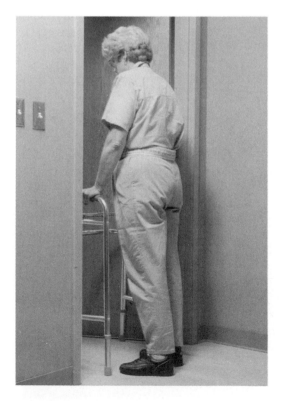

Figure 9.10–60. Walker tips used to block door closing.

9.11   AXILLARY CRUTCHES

Fitting

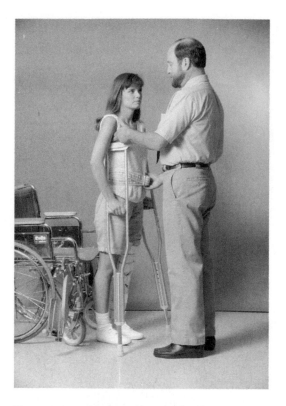

Figure 9.11–1. Measuring length of axillary crutches.

LO-15

Axillary crutches are fitted with a patient standing, and the shoulders relaxed. Proper adjustment requires appropriate posture because of the potential for injury. When improperly adjusted crutches are too long, or when a patient rests on the tops of the crutches, the crutch tops are forced into the axillae. Injury to nerves and blockage of blood vessels in the axillae can result from improper adjustment or use of crutches. The patient may report pain or tingling in the upper extremities, and muscle weakness or paralysis may occur.

The first adjustment is the overall length of the crutch. The crutches are positioned with the crutch tip on the floor, approximately 6 inches away from the toes at a 45-degree angle anterior and lateral to the small toe. With the patient's shoulders in a relaxed position, the therapist should be able to put two or three fingers between the patient's axilla and the top of the crutch on each side. When a pad is to be used on the crutch top, it should be in place during the fitting. In some styles of crutches, the nuts should not be tightened completely until after all adjustments are completed.

The handgrip height is adjusted after the overall length of the crutch is determined. The handgrip height of each crutch is adjusted to the level of the ulnar styloid process when the upper extremity is in a relaxed position at the patient's side. This provides 20 to 30 degrees of elbow flexion when the handgrip is grasped.

When all length and height adjustments have been completed, all nuts and button locks should be checked to ensure that they have been tightened or fully positioned to maintain crutch integrity during ambulation.

Figure 9.11–2. Measuring handgrip height.

In and Out of a Wheelchair

 LO-15 The wheelchair is prepared, and the patient positioned, in the manner described earlier in this chapter under "Assumption of Standing and Sitting." The therapist is positioned in the manner described earlier in this chapter under "Guarding."

Assuming Standing—Therapist on Involved Side

The wheelchair is locked and the footrest for the uninvolved lower extremity is moved out of the way. The crutches must be placed within reach of the therapist or patient before the patient starts this procedure.

The patient moves to the front edge of the seat. Assistance of the therapist to support the involved lower extremity may be necessary as the patient moves to the front edge of the seat. To provide assistance in supporting the involved lower extremity, the therapist squats in front and to the involved side of the patient.

When a patient is unable to flex the involved knee, an elevating legrest is used to support the involved lower extremity during sitting. This legrest must be removed or lowered and pivoted to the side before the patient's involved lower extremity is lowered to the floor. The therapist supports the involved lower extremity with one hand and arm while removing the legrest with the other hand.

The involved lower extremity is lowered carefully to the floor before the patient attempts to stand.

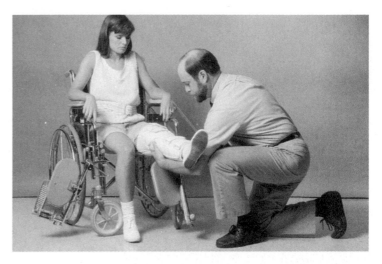

Figure 9.11–3. Therapist supporting involved lower extremity.

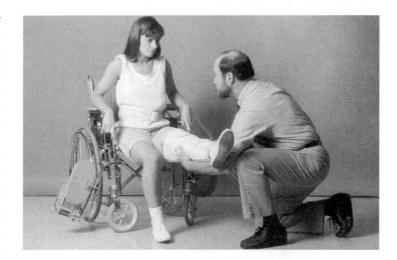

Figure 9.11–4. Legrest swung to side.

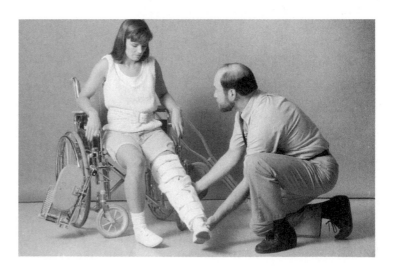

Figure 9.11–5. Lowering involved lower extremity.

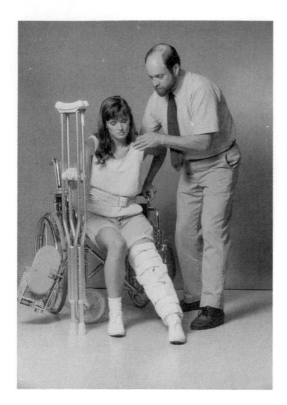

Figure 9.11–6. Starting position to assume standing with therapist on involved side.

The crutches are placed together in front of, and slightly lateral to, the patient's foot on the uninvolved side. Using the handgrips, the patient grasps both crutches with the hand on the uninvolved side. Positioned in stride to one side of the patient, the therapist grasps the patient's gait belt and shoulder.

The patient pushes to standing using the crutches on the uninvolved side and the armrest of the wheelchair on the other side.

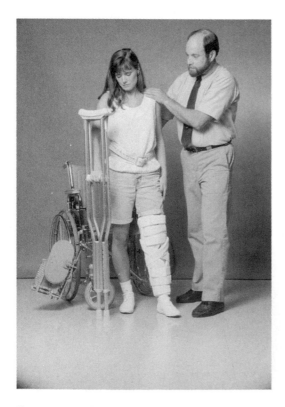

Figure 9.11–7. Assumption of standing.

When the patient has assumed the standing position, the therapist should ensure that the patient can control balance. The patient reaches across with the hand on the involved side for a crutch.

One at a time the crutches are positioned properly under the axillae. The crutch that was retrieved by the hand on the involved side is positioned under the axilla first. The crutch that remains in the hand on the uninvolved side is positioned second.

The patient is ready to ambulate.

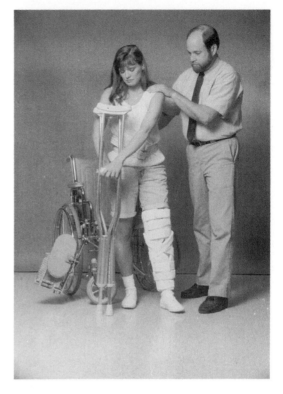

Figure 9.11–8. Reaching for crutch.

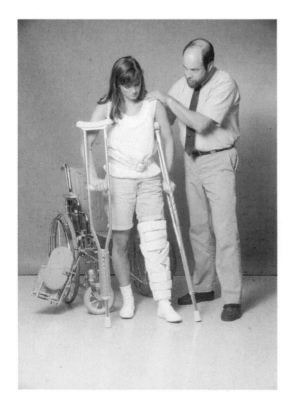

Figure 9.11–9. Positioning first crutch.

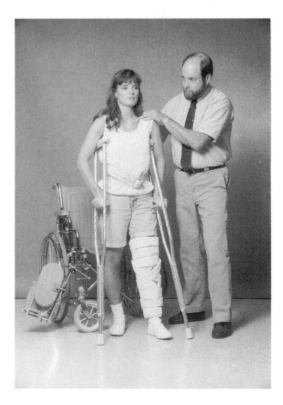

Figure 9.11–10. Both crutches positioned for ambulation.

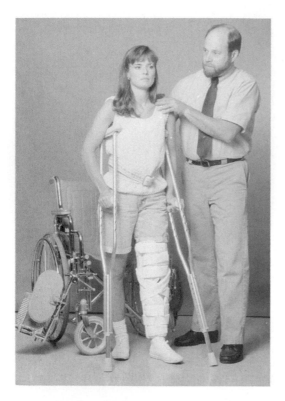

Figure 9.11–11. Starting position to assume sitting with therapist on involved side.

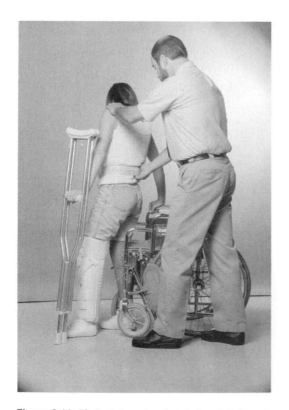

Figure 9.11–12. Both crutches in one hand and grasping armrest.

Assuming Sitting—Therapist on Involved Side

LO-15

The wheelchair is locked and the footrests moved out of the way. To sit, the patient positions herself at the front edge of the wheelchair seat, facing away from the wheelchair. The front edge of the wheelchair seat is felt against the back of the lower extremities. The patient's feet are positioned in stride, with the involved lower extremity far enough forward so the patient may sit. Positioned in stride, and behind and to one side of the patient, the therapist grasps the patient's gait belt and shoulder.

The crutch on the patient's involved side is removed from the axilla and held by the handgrip only. The crutch on the uninvolved side is removed from the axilla and passed to the hand on the involved side. Both crutches are held by the handgrips only. They are placed in front of, and slightly lateral to, the patient's foot on the involved side. The patient's hand on the uninvolved side reaches back and grasps the armrest.

The patient lowers herself to sitting.

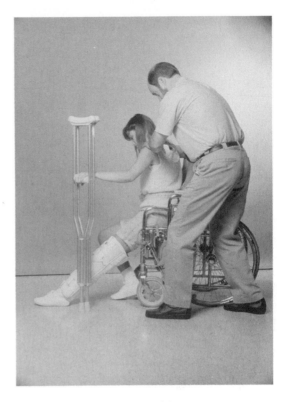

Figure 9.11–13. Lowering to sitting.

Setting the crutches aside, the patient grasps both arm-rests and moves back completely into the seat. The therapist may or may not need to provide assistance for the involved lower extremity.

When necessary, the patient's involved lower extremity is placed on the elevating legrest.

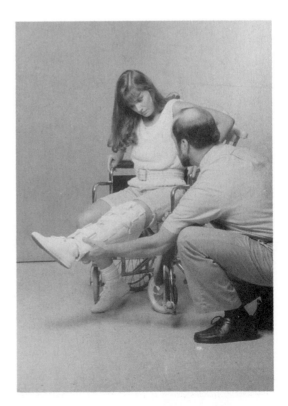

Figure 9.11–14. Adjusting final sitting position.

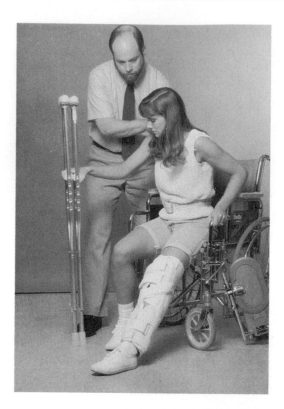

Figure 9.11–15. Starting position to assume standing with therapist on uninvolved side.

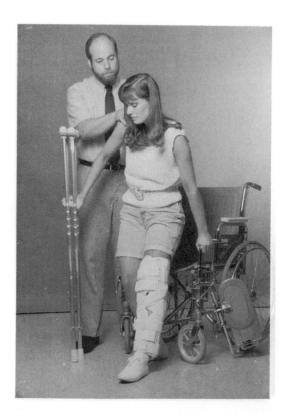

Figure 9.11–16. Assumption of standing.

Assuming Standing—Therapist on Uninvolved Side

LO-15 When a patient can control her involved lower extremity, the therapist assists the patient to standing from the patient's uninvolved side. The wheelchair is locked and the footrests moved out of the way. The patient is positioned at the front edge of the seat. Positioned in stride, and behind and to one side of the patient, the therapist grasps the patient's gait belt and shoulder.

The crutches are placed together to the front and side of the uninvolved foot. The patient grasps both crutches by the handgrips only. The patient's other hand is placed on the armrest of the wheelchair.

The patient pushes to standing.

When the patient has assumed the standing position, the therapist should ensure that the patient can control balance. Releasing her grasp on the armrest, the patient reaches for a crutch.

One at a time the crutches are positioned properly under the axillae. The crutch that was retrieved by the hand on the involved side is positioned under the axilla first. The crutch that remains in the hand on the uninvolved side is positioned second.

The patient is ready to ambulate.

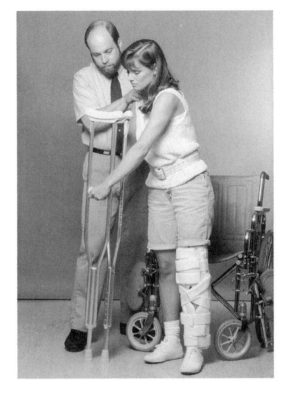

Figure 9.11–17. Reaching for crutch.

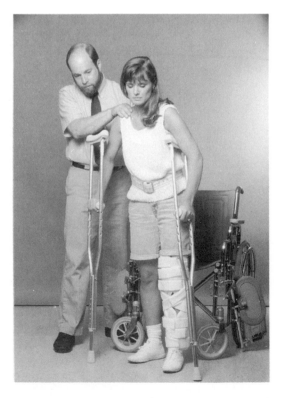

Figure 9.11–18. Positioning first crutch.

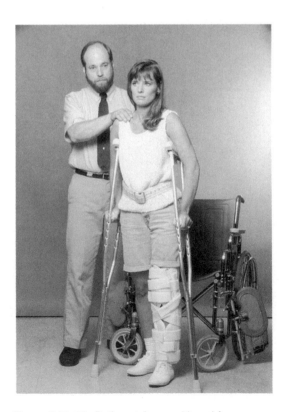

Figure 9.11–19. Both crutches positioned for ambulation.

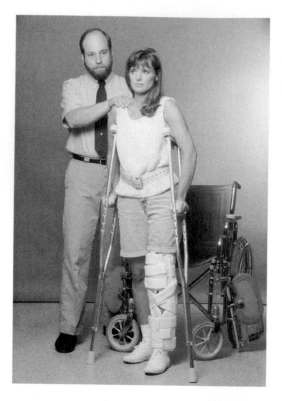

Figure 9.11–20. Starting position to assume sitting with therapist on uninvolved side.

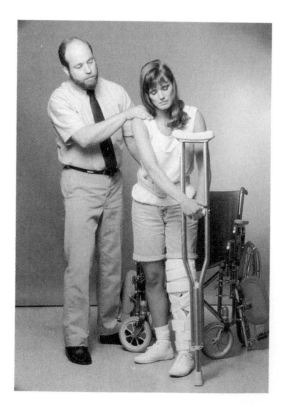

Figure 9.11–21. Positioning crutches.

Assuming Sitting—Therapist on Uninvolved Side

LO-15   The wheelchair is locked and the footrests moved out of the way. To sit, the patient positions herself at the front edge of the wheelchair seat, facing away from the wheelchair. The front edge of the wheelchair seat is felt against the back of the lower extremities. The patient's feet are positioned in stride, with the involved lower extremity far enough forward so that the patient may sit. Positioned in stride, and behind and to one side of the patient, the therapist grasps the patient's gait belt and shoulder.

The crutch on the patient's involved side is removed from the axilla and held by the handgrip only. The crutch on the uninvolved side is removed from the axilla and passed to the hand on the involved side.

Both crutches are held by the handgrips only on the patient's involved side. The patient's hand on the uninvolved side reaches back and grasps the armrest.

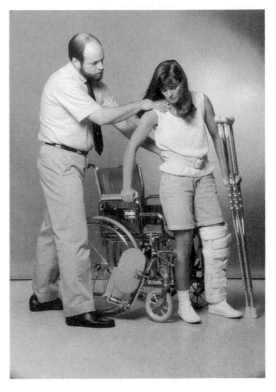

Figure 9.11–22. Both crutches in one hand and grasping armrest.

The patient lowers herself to sitting.

Setting the crutches aside, the patient grasps both armrests. The patient moves back completely into the seat. When necessary, the patient's involved lower extremity is placed on the elevating legrest.

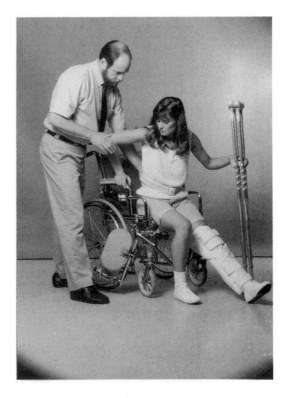

Figure 9.11–23. Lowering to sitting.

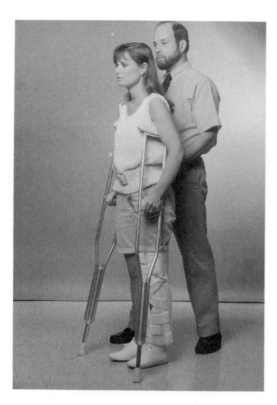

Figure 9.11–24. Starting position for ambulation using three-point gait pattern.

Ambulating Using a Three-Point Gait Pattern

Partial to Full Weight Bearing

LO-15

Positioned in stride, and behind and to one side of the patient, the therapist grasps the patient's gait belt and shoulder. In the starting position the patient stands with the crutches in the same position used for measuring crutch fit. The patient's feet are side by side.

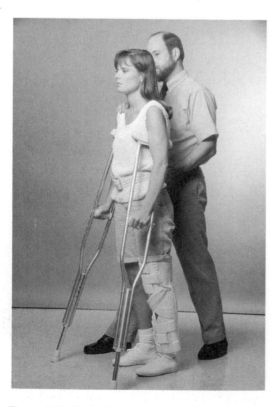

Figure 9.11–25. Both crutches moved forward.

To ambulate, both crutches are advanced simultaneously the same amount. The therapist advances his right, or outside, foot, either at the same time, or immediately after, the crutches are advanced.

The patient advances her involved lower extremity so the toes are even with the crutch tips.

As the patient improves, she may move the crutches and involved lower extremity at the same time, permitting a faster pace of gait.

Using her upper extremities to support her body weight, the patient advances her uninvolved lower extremity beyond the crutches. Initially, the patient may "step to" her involved lower extremity, rather than "step through." Stepping through is the normal gait pattern, and should be encouraged. The therapist advances his left, or inside, foot as the patient moves her uninvolved lower extremity.

The sequence is repeated for continued progression.

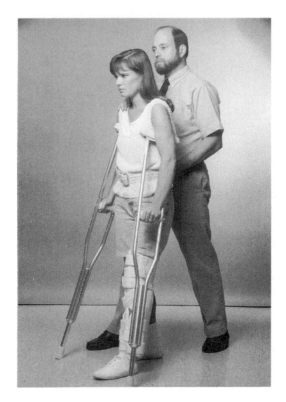

Figure 9.11–26. Involved lower extremity moved forward.

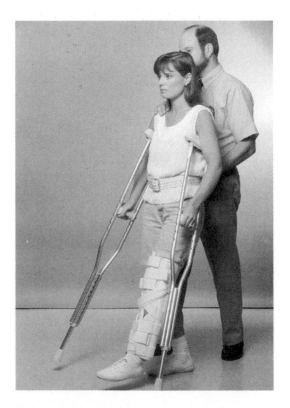

Figure 9.11–27. Crutches and involved lower extremity moved forward simultaneously.

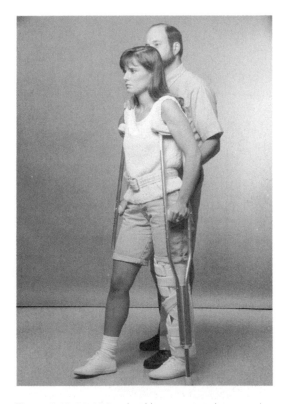

Figure 9.11–28. Uninvolved lower extremity moved forward.

Non-Weight Bearing

LO-15

Positioned in stride, and behind and to one side of the patient, the therapist grasps the patient's gait belt and shoulder. In the starting position the patient stands with the crutches in the same position used for measuring crutch fit. The involved lower extremity is not on the floor. Generally patients hold the involved lower extremity in front when the knee cannot be flexed, and behind when the knee can be flexed.

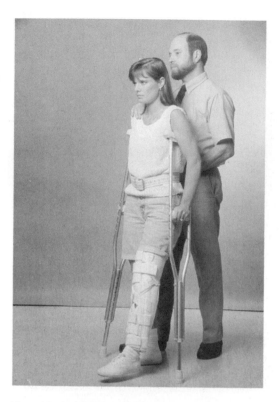

Figure 9.11–29. Starting position for ambulation using three-point non-weight bearing gait pattern.

To ambulate, both crutches and the involved lower extremity are advanced simultaneously the same amount. The therapist advances his right, or outside, foot, either at the same time, or immediately after, the crutches are advanced.

Figure 9.11–30. Both crutches and involved lower extremity moved forward simultaneously.

Using her upper extremities to support her body weight,

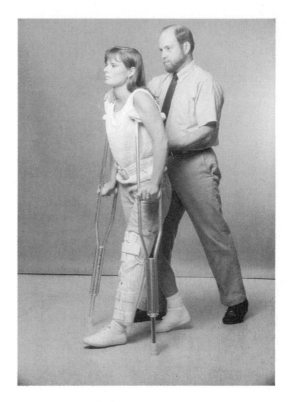

Figure 9.11–31. Shifting weight onto crutches.

the patient advances her uninvolved lower extremity beyond the crutches. Initially, the patient may "step to" her involved lower extremity, rather than "step through." Stepping through is the normal gait pattern, and should be encouraged. The therapist advances his left, or inside, foot as the patient moves her uninvolved lower extremity.

The sequence is repeated for continued progression.

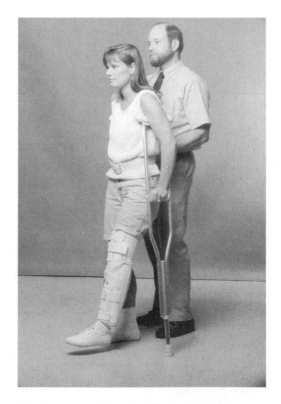

Figure 9.11–32. Uninvolved lower extremity moved forward.

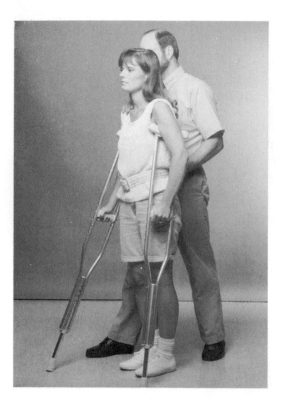

Figure 9.11–33. Right crutch moved forward.

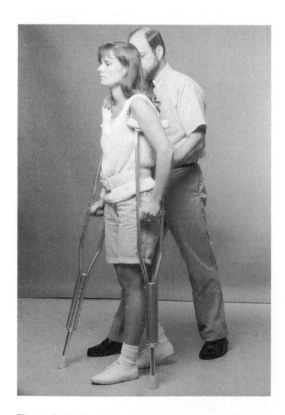

Figure 9.11–34. Left lower extremity moved forward.

Ambulating Using a Four-Point Gait Pattern

LO-15 Positioned in stride, and behind and to one side of the patient, the therapist grasps the patient's gait belt and shoulder. In the starting position the patient stands with the crutches in the same position used for measuring crutch fit. The patient's feet are side by side.

To ambulate, the patient advances one crutch. In this example the right crutch is advanced first. The therapist advances his right, or outside, foot.

The patient then advances her opposite lower extremity to a point even with the tip of the right crutch.

The patient shifts her weight to the right crutch and left lower extremity. She advances her left crutch beyond the right crutch.

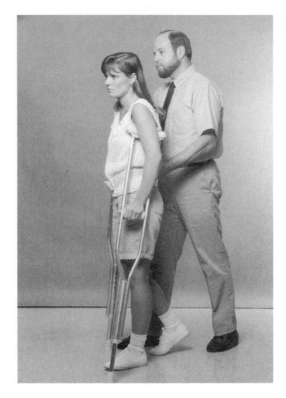

Figure 9.11–35. Left crutch moved forward.

The patient advances her right lower extremity to a point even with the tip of her left crutch. The therapist advances his left, or inside, foot.

The patient shifts her weight to her left crutch and right lower extremity. The sequence is repeated for continued progression.

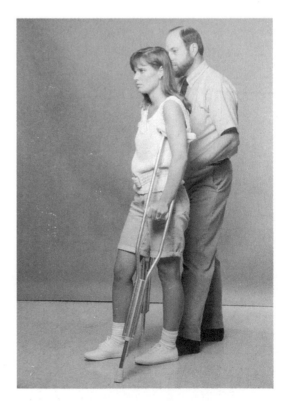

Figure 9.11–36. Right lower extremity moved forward.

Ambulating Using a Two-Point Gait Pattern

LO-15 Positioned in stride, and behind and to one side of the patient, the therapist grasps the patient's gait belt and shoulder. In the starting position the patient stands with the crutches in the same position used for measuring crutch fit. The patient's feet are side by side.

The patient advances one crutch and the opposite lower extremity simultaneously, placing the toes even with the tip of the crutch. Her weight is shifted onto this crutch and lower extremity. In this example, the right crutch and left foot have been advanced together. The therapist moves his right, or outside, foot at this time.

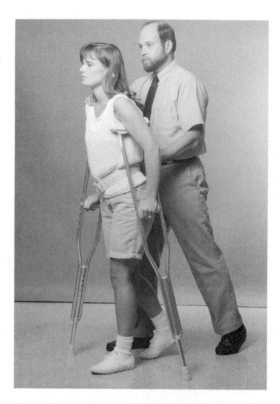

Figure 9.11–37. Right crutch and left lower extremity moved forward simultaneously.

The patient advances her left crutch and right lower extremity together. This crutch and lower extremity are advanced beyond the other crutch and lower extremity in a normal stride length. The patient shifts her weight onto the just advanced crutch and lower extremity. The therapist moves his left, or inside, foot at this time.

The sequence is repeated for continued progression.

Figure 9.11–38. Left crutch and right lower extremity moved forward simultaneously.

Falling

When a patient starts to fall, the therapist must decide whether to prevent the fall, or to permit a controlled fall in a manner that will prevent injury to the patient or himself. The therapist must be alert to a patient's movements at all times, and be able to react quickly to prevent or control a fall. Proper guarding and attention focused on the patient are required at all times.

The therapist prevents a fall by using the biomechanical advantages of standing in stride, behind and slightly to the side of the patient. By standing in stride the therapist is able to shift his weight onto his back foot and pull the patient into his base of support.

When the therapist cannot prevent the fall, he must control the fall. Falls usually occur when the patient loses control of a crutch.

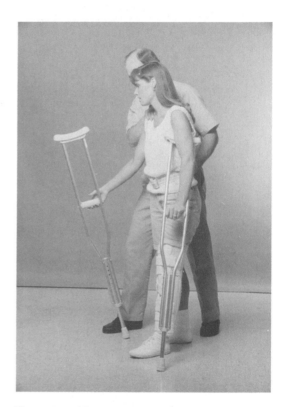

Figure 9.11–39. Losing control of crutch.

The patient is instructed to let the crutches fall to the sides, away from the area in which the patient will land, when possible, to avoid injury from landing on the crutches. The therapist steps forward in his stride position to widen his base of support as he slows the rate at which the patient falls.

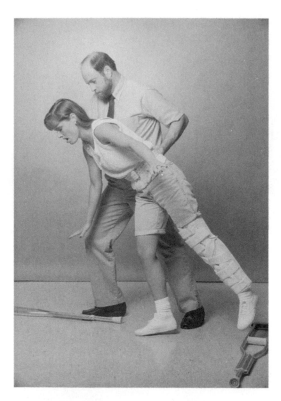

Figure 9.11–40. Crutches fall to sides.

The patient catches herself on her outstretched upper extremities, making sure that the elbows flex to absorb the impact. When elbow flexion is not permitted, injury to the patient's upper extremities may occur.

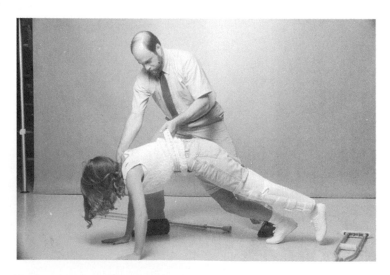

Figure 9.11–41. Patient lands on upper extremities with elbow flexion.

The therapist continues to lower the patient to the floor slowly, and the patient turns onto the side of the uninvolved lower extremity.

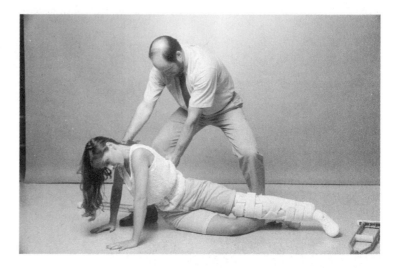

Figure 9.11–42. Therapist lowers patient to floor.

By turning from the side of the uninvolved lower extremity into a long sitting position, the patient is in a position to initiate getting up from the floor.

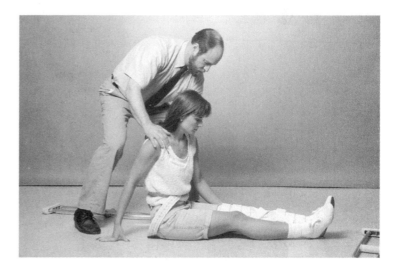

Figure 9.11–43. Patient assumes long sitting position.

The method used to rise from the floor depends on the patient's initial problem, and any additional injury the fall may have caused. When the patient is unsure of her ability to arise after having fallen, assistance should be summoned. Usually a patient can move on the floor in a sitting position to a chair or couch. Using furniture for stability and assistance, patients can usually assume standing again. Methods of moving from the floor to a sitting position in a chair are described in Chapter 8, "Independent Transfer From Wheelchair to Floor and Return."

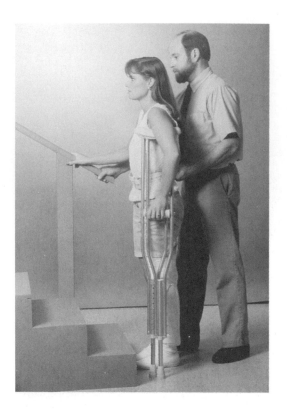

Figure 9.11–44. Both crutches together under upper extremity for stairs.

Stairs

Holding the Crutches

Ambulation on stairs can be performed using two crutches, without the use of a handrail. Use of a handrail, however, provides stability, and thus is an added safety factor. When using a handrail, the handrail takes the place of the crutch on one side. There are several methods of holding crutches when using a handrail. Whatever method of holding crutches is used, however, the sequence of movements for the lower extremities and assistive devices is the same.

A practical method of holding two crutches while using a handrail is to place both crutches together under the upper extremity on the side opposite the handrail.

A second method of holding two crutches while using a handrail is to hold the crutch on the side of the handrail in the hand that grasps the handrail. This crutch is held by one of its uprights, parallel to the handrail. The crutch on the side opposite the handrail is used in the usual manner.

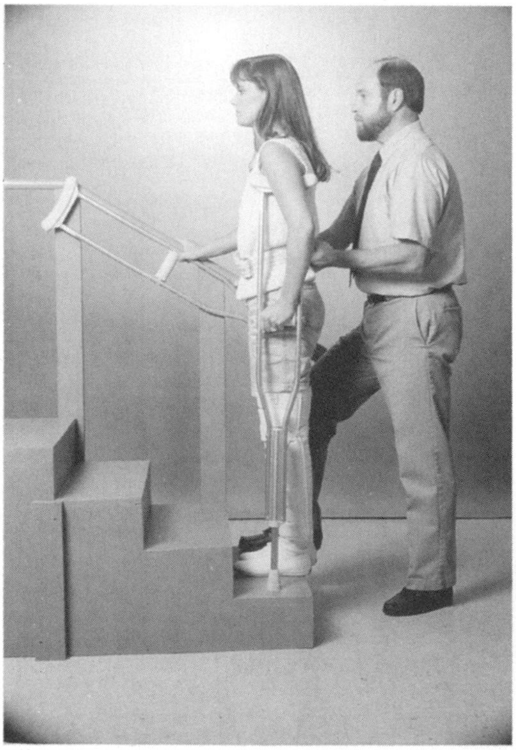

Figure 9.11–45. One crutch held parallel to handrail for stairs.

A third method of holding two crutches while using a handrail is to hold the handrail with one hand. The hand on the side opposite the handrail holds both crutches, one in the usual manner, and the other by one of its uprights, perpendicular to the first crutch.

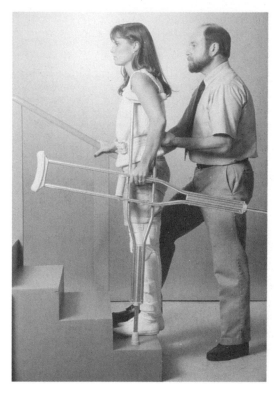

Figure 9.11–46. Crutches perpendicular to each other for stairs.

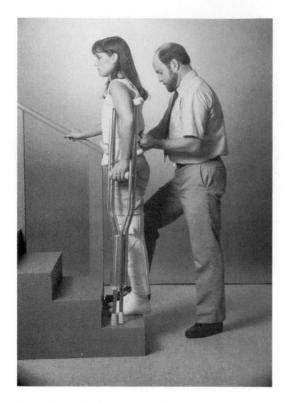

Figure 9.11–47. Starting position to ascend stairs.

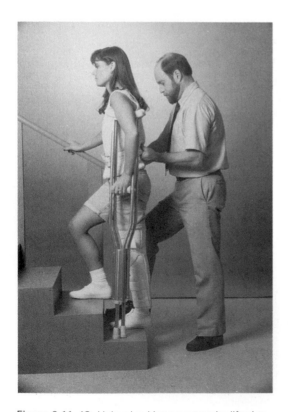

Figure 9.11–48. Uninvolved lower extremity lifted to next stair.

Ascending Using a Handrail

LO-15

To ascend stairs, for any of the methods of holding the crutches, the patient stands facing up the stairs. Positioned in stride behind the patient, the therapist grasps the patient's gait belt and the handrail. For the method illustrated in this section, the patient places both crutches under the upper extremity on the side opposite the handrail and grasps the handrail with the other hand.

The patient's uninvolved lower extremity is placed on the next higher stair while the body weight is supported by the upper extremities.

Weight is shifted to the uninvolved lower extremity on the next higher stair.

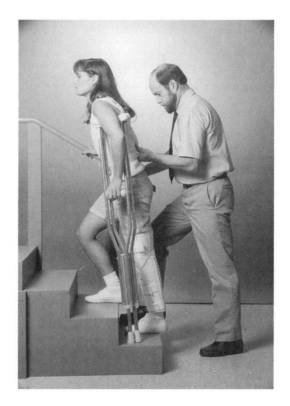

Figure 9.11–49. Weight shifted to uninvolved lower extremity.

Extending her uninvolved lower extremity, the patient lifts her body to the next higher stair. The crutches and involved lower extremity are advanced to the same stair at the same time. The crutches must be properly placed on the stair for stability, and to provide room for the patient to maneuver.

The therapist ascends with the patient.

This sequence is repeated to ascend an entire flight of stairs.

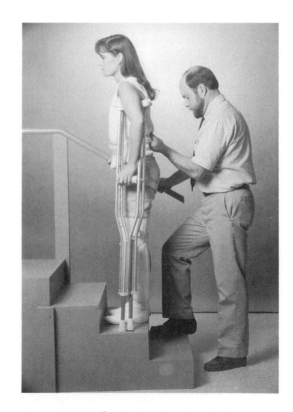

Figure 9.11–50. Crutches and involved lower extremity lifted to same stair.

Descending Using a Handrail

LO-15 To descend stairs, for any of the methods of holding the crutches, the patient stands facing down the stairs. Positioned in stride in front of the patient, the therapist grasps the patient's gait belt and the handrail. For the method illustrated in this section, the patient places both crutches under the upper extremity on the side opposite the handrail and grasps the handrail with the other hand.

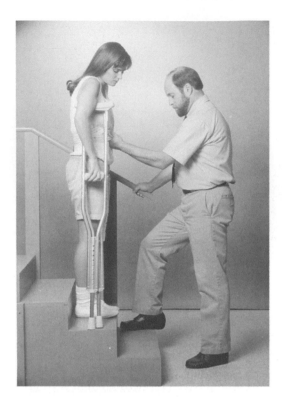

Figure 9.11–51. Starting position to descend stairs.

Flexing the uninvolved lower extremity to lower the body, the patient places the crutches and involved lower extremity on the next lower stair. The crutches are placed securely on the next lower stair, and must be spaced widely enough to permit the patient to move between the crutches.

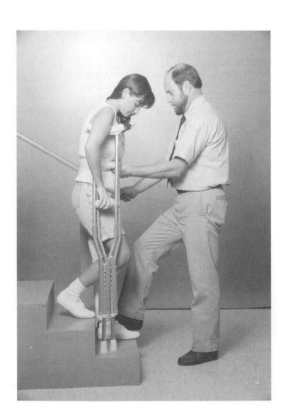

Figure 9.11–52. Crutches and involved lower extremity lowered to next stair.

With the body supported by the upper extremities, the uninvolved lower extremity is moved to the same stair.

The therapist descends with the patient.

This sequence is repeated to descend an entire flight of stairs.

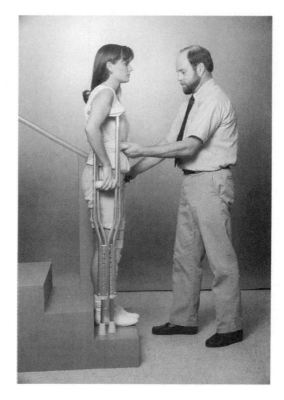

Figure 9.11–53. Uninvolved lower extremity lowered to same stair.

Ascending and Descending Stairs Without a Handrail

LO-15

To ascend or descend stairs without using a handrail, the crutches are retained in the same position used for walking. Rather than using a handrail for support on one side, the crutches are used for support on both sides. The position of the therapist, and the sequence of moving the crutches and lower extremities remains the same as for ascending stairs using a handrail and descending stairs using a handrail. The therapist holds onto the handrail, when available, whether the patient is using it or not.

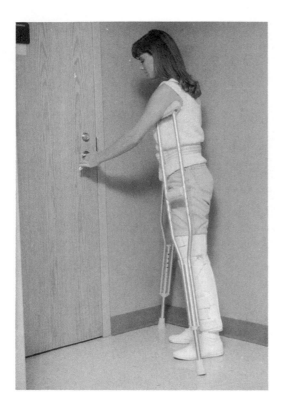

Figure 9.11–54. Positioned beyond door's arc of motion.

Doorways With Automatic Door Closers

Door Opens Toward the Patient

LO-15 The patient approaches the latch edge of the door, standing outside the arc through which the opening door will move. The patient shifts her weight onto the crutch on the side away from the hand that will be placed on the door handle. The unweighted hand is then placed on the door handle. Preferably, weight is shifted to the side closest to the door handle, and the hand farthest from the door handle is used to pull open the door.

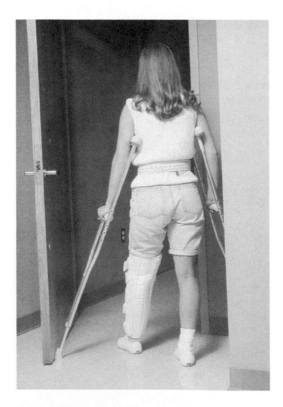

Figure 9.11–55. Crutch tip used to block door closing.

Using a pulling motion, the door is opened wider than the width of the patient. Opening the door wider than the patient is necessary because the door will start to close automatically before the patient can progress through the doorway. The hand used to open the door is quickly returned to the crutch. To block the automatic closing of the door, the patient turns into the doorway and places the tip of the crutch closest to the door on the floor in the path of the door. This acts as a door stop, permitting the patient to progress into the doorway without being struck by the closing door.

Continuing to use the tip of the crutch as a door stop, the patient ambulates through the doorway using the appropriate gait pattern.

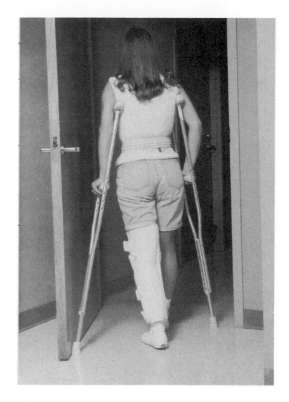

Figure 9.11–56. Moving through doorway.

As the patient moves through the doorway, the crutch tip used as a door stop is placed progressively closer to the hinge edge of the door. The therapist and patient must be aware that as the crutch tip gets closer to the hinge edge of the door, it becomes more difficult to hold open the door.

Once the patient has moved completely through the doorway, the door closes behind the patient.

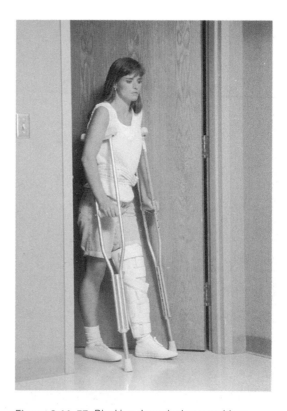

Figure 9.11–57. Blocking door closing near hinge edge.

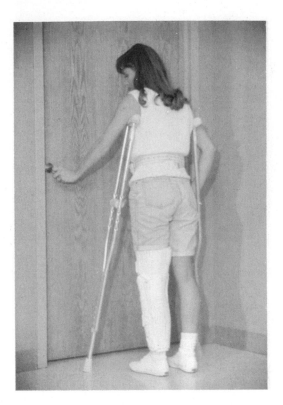

Figure 9.11–58. Grasping door handle.

Door Opens Away from the Patient

LO-15 The patient faces the door and shifts her weight onto the crutch away from the hand that is closest to the door handle. The unweighted hand is then placed on the door handle.

Using a pushing motion, the door is opened wider than the width of the patient. Opening the door wider than the patient is necessary because the door will start to close automatically before the patient can move through the doorway. The automatic closing of the door must be blocked by the tip of the crutch closest to the door, permitting the patient time to progress through the doorway. The hand used to open the door is quickly returned to the crutch. The opposite crutch is then advanced into the doorway to act as a door stop.

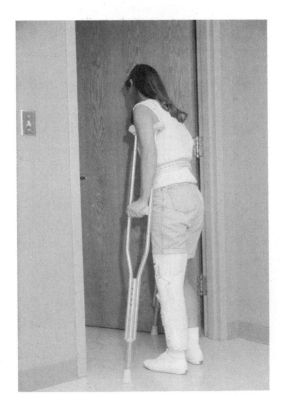

Figure 9.11–59. Crutch tip used to block door closing.

Continuing to use the tip of the crutch as a door stop, the patient ambulates through the doorway using the appropriate gait pattern.

As the patient moves through the doorway, the crutch tip used as a door stop is placed progressively closer to the latch edge of the door.

Once the patient has moved completely through the doorway, the door closes behind the patient.

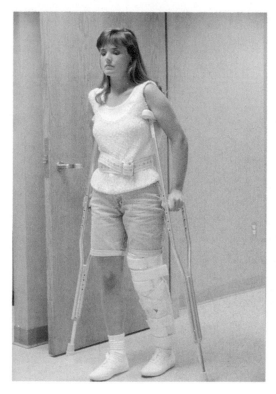

Figure 9.11–60. Blocking door closing near latch edge.

Doorways Without Automatic Door Closers

LO-15

When the door does not have an automatic closer, the initial rapid movement to place the crutch tip on the ground as a doorstop is not necessary. The extra wide opening of the door is also not necessary. Movement of the crutches can be performed more slowly, and placement of the crutch tip as a doorstop between the door and the patient is not required. The patient must turn to close the door because the door will not close automatically.

9.12   FOREARM (LOFSTRAND) CRUTCHES

Introduction

LO-15

Forearm crutches can be used for the same patients and with the same gait patterns as axillary crutches. The illustrations in this section present the use of forearm crutches for a patient with paraplegia. Patients with paraplegia have paralysis of the musculature of the lower extremities. Many patients with paraplegia lack lower extremity and lower trunk muscle strength to support themselves in an upright posture. To overcome this lack of strength, a greater degree of upper trunk and upper extremity strength is required. Ambulation for patients with paraplegia requires upper body movement to control paretic or paralyzed lower extremities.

Patients with paraplegia usually use a swing-to or swing-through gait pattern. They will use bilateral knee–ankle–foot orthoses (KAFOs). KAFOs lock at the knee and ankle joints, maintaining the patient's knees in extension and the ankles in slight dorsiflexion during ambulation. Initially patients may use a swing-to gait pattern. As ability improves, patients may progress to the swing-through pattern. The swing-through gait pattern is more efficient, permitting patients to move faster.

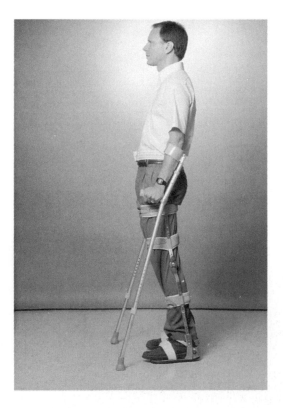

Figure 9.12–1. Fitting forearm crutches.

Fitting

LO-11

Setting the length of forearm crutches determines handgrip height. The crutches are positioned with the crutch tip on the floor, approximately 6 inches away from the toes at a 45-degree angle anterior and lateral to the small toe. The handgrip is level with the ulnar styloid process when the upper extremity is relaxed at the side. When the handgrips are held with the shoulders relaxed, the elbows should be in 20 to 30 degrees of flexion. Forearm cuff height is adjusted after crutch length has been adjusted. Cuff height should be adjusted to a point as high as possible on the forearm without interfering with elbow flexion. Cuff width should be tight enough to stay on the upper extremity when the handgrip is released, but loose enough not to bind. Cuff width is adjusted by squeezing the cuff together, or spreading it apart.

In and Out of a Wheelchair

 LO-15 Two methods, the turn around method and the power method, may be used to assume standing using forearm crutches and KAFOs. The turn around method requires less strength than the power method.

The wheelchair is locked and the footrests moved out of the way. The patient is positioned at the front edge of the seat. Positioned in stride, and behind and to one side of the patient, the therapist grasps the patient's gait belt and shoulder.

One forearm crutch is placed on either side of the wheelchair. The crutches must be supported securely enough so they will not fall as the patient moves, yet be accessible to the patient.

The patient moves forward on the seat of the wheelchair and secures the knee locks of his KAFOs in knee extension.

Assuming Standing Using the Turn Around Method

 LO-15 For this method, the therapist initially assumes the proper position on the side from which the patient will turn. In the illustrations for this section, this is on the patient's right side. The therapist must be prepared to move with the patient so as not to inhibit the patient's fluid motion. Initially, the therapist may assist by lifting or guiding the patient.

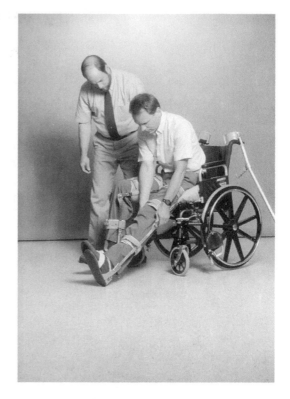

Figure 9.12–2. Securing knee locks on KAFOs.

When the patient turns to his left, he begins by hooking the medial upright of the right orthosis over the medial upright of the left orthosis. This aids in placement of the lower extremities as the patient stands. The patient then turns onto his left side. As the patient turns, he reaches behind with his left hand to grasp the right armrest, and in front with his right hand to grasp the left armrest.

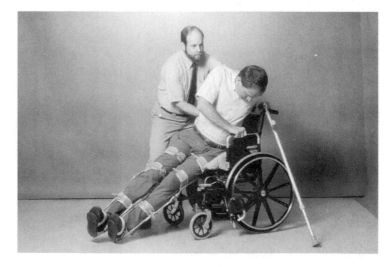

Figure 9.12–3. Initial turn to grasp armrests.

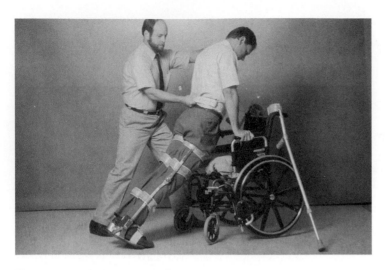

Figure 9.12–4. Pushing to standing.

Using his upper extremities, the patient pushes to standing. He completes the turn as he assumes a standing position facing the wheelchair.

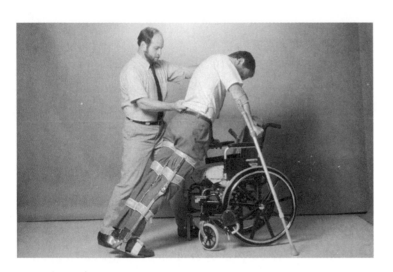

Figure 9.12–5. Grasping and positioning first forearm crutch.

Using the armrests for support, the patient performs a push-up while lifting his body to position his lower extremities. The feet must be positioned so the patient is centered in front of the wheelchair at a distance that will permit him to support himself with one upper extremity as the crutches are retrieved. The patient shifts his weight to one side, and grasps and positions the forearm crutch on the side that has been unweighted.

Shifting his weight onto the forearm crutch, the patient grasps the second forearm crutch and places it properly.

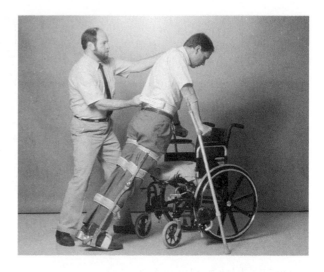

Figure 9.12–6. Grasping and positioning other forearm crutch.

Using both crutches for support, the patient pushes to the fully upright position. His shoulders are behind his hips to maintain hip extension. This posture is called a "C" curve.

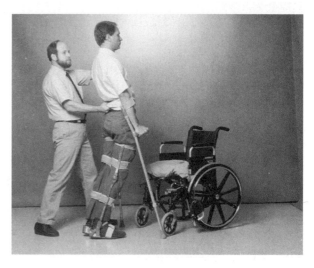

Figure 9.12–7. "C" curve in upright position.

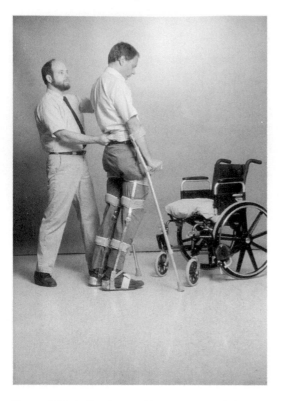

Figure 9.12–8. Starting position to assume sitting using turn around method.

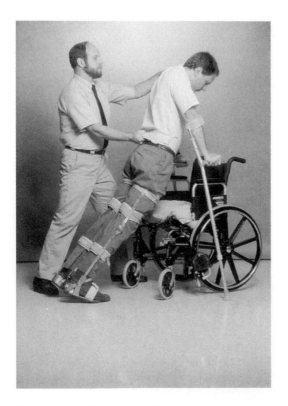

Figure 9.12–9. Crutches positioned.

Assuming Sitting Using the Turn Around Method

LO-15 The wheelchair is locked and the footrests moved out of the way. Positioned in stride, slightly behind and to the side to which the patient will turn, the therapist grasps the patient's gait belt and shoulder. The therapist must be prepared to move as the patient moves to avoid interfering with the patient's fluid motion. Initially, the therapist may guide or control the rate at which the patient turns and lowers himself into the seat.

To assume sitting using the turn around method, the patient approaches the wheelchair.

The patient faces the wheelchair with his crutches placed on either side of the wheelchair.

Shifting his weight onto one forearm crutch, the patient removes the other forearm crutch. The crutch that has been removed is placed against the wheelchair. The patient then grasps the armrest with his free hand.

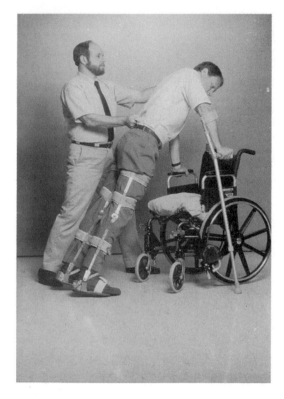

Figure 9.12–10. Grasping one armrest.

Shifting his weight onto the upper extremity that is grasping the armrest, the patient removes the remaining crutch and places it against the wheelchair. He is then able to grasp the remaining armrest.

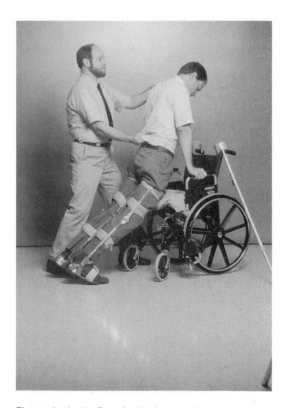

Figure 9.12–11. Grasping both armrests.

The patient turns and lowers himself into the wheelchair.

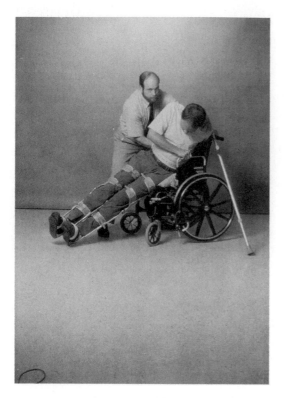

Figure 9.12–12. Turning and lowering onto wheelchair.

Repositioning his upper extremities, the patient adjusts his position in the wheelchair.

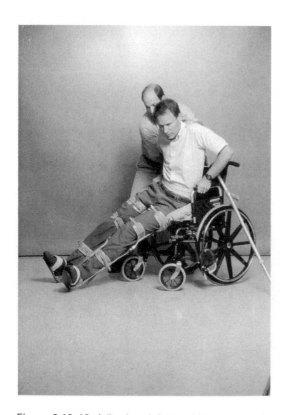

Figure 9.12–13. Adjusting sitting position.

The knee locks on the KAFOs are released.

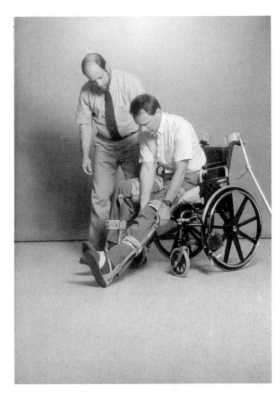

Figure 9.12–14. Unlocking knee locks on KAFOs.

Once the knee locks on the KAFOs are released, the patient can adjust his position further.

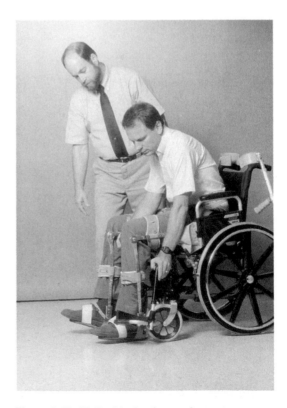

Figure 9.12–15. Positioning feet on footrests.

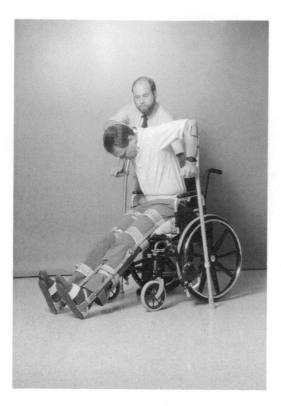

Figure 9.12–16. Crutches positioned.

Assuming Standing Using the Power Method

LO-15 The wheelchair is locked and the footrests moved out of the way. The patient is positioned toward the front edge of the seat. Positioned in stride, and behind and to one side of the patient, the therapist grasps the patient's gait belt and shoulder. The therapist must be prepared to move as the patient moves to avoid interfering with the patient's fluid motion.

With the knee locks of the KAFOs secured, the patient grasps one crutch in each hand. The tips of the crutches are placed on the floor even with his hips on either side of the wheelchair.

Pushing on the crutches, the patient extends his upper extremities and depresses his shoulders to produce a quick thrusting movement that propels his body upward and forward into a standing position.

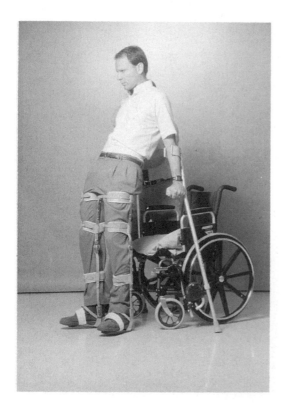

Figure 9.12–17. Assuming standing.

The patient must move the crutches forward quickly to halt the forward momentum of his body.

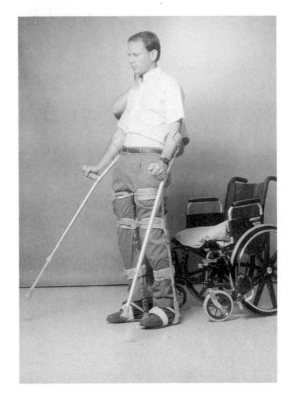

Figure 9.12–18. Moving crutches forward.

The patient places the crutches slightly ahead, and to the side, of his toes, and assumes a "C" curve. The therapist can assist the patient into the "C" curve position by pushing forward on the gait belt and pulling backward on the patient's shoulder.

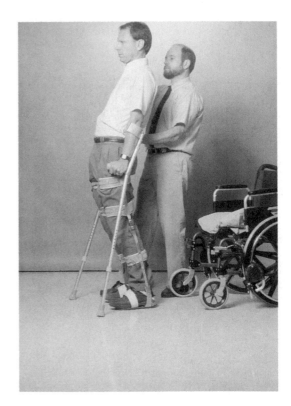

Figure 9.12–19. Crutches positioned for ambulation.

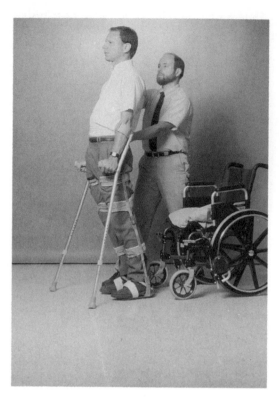

Figure 9.12–20. Starting position to assume sitting.

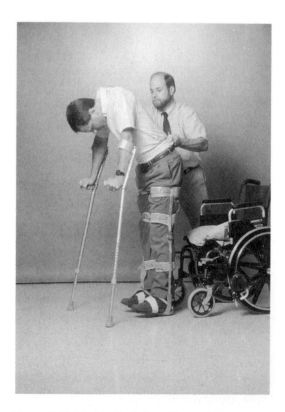

Figure 9.12–21. "Jackknife" position to initiate lowering.

Assuming Sitting Using the Power Method

LO-15   The wheelchair is locked and the footrests moved out of the way. Positioned in stride, slightly behind and to the side, the therapist grasps the patient's gait belt and shoulder. The therapist must be prepared to move as the patient moves to avoid interfering with the patient's fluid motion.

To sit, the patient stands facing away from the wheelchair with his feet approximately 12 to 18 inches in front of the front edge of the seat. The position of the feet must permit the patient to end up sitting securely in the seat as he lowers himself with the knee locks of the KAFOs locked.

Moving his shoulders anterior to his hips, the patient flexes at the hips into a "jackknife" position. The patient permits himself to start falling backward, initiating lowering into the wheelchair.

As the patient sits, the crutches are lifted.

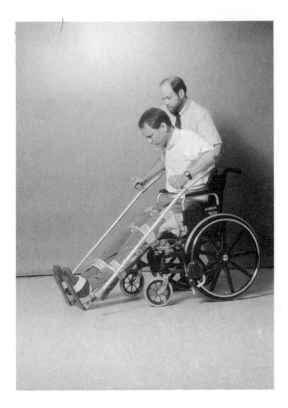

Figure 9.12–22. Lowering to sitting and lifting crutches.

After the patient is seated, the knee locks on the KAFOs are released. Once the KAFOs have been unlocked the patient can adjust his position further.

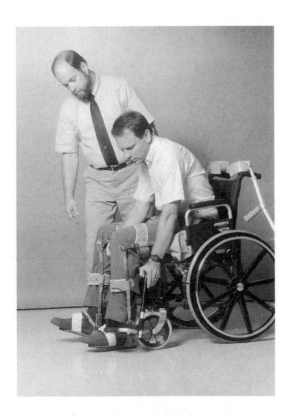

Figure 9.12–23. Positioning feet on footrests.

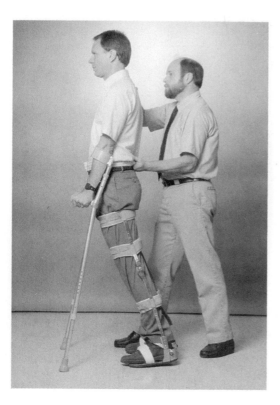

Figure 9.12–24. Starting position for ambulation using swing-to gait pattern.

Ambulating Using a Swing-To Gait Pattern

LO-15 Positioned in stride, slightly behind and to the side, the therapist grasps the patient's gait belt and shoulder. The therapist must be prepared to move as the patient moves to avoid interfering with the patient's fluid motion.

In the starting position the patient's hips are maintained in extension by keeping his shoulders behind his hips in a "C" curve. The therapist can assist in maintaining a "C" curve by pushing forward with the hand on the gait belt while pulling backward with the hand on the shoulder.

To initiate the swing-to gait pattern, the patient advances the crutches one stride length beyond the patient's toes. The therapist advances his right, or outside, foot.

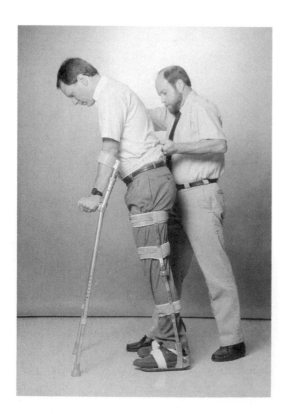

Figure 9.12–25. Initiating lift.

Pushing down on the crutches, the patient extends his upper extremities and depresses his shoulders. At the same time he flexes his trunk to lift his feet off the ground. The therapist may assist by lifting with the hand on the gait belt.

With his feet off the ground and his trunk flexed, gravity will swing the patient's lower extremities forward. As his lower extremities swing forward, the patient begins to extend his neck and trunk to regain the "C" curve. With his feet placed on the floor between the crutches, momentum continues to move the patient's hips anterior to his shoulders. As the patient swings forward the therapist steps forward with his left, or inside, foot. The therapist may assist the patient to regain a "C" curve by pushing forward with the hand on the gait belt and pulling backward with the hand on the patient's shoulder.

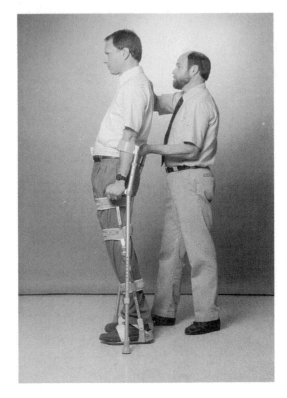

Figure 9.12–26. Regaining "C" curve.

Once the "C" curve is regained, the crutches are advanced.

The sequence is repeated for continued progression.

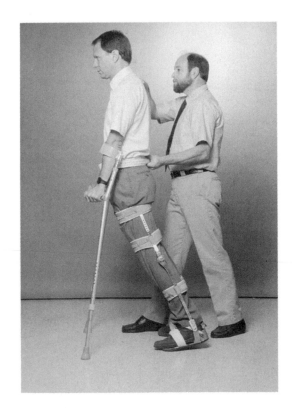

Figure 9.12–27. Crutches moved forward.

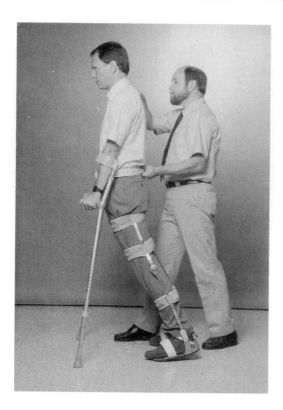

Figure 9.12–28. Starting position for ambulation using swing-through gait pattern.

Ambulating Using a Swing-Through Gait Pattern

LO-15

The swing-through gait pattern is essentially the same as the swing-to gait pattern. The role and position of the therapist are the same. The difference is that during the swing phase of the swing-through gait pattern the patient swings beyond the crutches, and lands anterior to the placement of the crutch tips.

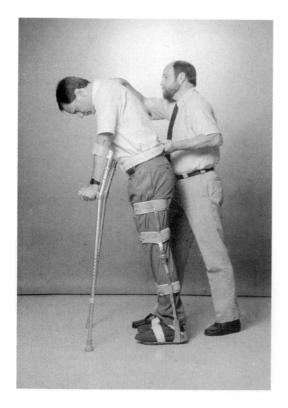

Figure 9.12–29. Initiating lift.

Pushing down on the crutches, the patient extends his upper extremities and depresses his shoulders. At the same time, he flexes his trunk to lift his feet off the ground. The therapist may assist by lifting with the hand on the gait belt.

With his feet off the ground and his trunk flexed, gravity will swing the patient's lower extremities forward. As his lower extremities swing forward, the patient extends his neck and trunk to regain the "C" curve. He lands with his feet anterior to the crutches. As the patient swings forward the therapist steps forward with his left, or inside, foot.

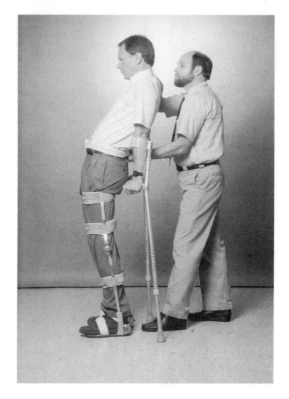

Figure 9.12–30. Completing swing-through into "C" curve.

Because of the momentum generated by the larger swing, the crutches must be advanced quickly to prevent the patient from falling. As the crutches are advanced, the therapist steps forward with his right, or outside, foot.

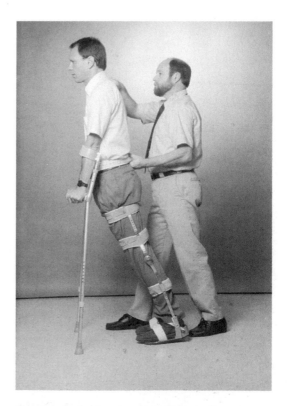

Figure 9.12–31. Crutches moved forward.

Falling

LO-15 When a patient starts to fall, the therapist must decide whether to prevent the fall, or to permit a controlled fall in a manner that will prevent injury to the patient or himself. The therapist must be alert to a patient's movements at all times, and be able to react quickly to prevent or control a fall. Proper guarding and attention focused on the patient are required at all times.

Patients with paraplegia tend to fall because they lose their "C" curve, or momentum into the "C" is interrupted, causing them to "jackknife."

The most effective method of preventing a fall in these situations is for the therapist to assist the patient in regaining the "C" curve. This is achieved by pulling the patient's shoulders backward while pushing forward with the hand on the gait belt.

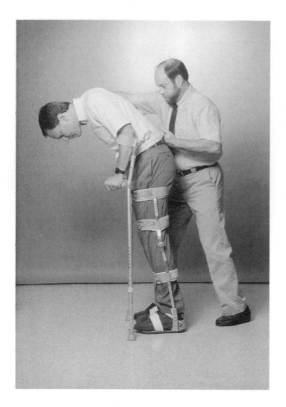

Figure 9.12–32. Loss of "C" curve.

When the therapist cannot prevent the fall, he must control the fall. The patient is instructed to let the crutches fall to the sides, away from the area in which the patient will land, to avoid injury from landing on the crutches. The therapist steps forward in his stride position to widen his base of support as he slows the rate at which the patient falls.

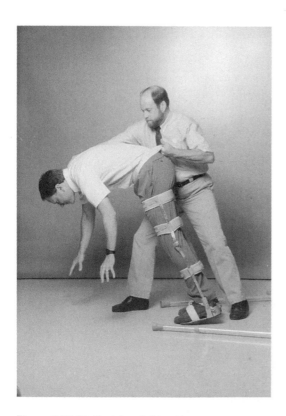

Figure 9.12–33. Crutches fall to side.

The patient catches himself on his outstretched hands, making sure that the elbows flex to absorb the impact. When elbow flexion is not permitted, injury to the patient's upper extremities may occur.

The therapist continues to lower the patient to the floor slowly.

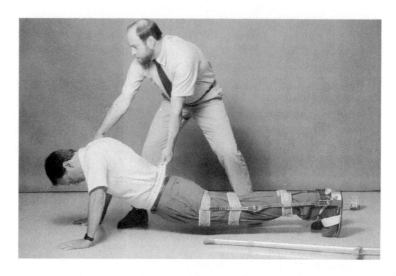

Figure 9.12–34. Patient lands on upper extremities with elbow flexion.

Assuming Standing from the Floor

LO-15

It is a difficult maneuver for a patient with KAFOs and forearm crutches to assume standing from the floor independently. The most practical method is to move along the floor to a chair or other sturdy object, and use the object as support to arise from the floor. Methods of moving from the floor to a sitting position in a chair are described in the Chapter 8 section, "Independent Transfer From Wheelchair to Floor and Return."

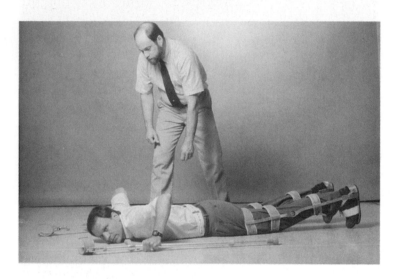

Figure 9.12–35. Crutches positioned at sides.

To assume standing directly from a prone position on the floor, the patient must first retrieve his crutches. The crutches are positioned with the tips toward his feet and with the handgrips approximately at the level of his shoulders.

Grasping one crutch below the handgrip, the patient places it upright with the tip of the crutch on the floor. The patient's other hand is placed on the floor at the level of the shoulder. Pushing with the hand on the floor and pulling with the hand on the crutch, the patient raises his trunk. Positioned in stride, slightly behind and to the side, the therapist grasps the patient's gait belt and shoulder. The therapist may assist by lifting with the hand on the gait belt.

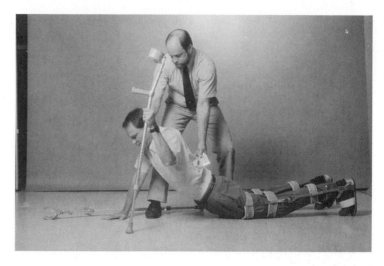

Figure 9.12–36. Grasping one crutch.

With his weight shifted onto the upper extremity that is on the floor, the patient shifts his grasp on the crutch to the handgrip. Pushing down on the handgrip and floor, the patient assumes a "jackknife" position. The therapist may assist by lifting on the gait belt. The therapist may also need to block the patient's feet to prevent them from sliding posteriorly.

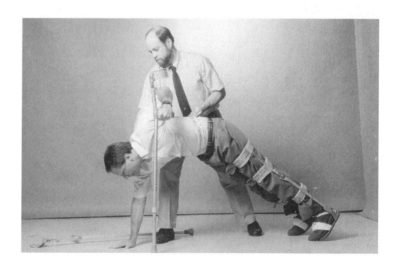

Figure 9.12–37. Pushing on handgrip and floor to assume "jackknife" position.

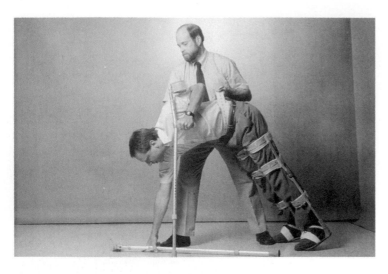

After shifting his weight onto the upright crutch, the patient grasps the handgrip of remaining crutch.

Figure 9.12–38. Retrieving second crutch.

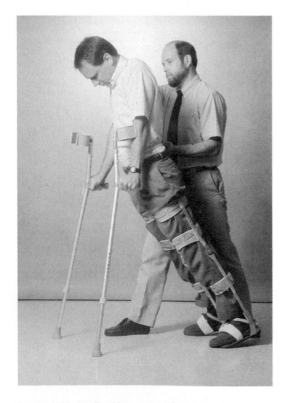

The second crutch is positioned upright with the tip on the floor in line with the tip of the first crutch. The patient then uses both crutches to push through an upright position, into a "C" curve.

Figure 9.12–39. Pushing on two handgrips to assume "C" curve.

The crutches are properly positioned one at a time.

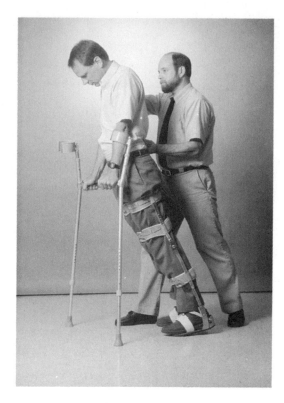

Figure 9.12–40. Left crutch positioned.

The patient is ready to ambulate.

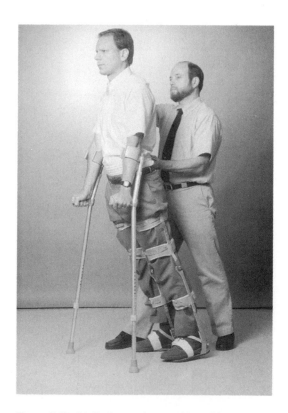

Figure 9.12–41. Both crutches positioned for ambulation.

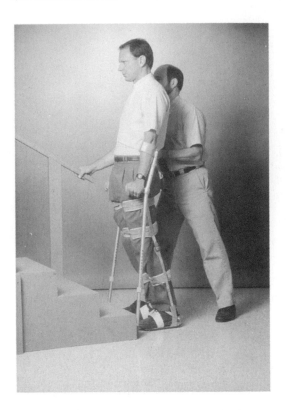

Figure 9.12–42. Starting position to ascend stairs forward.

Stairs

LO-15

There are two basic methods for a patient using KAFOs and forearm crutches to ambulate on the stairs, the forward and the backward methods. In both methods, patients may use a handrail and one crutch, or two crutches. In both methods, the therapist is positioned in stride on the stairs below the patient, and grasps the patient's gait belt and the handrail. Initially, gait training on stairs may require the assistance of two people to ensure patient safety.

Ascending—Forward Method

To ascend stairs using the forward method, the patient starts in a "C" curve position while facing up the stairs. The feet and crutch tips are parallel with the base of the stair.

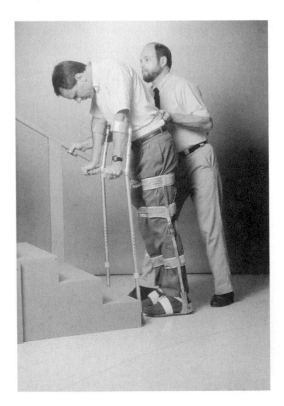

Figure 9.12–43. Initiating lift.

The same motion used to initiate ambulation on level surfaces is used to initiate ambulation on stairs. Flexing his neck and upper trunk, the patient extends his upper extremities and depresses his shoulders to lift his body. The therapist may assist by lifting on the gait belt as the patient raises his body.

As his feet are lifted from the ground, gravity swings his lower extremities forward onto the next higher stair. The patient extends his neck and trunk to regain a "C" curve as he places his lower extremities onto the next higher stair. The therapist may assist the patient in regaining the "C" curve by pushing forward on the gait belt.

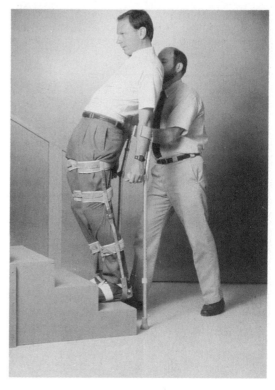

Figure 9.12–44. Lower extremities lifted to next stair.

The crutches are advanced to the same stair as the feet.
The sequence is repeated to ascend an entire flight of stairs.

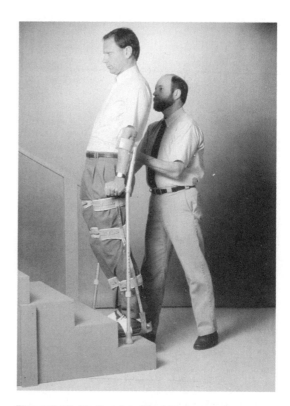

Figure 9.12–45. Crutches lifted to same stair.

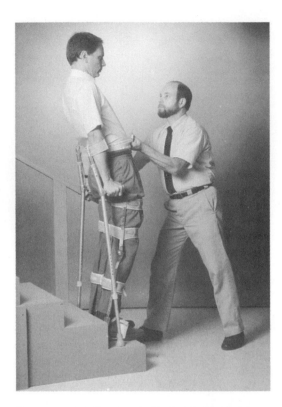

Figure 9.12–46. Starting position to descend stairs forward.

Descending—Forward Method

LO-15

To descend stairs using the forward method, the patient starts in a "C" curve position facing down the stairs. The feet and crutch tips are parallel with the base of the stair.

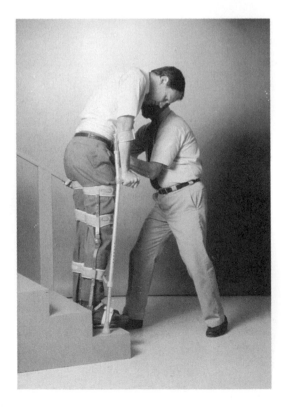

Figure 9.12–47. Initiating lift.

The same motion used to initiate ambulation on level surfaces is used to initiate ambulation on stairs. Flexing his neck and upper trunk, the patient extends his upper extremities and depresses his shoulders to lift his body. The therapist may assist by lifting on the gait belt as the patient raises his body.

As his feet are lifted from the ground, gravity swings his lower extremities forward over the next lower stair. As his lower extremities swing over the stair, the patient uses his upper extremities to lower himself in a controlled manner onto the next lower stair. Extending his neck and trunk, the patient regains a "C" curve as he places his lower extremities on the next lower stair. The therapist may assist the patient in regaining the "C" curve by pulling forward on the gait belt.

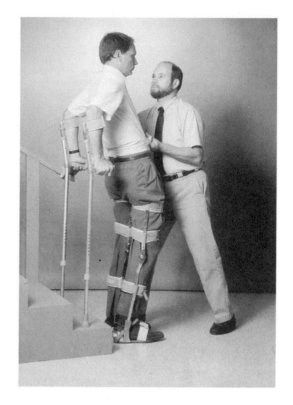

Figure 9.12–48. Lower extremities lowered to next stair.

The crutches are advanced onto the same stair as his lower extremities.

The patient often descends two steps at a time. The sequence is repeated to descend an entire flight of stairs.

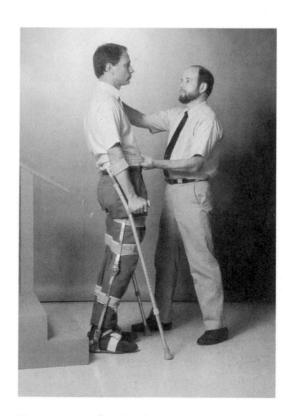

Figure 9.12–49. Crutches lowered to same stair.

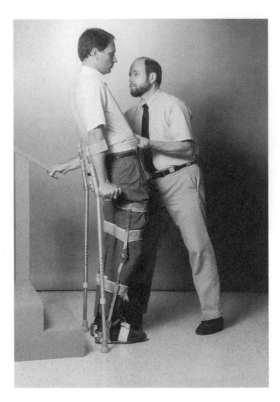

Figure 9.12–50. Starting position to ascend stairs backward.

Ascending—Backward Method

LO-15

To ascend stairs using the backward method, the patient starts in a "C" curve position while facing away from the stairs. The feet and crutch tips are parallel with the base of the stair.

The same motion used to initiate ambulation on level surfaces is used to initiate ambulation on stairs. Flexing his neck and upper trunk, the patient extends his upper extremities and depresses his shoulders to lift his body. The therapist may assist by lifting and pushing on the gait belt as the patient raises his body. Because the therapist's push is into the abdominal area, the therapist must be careful not to injure the patient.

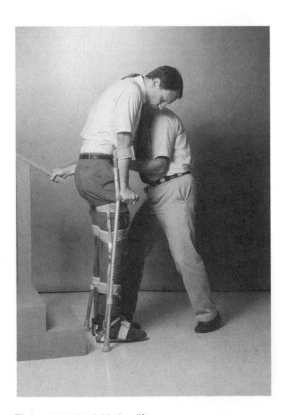

Figure 9.12–51. Initiating lift.

As the patient lifts into a "jackknife" position, the backward momentum of his lower extremities moves them up and over the next higher stair. The patient uses his upper extremities to lower himself onto the next higher stair.

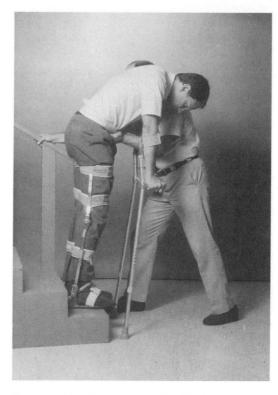

Figure 9.12–52. Lower extremities lifted to next stair.

Once the patient's lower extremities are on the next higher stair, the patient permits his pelvis to move forward. As this movement occurs, he extends his neck and trunk to regain a "C" curve, and moves his crutches onto the same stair as his lower extremities. The therapist may assist the patient in regaining the "C" curve by pulling forward on the gait belt.

The sequence is repeated to ascend an entire flight of stairs.

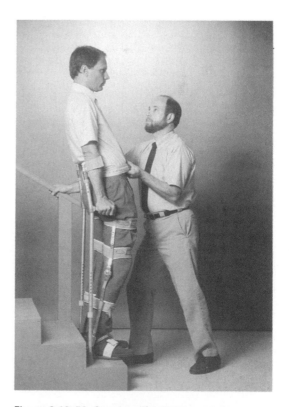

Figure 9.12–53. Crutches lifted to same stair.

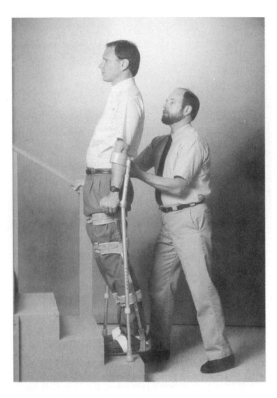

Figure 9.12–54. Starting position to descend stairs backward.

Descending—Backward Method

LO-15

To descend stairs using the backward method, the patient starts in a "C" curve position while facing up the stairs. The feet and crutch tips are parallel with the base of the stair.

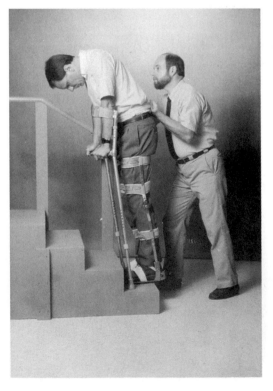

Figure 9.12–55. Initiating lift.

The same motion used to initiate ambulation on level surfaces is used to initiate ambulation on stairs. Flexing his neck and upper trunk, the patient extends his upper extremities and depresses his shoulders to lift his body. The therapist may assist by lifting on the gait belt as the patient raises his body.

As the patient lifts into a "jackknife" position, the backward momentum of his lower extremities moves them over the next lower stair. Once the patient's lower extremities are over the stair, the patient uses his upper extremities to lower himself in a controlled manner onto the next lower stair.

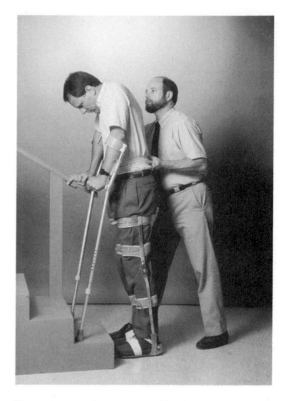

Figure 9.12–56. Lower extremities lowered to next stair.

After his lower extremities are on the next lower stair, the patient permits his pelvis to move forward. As this movement occurs, he extends his neck and trunk to regain a "C" curve and moves his crutches onto the same stair as his lower extremities. The therapist may assist the patient in regaining the "C" curve by pushing forward on the gait belt.

The sequence is repeated to descend an entire flight of stairs.

Doorways

Patients using forearm crutches maneuver through doorways in the same manner as do patients using axillary crutches.

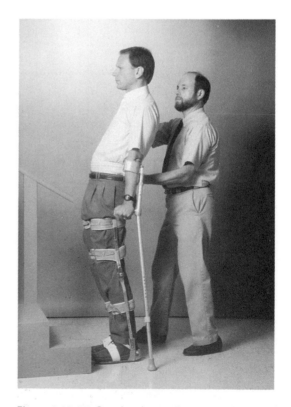

Figure 9.12–57. Crutches lowered to same stair.

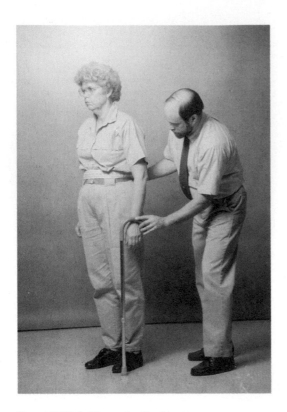

Figure 9.13–1. Measuring fit of cane.

9.13   ONE CANE

Fitting

LO-11

Canes are fitted with the patient standing and the shoulders relaxed. The cane is positioned upright, with the tip on the floor alongside the small toe. With the cane in this position, the top of the cane is adjusted to be at the level of the patient's ulnar styloid process. This permits 20 to 30 degree elbow flexion when the cane is held in the patient's hand. When used properly, the force on the cane should be exerted directly downward.

Figure 9.13–2. Checking amount of elbow flexion.

When using a quad cane, the longer legs of the cane are positioned away from the patient. This reduces the risk of a patient's foot becoming entangled in the legs of the quad cane. A quad cane is measured and used in the same manner as the standard cane.

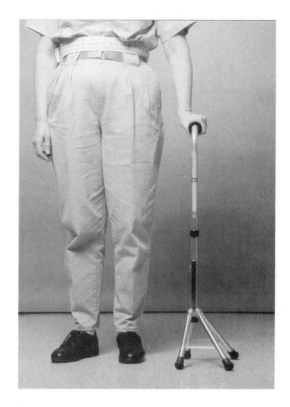

Figure 9.13–3. Position of quad cane base for ambulation.

In and Out of a Wheelchair

Assuming Standing—Quad Cane and Armrests

LO-15

The wheelchair is locked and the footrests moved out of the way. The patient is positioned at the front edge of the seat, with her feet in stride or side by side. Positioned in stride, and behind and to one side of the patient, the therapist grasps the patient's gait belt and shoulder.

The quad cane is positioned alongside the foot on the side on which it will be held. Both hands are placed on their respective armrests and used by the patient to push downward to assume standing. When the patient has only one functional upper extremity, that upper extremity is used on the armrest to push to standing. In the illustrations for this section, the patient is demonstrating the use of only one functional upper extremity.

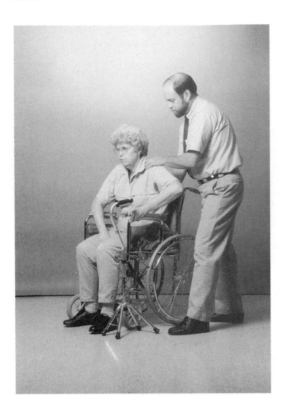

Figure 9.13–4. Starting position to assume standing using armrest.

The patient pushes to standing, making sure she is erect and balanced.

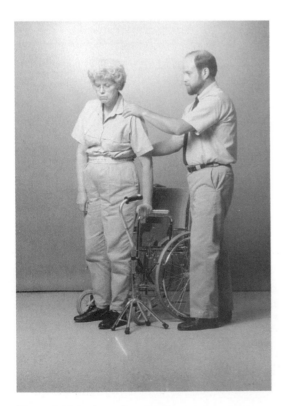

Figure 9.13–5. Assuming standing.

Once standing, she grasps the quad cane.
The patient is ready to ambulate.

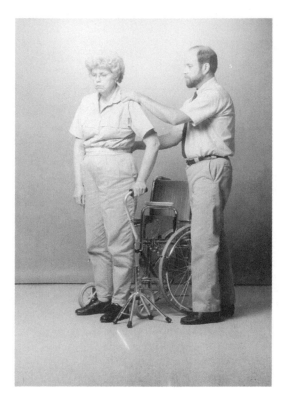

Figure 9.13–6. Grasping quad cane for ambulation.

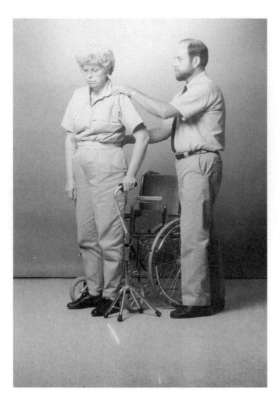

Figure 9.13–7. Starting position to assume sitting using armrest.

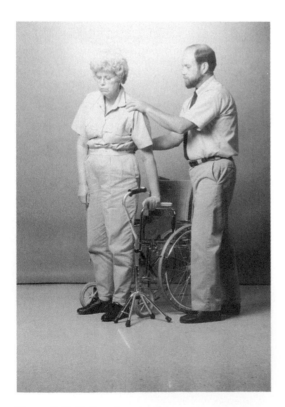

Figure 9.13–8. Grasping armrest.

Assuming Sitting—Quad Cane and Armrests

LO-15

The wheelchair is locked and the footrests moved out of the way. To sit, the patient positions herself at the front edge of the wheelchair seat, facing away from the wheelchair. The front edge of the wheelchair seat is felt against the back of the lower extremities. The patient's feet are positioned in stride or side by side. Positioned in stride, and behind and to one side of the patient, the therapist grasps the patient's gait belt and shoulder.

When the patient has only one functional upper extremity, she releases the quad cane, and grasps the armrest on that side of the wheelchair.

While grasping the armrest, the patient lowers herself in a controlled manner onto the seat.

The patient moves completely into the seat and positions herself appropriately.

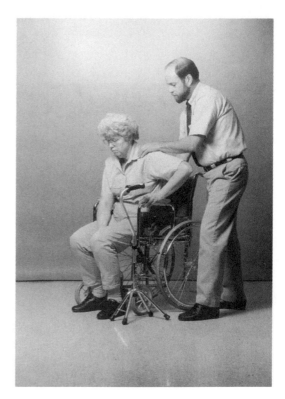

Figure 9.13–9. Lowering to sitting.

Assuming Standing—Quad Cane Only

LO-15
Patients with sufficient strength and balance may assume standing using the quad cane instead of the armrest for support.

The wheelchair is locked and the footrests moved out of the way. The patient is positioned at the front edge of the seat, with her feet in stride or side by side. Positioned in stride, and behind and to one side of the patient, the therapist grasps the patient's gait belt and shoulder.

The quad cane is positioned alongside the foot on the side on which it will be held. One hand is placed on the armrest and the other hand is placed on the quad cane. When the patient has only one functional upper extremity, that upper extremity is used on the quad cane to push to standing. The patient must push directly downward to prevent the cane from tipping. In the illustrations for this section, the patient is demonstrating the use of only one functional upper extremity.

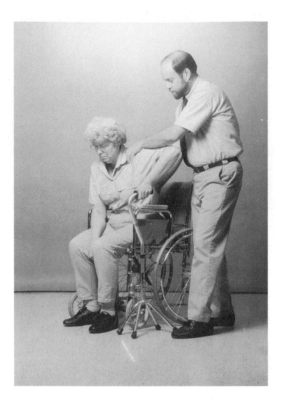

Figure 9.13–10. Starting position to assume standing using quad cane.

The patient pushes to standing, making sure she is erect and balanced.

The patient is ready to ambulate.

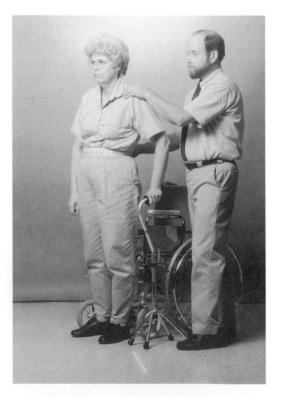

Figure 9.13–11. Assuming standing.

8

Assuming Sitting—Quad Cane Only

LO-15 The wheelchair is locked and the footrests moved out of the way. To sit, the patient positions herself at the front edge of the wheelchair seat, facing away from the wheelchair. The front edge of the wheelchair seat is felt against the back of the lower extremities. The patient's feet are positioned in stride or side by side. Positioned in stride, and behind and to one side of the patient, the therapist grasps the patient's gait belt and shoulder.

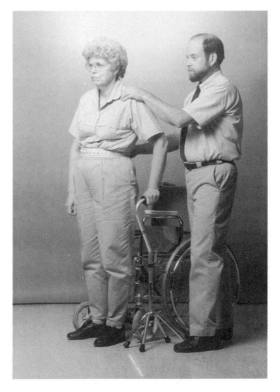

Figure 9.13–12. Starting position to assume sitting using quad cane.

While grasping the quad cane, the patient lowers herself in a controlled manner onto the seat.

Setting the quad cane aside, the patient moves completely into the seat and positions herself appropriately.

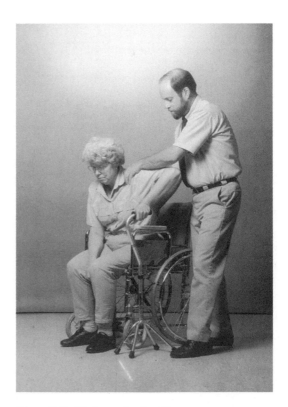

Figure 9.13–13. Lowering to sitting.

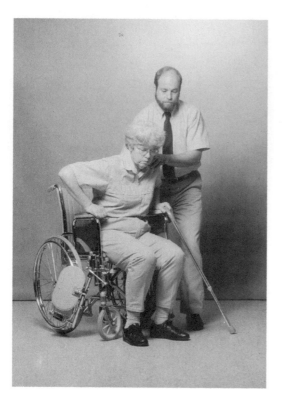

Figure 9.13–14. Starting position to assume standing using armrests and cane.

Assuming Standing—Standard Cane and Armrests

LO-15

The wheelchair is locked and the footrests moved out of the way. The patient is positioned at the front edge of the seat with her feet in stride or side by side. Positioned in stride, and behind and to one side of the patient, the therapist grasps the patient's gait belt and shoulder.

When using a standard cane, both hands are placed on their respective armrests. The cane is grasped in the same hand as it will be used for ambulation. Thus, the patient must grasp both the cane and armrest at the same time with this hand. In the illustrations for this section, the patient is demonstrating the use of two functional upper extremities.

Pushing downward on both armrests, the patient pushes to standing.

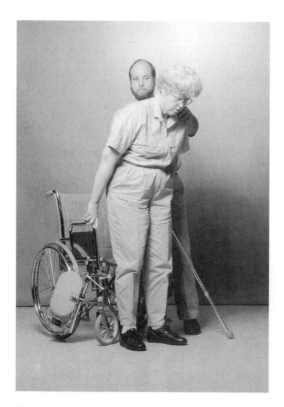

Figure 9.13–15. Assuming standing.

Once standing, the patient releases her grasp on the arm-rests, stands erect, and positions the cane.

The patient is ready to ambulate.

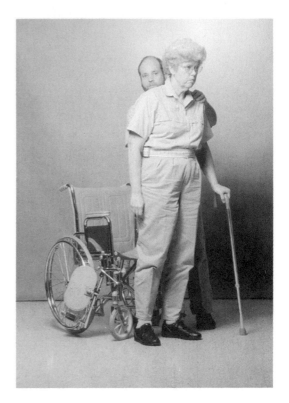

Figure 9.13–16. Positioning cane for ambulation.

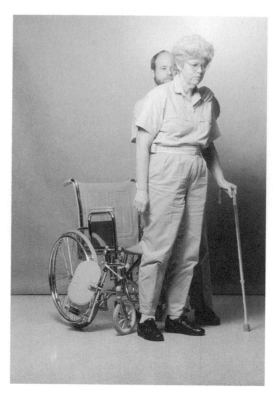

Figure 9.13–17. Starting position to assume sitting using armrests and cane.

Assuming Sitting—Standard Cane and Armrests

LO-15 The wheelchair is locked and the footrests moved out of the way. To sit, the patient positions herself at the front edge of the wheelchair seat, facing away from the wheelchair. The front edge of the wheelchair seat is felt against the back of the lower extremities. The patient's feet are positioned in stride or side by side. Positioned in stride, and behind and to one side of the patient, the therapist grasps the patient's gait belt and shoulder.

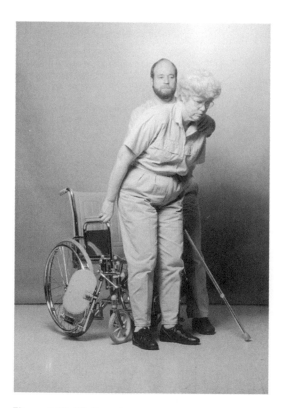

Figure 9.13–18. Grasping armrests.

The patient grasps the armrests with both hands. This may be performed with both hands simultaneously, or the hands may be moved one at a time. The cane is grasped in the same hand in which it was used for ambulation. The cane and armrest are held together by the hand that grasps the cane.

The patient lowers herself in a controlled manner onto the seat.

Setting the cane aside, the patient moves completely into the seat and positions herself appropriately.

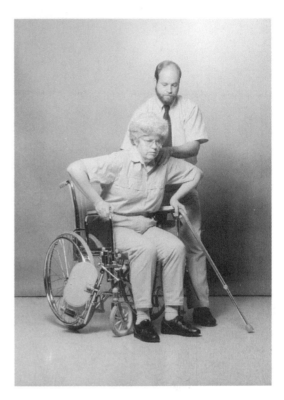

Figure 9.13–19. Lowering to sitting.

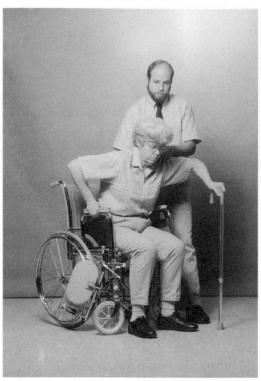

Figure 9.13–20. Starting position to assume standing using cane and one armrest.

Assuming Standing—Standard Cane and Armrest

LO-15 The wheelchair is locked and the footrests moved out of the way. The patient is positioned at the front edge of the seat, with her feet in stride or side by side. Positioned in stride, and behind and to one side of the patient, the therapist grasps the patient's gait belt and shoulder.

The cane is positioned alongside the foot on the side on which it will be held. One hand is placed on the armrest and the other hand is placed on the cane. The patient must push directly downward on the cane to prevent the cane from tipping. When the patient has only one functional upper extremity, that upper extremity is used on the cane to push to standing. In the illustrations for this section, the patient is demonstrating the use of two functional upper extremities.

The patient pushes to standing.

Figure 9.13–21. Assuming standing.

Once standing and balanced, the patient releases her grasp on the armrest and stands erect.

The patient is ready to ambulate.

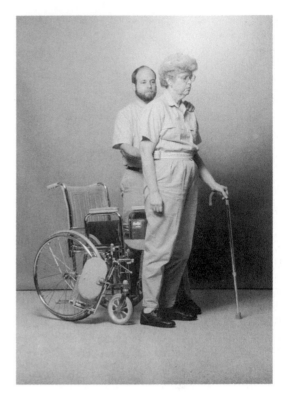

Figure 9.13–22. Releasing armrest and positioning cane for ambulation.

Assuming Sitting—Standard Cane and Armrest

 LO-15 The wheelchair is locked and the footrests moved out of the way. To sit, the patient positions herself at the front edge of the wheelchair seat, facing away from the wheelchair. The front edge of the wheelchair seat is felt against the back of the lower extremities. The patient's feet are positioned in stride or side by side. Positioned in stride, and behind and to one side of the patient, the therapist grasps the patient's gait belt and shoulder.

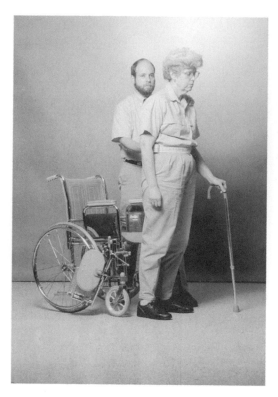

Figure 9.13–23. Starting position to assume sitting using cane and one armrest.

While continuing to use the cane, the patient reaches back and grasps the armrest with the opposite hand.

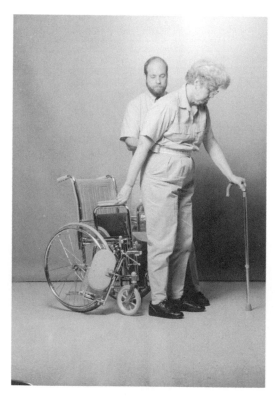

Figure 9.13–24. Grasping armrest.

The patient lowers herself in a controlled manner onto the seat.

Setting the cane aside, the patient moves completely into the seat and positions herself appropriately.

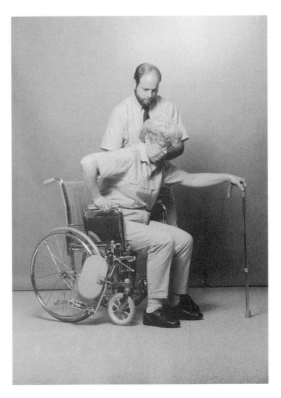

Figure 9.13–25. Lowering to sitting.

Ambulating Using One Cane

LO-15

The gait pattern and sequence when using one standard cane or one quad cane are the same.

Positioned in stride, behind and to one side of the patient, the therapist grasps the patient's gait belt and shoulder. The patient's feet are side by side, with the cane next to the small toe.

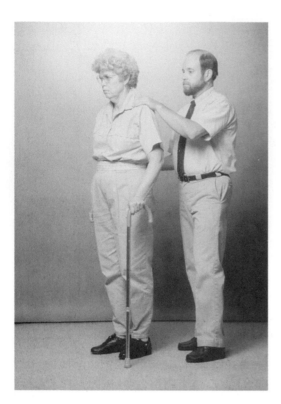

Figure 9.13–26. Starting position for ambulation using one cane.

The cane is advanced first, approximately one stride length ahead. The therapist steps forward with his left, or outside, foot.

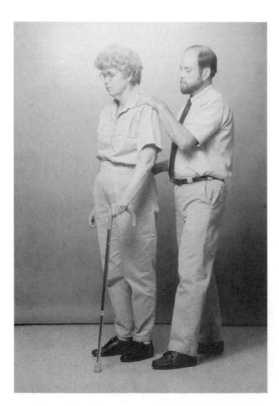

Figure 9.13–27. Cane moved forward.

The patient advances the lower extremity on the side op-posite the cane up to the cane.

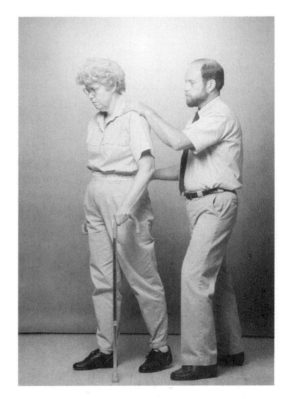

Figure 9.13–28. Lower extremity opposite cane moved forward.

The patient advances the lower extremity on the same side as the cane. The therapist advances his right, or inside, foot as the patient moves her lower extremity. Initially, the patient may only step to the other lower extremity and cane, but should be encouraged to step beyond the other lower extremity and cane. This encourages the patient to develop a more normal rhythm and pattern of gait.

The sequence is repeated for continued progression.

As the patient improves, she may move the cane and in-volved lower extremity at the same time, permitting a faster pace of gait.

As the patient is able, she uses the cane on the involved side, moving the cane and involved lower extremity simul-taneously.

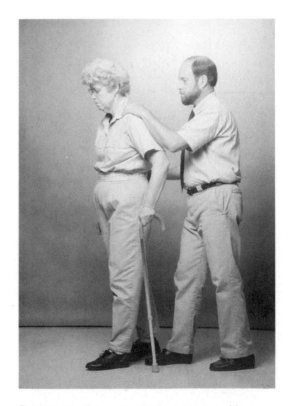

Figure 9.13–29. Lower extremity on same side as cane moved forward.

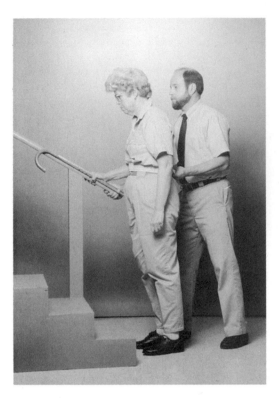

Figure 9.13–30. Cane held parallel to handrail for stairs.

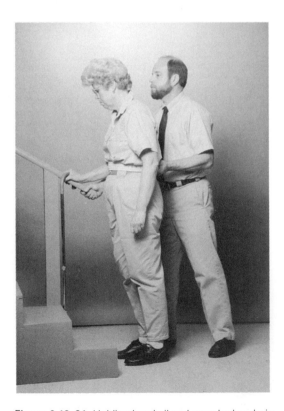

Figure 9.13–31. Holding handrail and cane by handgrip for stairs.

Stairs

Holding the Cane

LO-15

Initially, patients should be taught to use a handrail for more stability. A patient who uses a cane on the left side continues to grasp the cane with the left hand, and grasps the handrail with the right hand. A patient who uses the cane in the right hand must do one of three things: 1) continue to use the cane in the right hand and not use the handrail, 2) switch the cane to the left hand and grasp the handrail with the right hand, or 3) grasp both the handrail and cane with the right hand. Patients with a functional right upper extremity only must either continue to use the cane without using the handrail, or grasp both the handrail and cane with the right hand.

There are two methods for grasping both the cane and handrail in the right hand. In one method the cane is held at midshaft, parallel to the handrail.

In the second method the cane is held at the handgrip and remains in a vertical position.

The base of a quad cane may be larger than a stair tread. In some cases, turning the quad cane sideways permits all four legs of the quad cane to be supported on the stair.

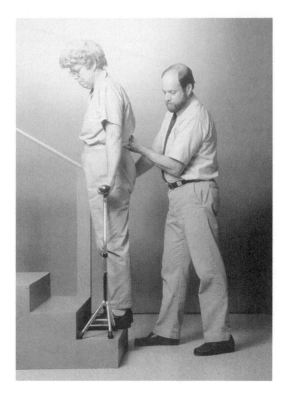

Figure 9.13–32. Position of quad cane for stairs.

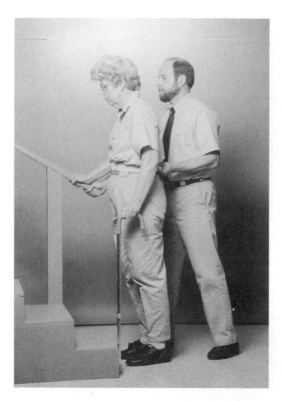

Figure 9.13–33. Starting position to ascend stairs using handrail and cane.

Ascending Using a Cane and Handrail

LO-15

Positioned in stride behind the patient, the therapist grasps the patient's gait belt and the handrail.

To ascend stairs, the patient stands facing up the stairs with her feet and cane parallel to the base of the first stair. In the illustrations for this section, the patient demonstrates the use of two functional upper extremities, permitting use of the cane in the left hand while grasping the handrail with the right hand.

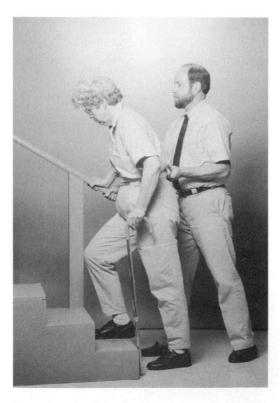

Figure 9.13–34. Uninvolved lower extremity lifted to next stair.

The uninvolved lower extremity is moved to the next higher stair, and weight is shifted onto this extremity.

Extending her uninvolved lower extremity, the patient lifts her body. The involved lower extremity is placed on the same stair as the uninvolved lower extremity.

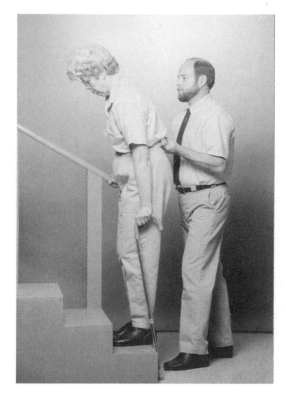

Figure 9.13–35. Involved lower extremity lifted to same stair.

The cane is advanced to the same stair as the lower extremities, and placed securely on the stair tread. As the patient improves her balance and strength, the cane and involved lower extremity may be moved simultaneously.

The sequence is repeated to ascend the remaining stairs.

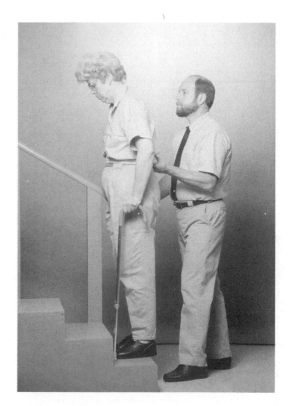

Figure 9.13–36. Cane lifted to same stair.

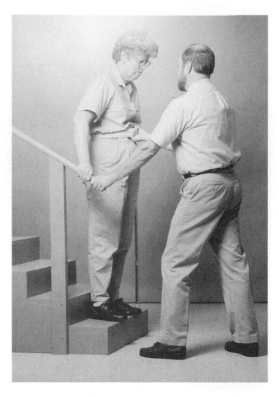

Figure 9.13–37. Starting position to descend stairs using handrail.

Descending Using a Cane and Handrail

LO-15   Positioned in stride in front of the patient, the therapist grasps the patient's gait belt and the handrail.

To descend stairs, the patient stands facing down the stairs, with her feet and cane parallel to the stair. In the illustrations for this section, the patient demonstrates the use of two functional upper extremities, permitting the use of the cane in the left hand while grasping the handrail with the right hand.

The cane is lowered to the next lower stair and placed securely on the stair tread.

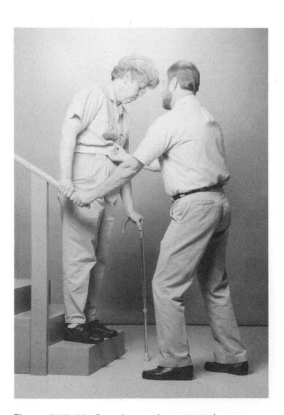

Figure 9.13–38. Cane lowered to next stair.

The patient lowers her involved lower extremity to the next lower stair by flexing her uninvolved lower extremity. As the patient improves her balance and strength, she may move the cane and involved lower extremity simultaneously.

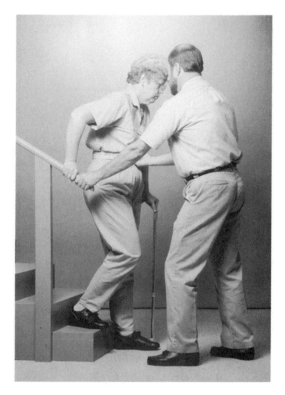

Figure 9.13–39. Involved lower extremity lowered to same stair.

Weight is shifted to the involved lower extremity and cane, and the uninvolved lower extremity is lowered to the same stair as the cane and involved lower extremity.

The sequence is repeated to descend the remaining stairs.

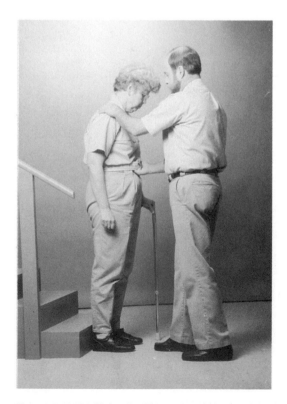

Figure 9.13–40. Uninvolved lower extremity lowered to same stair.

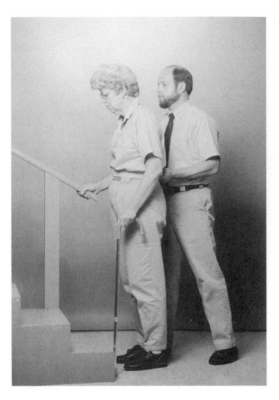

Figure 9.13–41. Starting position to ascend stairs using cane only.

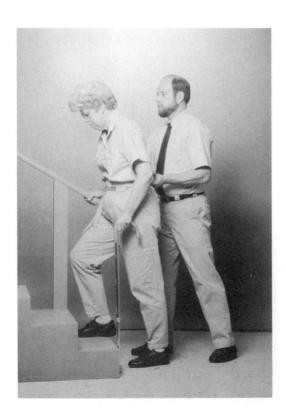

Figure 9.13–42. Uninvolved lower extremity lifted to next stair.

Ascending Using a Cane

LO-15 Positioned in stride behind the patient, the therapist grasps the patient's gait belt and the handrail.

To ascend stairs, the patient stands facing up the stairs with her feet and cane parallel to the base of the first stair. In the illustrations for this section, the patient demonstrates the use of only one cane without using a handrail. The hand seen on the handrail is that of the therapist.

The uninvolved lower extremity is moved to the next higher stair, and weight is shifted onto this extremity.

Extending her uninvolved lower extremity, the patient lifts her body. The involved lower extremity is placed on the same stair as the uninvolved lower extremity.

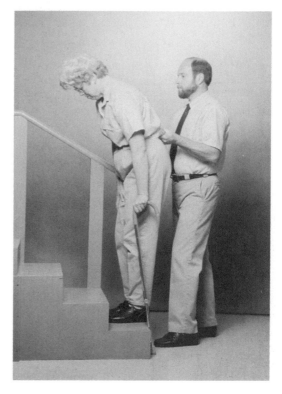

Figure 9.13–43. Involved lower extremity lifted to same stair.

The cane is advanced to the same stair as the lower extremities, and placed securely on the stair tread. As the patient improves her balance and strength, the cane and involved lower extremity may be moved simultaneously.

The sequence is repeated to ascend the remaining stairs.

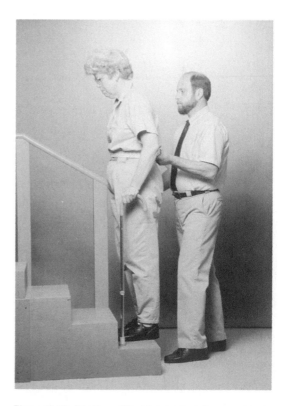

Figure 9.13–44. Cane lifted to same stair

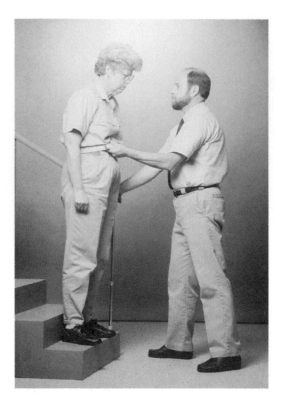

Figure 9.13–45. Starting position to descend stairs using cane only.

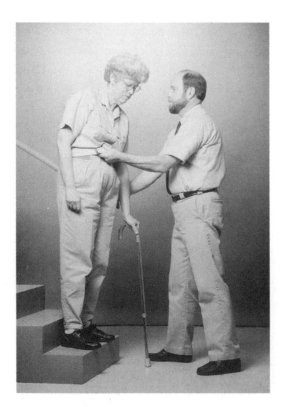

Figure 9.13–46. Cane lowered to next stair.

Descending Using a Cane

 Positioned in stride in front of the patient, the therapist grasps the patient's gait belt and the handrail.

LO-15 To descend stairs, the patient stands facing down the stairs, with her feet and cane parallel to the stair. In the illustrations for this section, the patient demonstrates the use of only one cane without using a handrail.

The cane is lowered to the next lower stair and placed securely on the stair tread.

The patient lowers her involved lower extremity to the next lower stair by flexing her uninvolved lower extremity. As the patient improves her balance and strength, she may move the cane and involved lower extremity simultaneously.

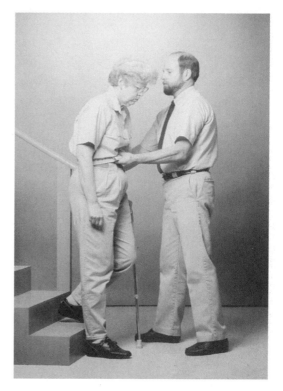

Figure 9.13–47. Involved lower extremity lowered to same stair.

Weight is shifted to the involved lower extremity and cane, and the uninvolved lower extremity is lowered to the same stair as the cane and involved lower extremity.

The sequence is repeated to descend the remaining stairs.

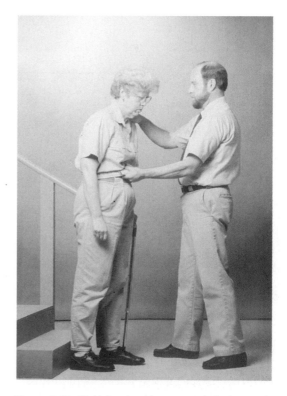

Figure 9.13–48. Uninvolved lower extremity lowered to same stair.

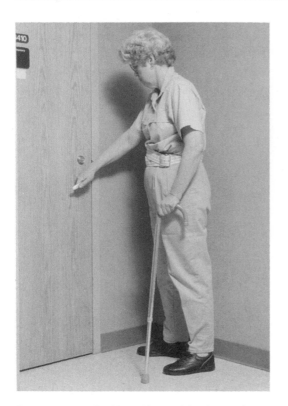

Figure 9.13–49. Positioned beyond door's arc of motion with cane toward hinge edge.

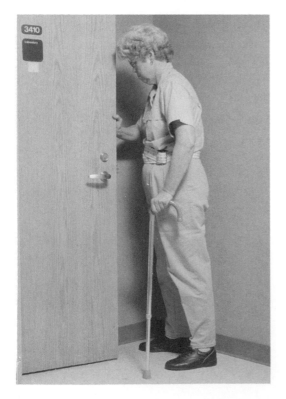

Figure 9.13–50. Opening door.

Doorways With Automatic Door Closers

LO-15

In each of the sections concerning ambulating through doorways with a cane, the patient is demonstrating the use of two functional upper extremities. When a patient has only one functional upper extremity, the cane must be held by the hand of the functional extremity while it manipulates the door handle and door.

Door Opens Toward the Patient—Cane at Hinge Edge

In the illustrations for this section, the cane is used in the patient's left hand, the hand closest to the hinge edge of the door as she faces the door.

The patient approaches the door and stands at the latch edge of the door, out of the arc of the opening door. The patient places her right hand on the door handle.

The door is opened wide enough to permit the patient to grasp the latch edge of the door before it closes. Unlike the sequences for a walker or crutches, the door is not opened completely in a single motion. Opening the door in a single motion when using one cane is often not possible when the patient must pull open the door by moving the upper extremity across the body. Attempting to do so can compromise the patient's safety.

The door is opened further, and the tip of the cane is placed on the floor in front to act as a door stop.

As the patient moves through the doorway, the tip of the cane is placed progressively closer to the hinge edge of the door to act as a door stop. The therapist and patient must be aware that as the tip of the cane is placed closer to the hinge edge of the door, the door becomes more difficult to block.

The patient continues to move through the doorway, using the tip of the cane as a door stop. Once the patient has moved completely through the doorway, the door closes behind her.

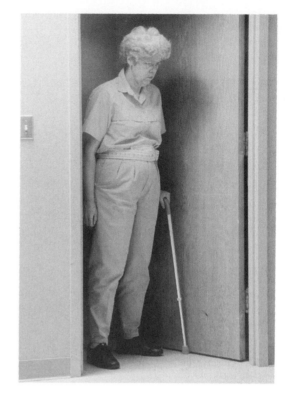

Figure 9.13–51. Tip of cane used to block door closing.

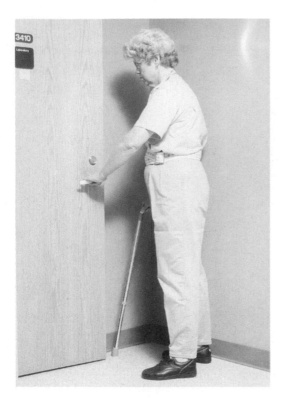

Figure 9.13–52. Positioned beyond door's arc of motion with cane toward latch edge.

Door Opens Toward the Patient—Cane at Latch Edge

LO-15

In the illustrations for this section, the cane is used in the patient's right hand, the hand closest to the latch edge of the door as she faces the door.

The patient approaches the door and stands at the latch edge of the door, out of the arc of the opening door. The patient places her left hand on the door handle and opens the door.

The door is opened wide enough to permit the patient to move into the doorway. The patient moves her left hand from the door handle to the door and uses this hand to hold open the door.

The patient continues to move through the doorway, using her hand to hold open the door. Once the patient has moved completely through the doorway, the door closes behind her.

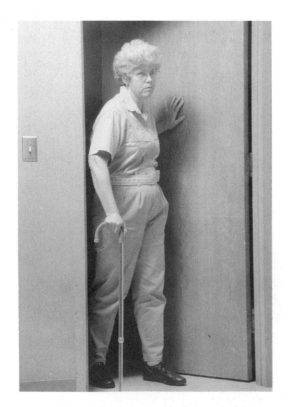

Figure 9.13–53. Hand used to block door closing.

Door Opens Away from the Patient—Cane at Hinge Edge

LO-15

In the illustrations for this section, the cane is used in the patient's right hand, the hand closest to the hinge edge of the door as she faces the door.

The patient approaches the door and places her left hand on the door handle.

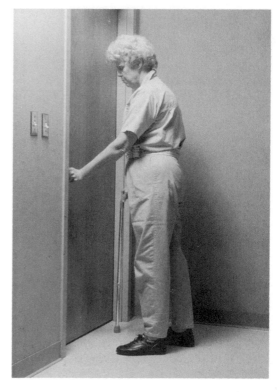

Figure 9.13–54. Approaching door with cane toward hinge edge.

The door is opened wide enough to permit the patient to enter the doorway. The tip of the cane is placed on the floor as a door stop. The door is not opened completely in a single motion.

As the patient moves through the doorway, the tip of the cane is placed progressively closer to the latch edge of the door to act as a door stop. Once the patient has moved completely through the doorway, the door closes behind her.

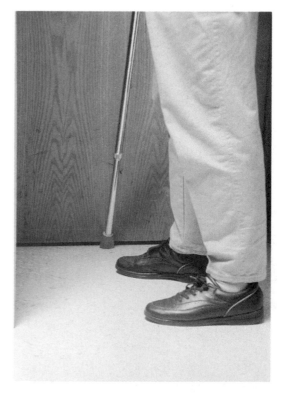

Figure 9.13–55. Tip of cane used to block door closing.

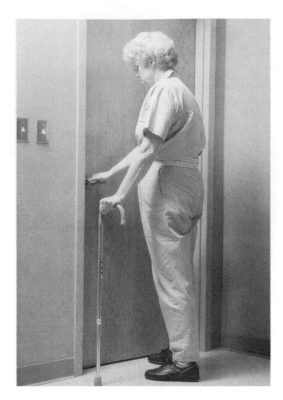

Figure 9.13–56. Approaching door with cane toward latch edge.

Door Opens Away from the Patient—Cane at Latch Edge

LO-15

In the illustrations for this section, the cane is used in the patient's left hand, the hand closest to the latch edge of the door as she faces the door.

The patient approaches the door and places her right hand on the door handle.

The door is pushed open wide enough to permit the patient to move into the doorway. The patient moves her right hand from the door handle to the door and uses this hand to hold open the door.

The patient continues to move through the doorway, using her hand to hold open the door. Once the patient has moved completely through the doorway, the door closes behind her.

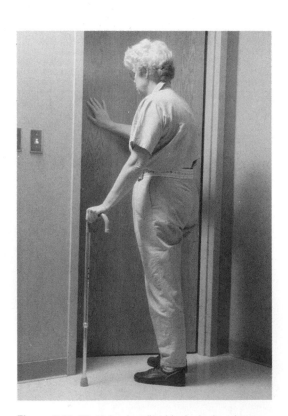

Figure 9.13–57. Using hand to block closing door.

9.14 TWO CANES

In and Out of a Wheelchair

Assuming standing and sitting using two canes is performed in a similar manner to these maneuvers when using one cane.

LO-15

Assuming Standing—Cane and Armrest in Each Hand

The wheelchair is locked and the footrests moved out of the way. The patient is positioned at the front edge of the seat, with her feet in stride or side by side. Positioned in stride, and behind and to one side of the patient, the therapist grasps the patient's gait belt and shoulder.

The tips of the canes are placed to the side, and slightly ahead of the patient's toes. The patient simultaneously grasps a cane and armrest in each hand. This places the shafts of the canes at an angle to the vertical.

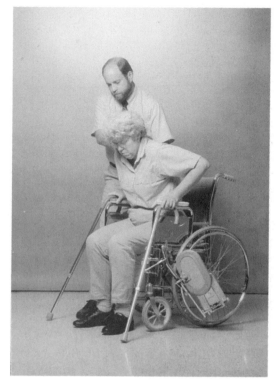

Figure 9.14–1. Starting position to assume standing using cane and armrest in each hand.

The patient assumes standing by extending her upper and lower extremities. During the initial phase of rising, the patient's upper extremity force is directed downward on the armrests. As the patient rises, she releases her grasp on the armrests, and completes the assumption of standing by supporting herself with the canes. Throughout the maneuver the tips of the canes remain in the same position on the floor, and the shafts of the canes move close to a vertical position when the patient is standing.

The patient is ready to ambulate.

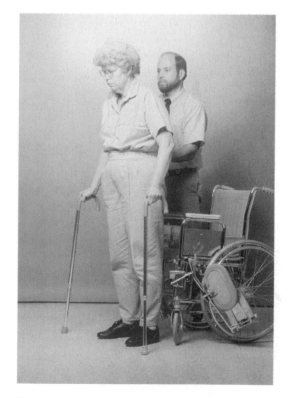

Figure 9.14–2. Assuming standing.

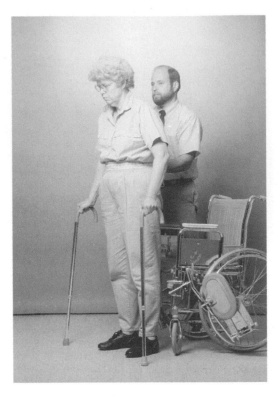

Figure 9.14–3. Starting position to assume sitting using cane and armrest in each hand.

Assuming Sitting—Cane and Armrest in Each Hand

LO-15

The wheelchair is locked and the footrests moved out of the way. To sit, the patient positions herself at the front edge of the wheelchair seat, facing away from the wheelchair. The front edge of the wheelchair seat is felt against the back of the lower extremities. The patient's feet are positioned in stride or side by side. Positioned in stride, and behind and to one side of the patient, the therapist grasps the patient's gait belt and shoulder.

While holding a cane in each hand, the patient reaches behind and grasps an armrest with each hand.

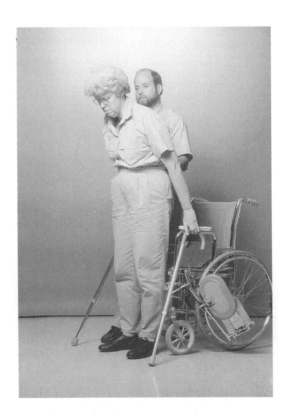

Figure 9.14–4. Grasping armrests and canes.

The patient lowers herself in a controlled manner onto the seat.

Setting the canes aside, the patient moves completely into the seat and positions herself appropriately.

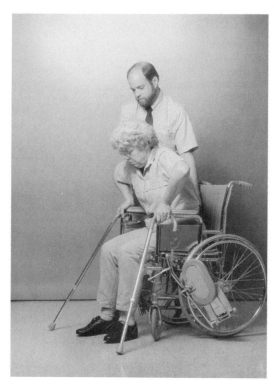

Figure 9.14–5. Lowering to sitting.

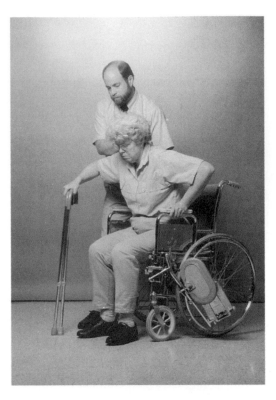

Figure 9.14–6. Starting position to assume standing using two canes in one hand.

Assuming Standing—Two Canes in One Hand

LO-15

The wheelchair is locked and the footrests moved out of the way. The patient is positioned at the front edge of the seat, with her feet in stride or side by side. Positioned in stride, and behind and to one side of the patient, the therapist grasps the patient's gait belt and shoulder.

The patient grasps both canes with one hand. The tips of the canes are placed on the floor to the side and slightly beyond the patient's toes. The opposite hand grasps the armrest.

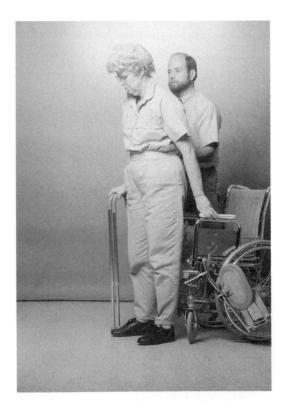

Figure 9.14–7. Assuming standing.

The patient pushes to standing, supporting and balancing on the two canes on one side and the armrest on the other side.

When the patient has assumed the standing position, the therapist should ensure that the patient can control balance. The patient releases the armrest, and when erect, reaches for a cane.

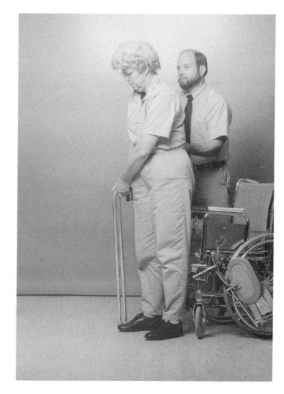

Figure 9.14–8. Reaching for cane.

One at a time the canes are positioned properly, one in each hand.

The patient is ready to ambulate.

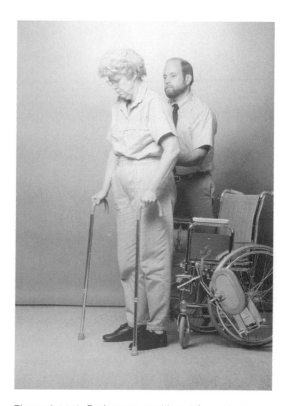

Figure 9.14–9. Both canes positioned for ambulation.

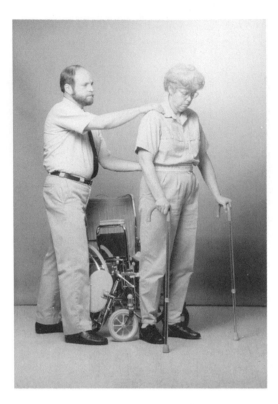

Figure 9.14–10. Starting position to assume sitting using two canes in one hand.

Assuming Sitting—Two Canes in One Hand

LO-15 The wheelchair is locked and the footrests moved out of the way. To sit, the patient positions herself at the front edge of the wheelchair seat, facing away from the wheelchair. The front edge of the wheelchair seat is felt against the back of the lower extremities. The patient's feet are positioned in stride or side by side. Positioned in stride, and behind and to one side of the patient, the therapist grasps the patient's gait belt and shoulder.

Both canes are placed together in one hand.

Figure 9.14–11. Placing both canes in one hand.

The patient advances her uninvolved lower extremity beyond the canes. Initially, the patient may "step to" her involved lower extremity, rather than "step through." Stepping through is the normal gait pattern, and should be encouraged. The therapist advances his right, or inside, foot as the patient moves her uninvolved lower extremity.

The sequence is repeated for continued progression.

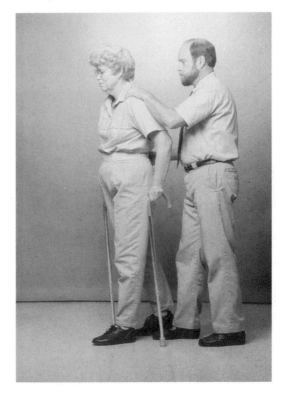

Figure 9.14–16. Uninvolved lower extremity moved forward beyond canes.

Four-Point Gait Pattern

LO-15 Positioned in stride, and behind and to one side of the patient, the therapist grasps the patient's gait belt and shoulder. In the starting position the patient stands with one cane in each hand in the same position used for measuring cane fit. The patient's feet are side by side.

To ambulate, the patient advances one cane. In this example the right cane is advanced first.

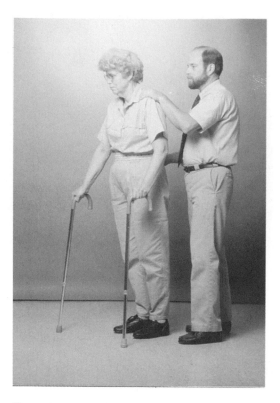

Figure 9.14–17. Right cane moved forward.

The patient then advances her opposite, or left, lower extremity to a point even with the tip of the right cane. The therapist advances his right, or inside, foot.

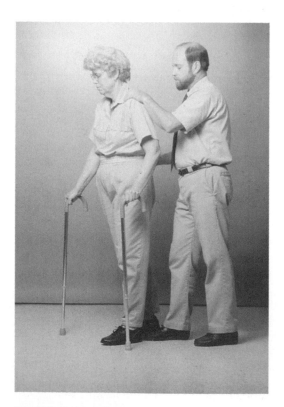

Figure 9.14–18. Left lower extremity moved forward.

The patient shifts her weight to the right cane and left lower extremity. She advances her left cane beyond the right cane.

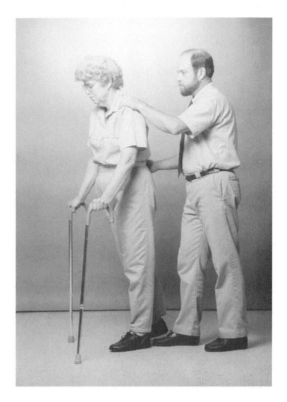

Figure 9.14–19. Left cane moved forward.

The patient advances her right lower extremity to a point even with the tip of her left cane. The therapist advances his left, or outside, foot.

The patient shifts her weight to her left cane and right lower extremity. The sequence is repeated for continued progression.

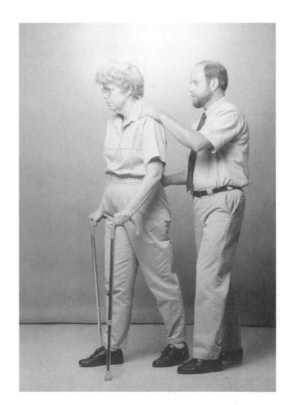

Figure 9.14–20. Right lower extremity moved forward.

Two-Point Gait Pattern

LO-15 Positioned in stride, and behind and to one side of the patient, the therapist grasps the patient's gait belt and shoulder. In the starting position the patient stands with one cane in each hand in the same position used for measuring cane fit. The patient's feet are side by side.

The patient advances one cane and the opposite lower extremity simultaneously, placing the toes even with the tip of the cane. Her weight is shifted onto this cane and lower extremity. In this example, the right cane and left foot have been advanced together. The therapist moves his right, or inside, foot at this time.

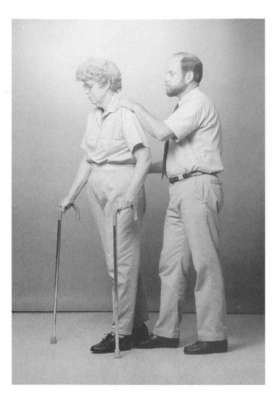

Figure 9.14–21. Right cane and left lower extremity moved forward.

The patient advances her left cane and right lower extremity together. This cane and lower extremity are advanced beyond the other cane and lower extremity in a normal stride length. The patient shifts her weight onto the just advanced cane and lower extremity. The therapist moves his left, or outside, foot at this time.

The sequence is repeated for continued progression.

Figure 9.14–22. Left cane and right lower extremity moved forward.

Stairs

Holding the Canes

LO-15

Ambulation on stairs can be performed using two canes, with or without the use of a handrail. Use of a handrail, however, provides stability, and thus is an added safety factor. When using a handrail, the handrail takes the place of the cane on one side. There are several methods of holding canes when using a handrail. Whatever method of holding canes is used, the sequence of movements for the lower extremities and assistive devices is the same.

A practical method of holding two canes while using a handrail is to place both canes in one hand.

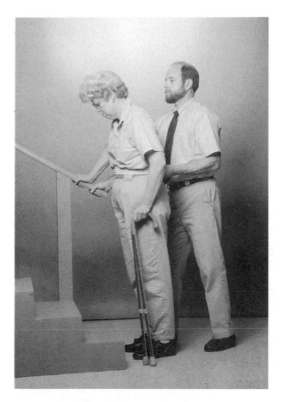

Figure 9.14–23. Holding two canes in one hand for stairs.

There are two methods of holding a cane in the hand that is grasping the handrail and the cane simultaneously. When grasping a cane and handrail in the same hand, the cane may be held in a vertical position by the hand-grip, or the cane may be held at midshaft, parallel to the handrail. These methods are illustrated in this chapter, in the section "One Cane/Stairs/ Holding the Cane." The cane on the side opposite the handrail is used in the usual manner.

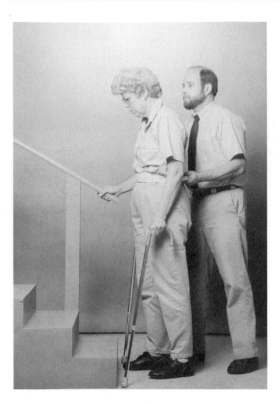

Figure 9.14–24. Starting position to ascend stairs using two canes and three-point gait pattern.

Ascending—Three-Point Gait Pattern

LO-15 To ascend the stairs, the patient stands facing up the stairs with her feet and canes parallel to the base of the first stair. Positioned in stride behind the patient, the therapist grasps the patient's gait belt and the handrail. For the method presented in this section, the patient grasps one cane in each hand. In the illustrations for this section, the hand that can be seen on the handrail is the therapist's hand.

The patient's uninvolved lower extremity is placed on the next higher stair, and weight is shifted onto this extremity.

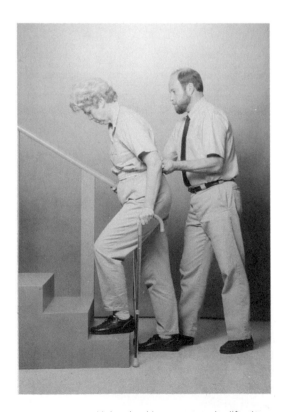

Figure 9.14–25. Uninvolved lower extremity lifted to next stair.

The uninvolved lower extremity is extended to raise the body to the next higher stair. The canes and involved lower extremity are advanced to the same stair at the same time. The canes must be properly placed on the stair for stability, and to provide room for the patient to maneuver.

The sequence is repeated to ascend the remaining stairs.

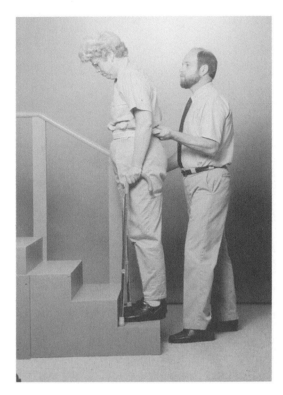

Figure 9.14–26. Canes and involved lower extremity lifted to same stair.

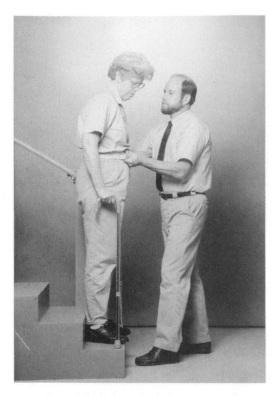

Figure 9.14–27. Starting position to descend stairs using two canes and three-point gait pattern.

Descending—Three-Point Gait Pattern

LO-15

To descend stairs, the patient stands facing down the stairs. Positioned in stride in front of the patient, the therapist grasps the patient's gait belt and the handrail. For the method presented in this section, the patient grasps one cane in each hand. In the illustrations for this section, the hand that can be seen on the handrail is the therapist's hand.

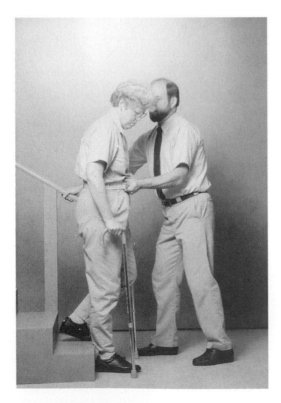

Figure 9.14–28. Canes and involved lower extremity lowered to next stair.

Flexing the uninvolved lower extremity to lower the body, the patient lowers the canes and involved lower extremity to the next lower stair.

Weight is shifted to the involved lower extremity and canes, and the uninvolved lower extremity is moved to the same stair.

The sequence is repeated to descend the remaining stairs.

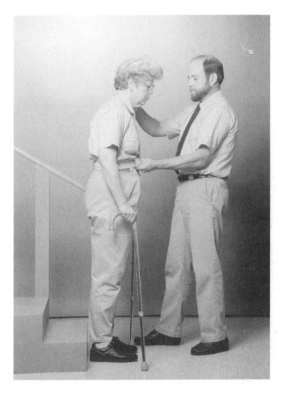

Figure 9.14–29. Uninvolved lower extremity lowered to same stair.

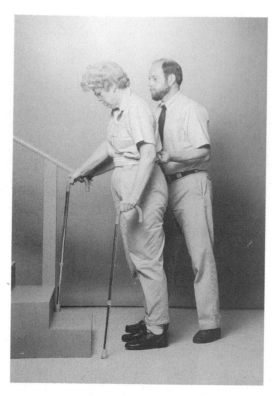

Figure 9.14–30. Right cane lifted to next stair.

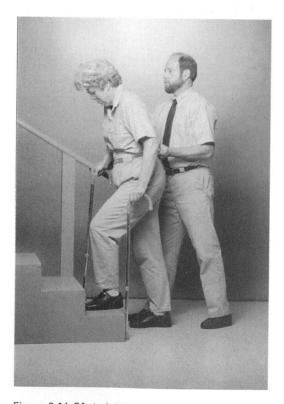

Figure 9.14–31. Left lower extremity lifted to same stair.

Ascending—Four-Point Gait Pattern

LO-15 To ascend stairs, the patient stands facing up the stairs with her feet and canes parallel to the base of the stair. Positioned in stride behind the patient, the therapist grasps the patient's gait belt and the handrail. For the method presented in this section, the patient grasps one cane in each hand. In the illustrations for this section, the hand that can be seen on the handrail is the therapist's hand.

The patient advances one cane to the next higher stair.

The patient advances the opposite lower extremity to the same stair, and weight is shifted onto the cane and lower extremity that have been placed on the higher stair.

The second cane is advanced to the same stair.

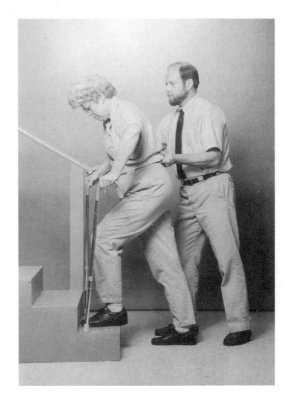

Figure 9.14–32. Left cane lifted to same stair.

The lower extremity on the higher stair is extended to lift the body to that stair. The second lower extremity is placed on the same stair. Thus, both lower extremities and both canes are on the same stair.

The sequence is repeated to ascend the remaining stairs.

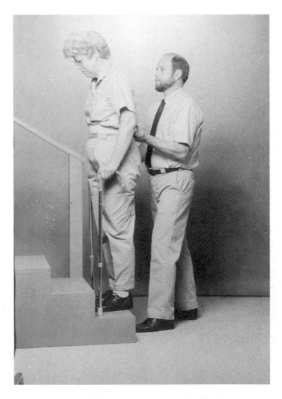

Figure 9.14–33. Right lower extremity lifted to same stair.

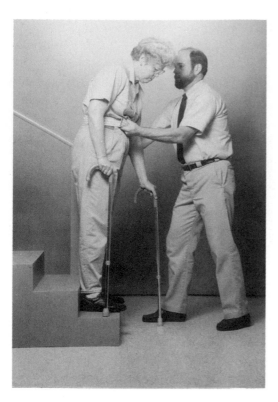

Figure 9.14–34. Left cane lowered to next stair.

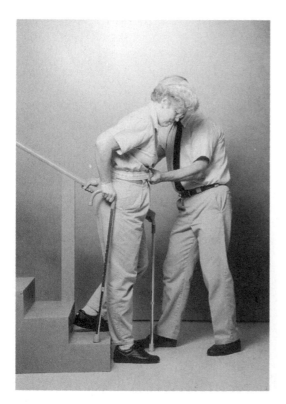

Figure 9.14–35. Right lower extremity lowered to same stair.

Descending—Four-Point Gait Pattern

LO-15 To descend stairs, the patient stands facing down the stairs. Positioned in stride in front of the patient, the therapist grasps the patient's gait belt and the handrail. For the method presented in this section, the patient grasps one cane in each hand. In the illustrations for this section, the hand that can be seen on the handrail is the therapist's hand.

The patient moves the left cane to the next lower stair.

The patient's left lower extremity is flexed to lower her body, placing her right lower extremity on the next lower stair.

Shifting weight onto the cane and lower extremity on the lower stair, the right cane is moved to the next lower stair.

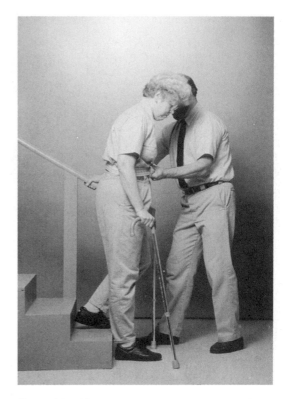

Figure 9.14–36. Right cane lowered to same stair.

The left lower extremity is placed on the next lower stair. Thus, both lower extremities and both canes are on the same stair.

The sequence is repeated to descend the remaining stairs.

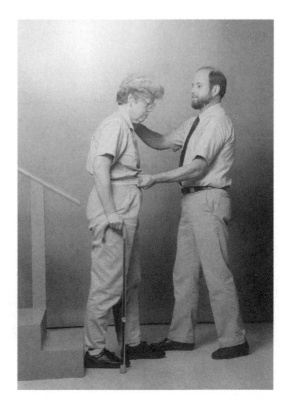

Figure 9.14–37. Left lower extremity lowered to same stair.

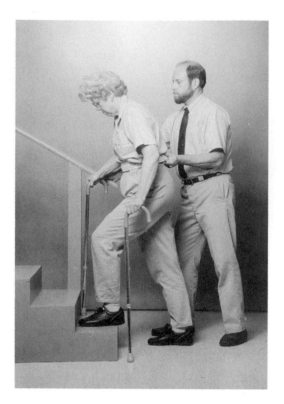

Figure 9.14–38. Right cane and left lower extremity lifted to next stair.

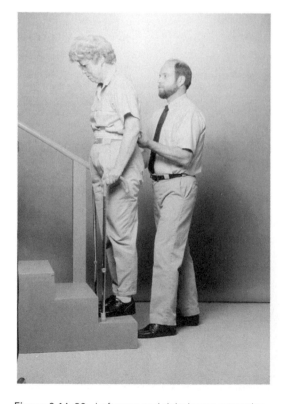

Figure 9.14–39. Left cane and right lower extremity lifted to same stair.

Ascending—Two-Point Gait Pattern

LO-15 To ascend stairs, the patient stands facing up the stairs, with her feet and canes parallel to the base of the stair. Positioned in stride behind the patient, the therapist grasps the patient's gait belt and the handrail. For the method presented in this section, the patient grasps one cane in each hand. In the illustrations for this section, the hand that can be seen on the handrail is the therapist's hand.

The patient advances one cane and the opposite lower extremity simultaneously to the next higher stair.

Weight is shifted onto the cane and lower extremity on the higher stair. The lower extremity on the higher stair is extended to lift the body to that stair. The patient places the remaining cane and lower extremity on the same stair. Thus, both lower extremities and both canes are on the same stair.

The sequence is repeated to ascend the remaining stairs.

Descending—Two-Point Gait Pattern

LO-15 To descend stairs, the patient stands facing down the stairs. Positioned in stride in front of the patient, the therapist grasps the patient's gait belt and the handrail. For the method presented in this section, the patient grasps one cane in each hand. In the illustrations for this section, the hand that can be seen on the handrail is the therapist's hand.

Flexing the right lower extremity, the patient lowers her body and moves the right cane and the left lower extremity to the next lower stair.

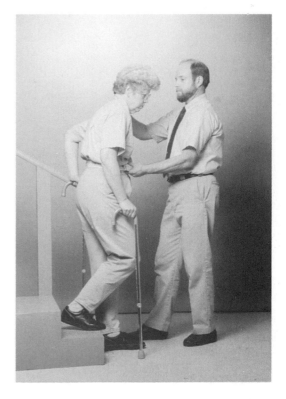

Figure 9.14–40. Right cane and left lower extremity lowered to next stair.

Shifting weight onto the cane and lower extremity on the lower stair, the patient places the left cane and right lower extremity on the same stair. Thus, both lower extremities and both canes are on the same stair.

The sequence is repeated to descend the remaining stairs.

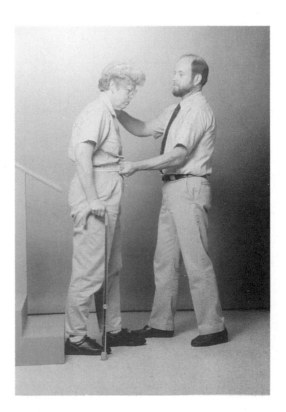

Figure 9.14–41. Left cane and right lower extremity lowered to same stair.

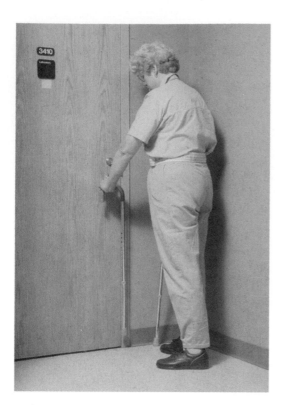

Figure 9.14–42. Positioned beyond the door's arc of motion while grasping door handle and cane.

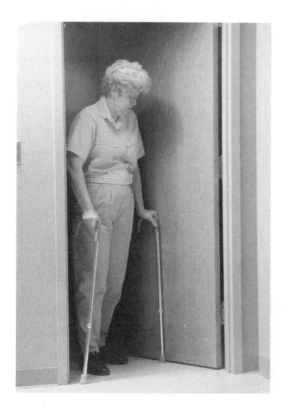

Figure 9.14–43. Tip of cane used to block door closing.

Doorways With Automatic Door Closers

LO-15 When moving through a doorway, the patient can use one cane in each hand, or may place both canes in one hand. The method of moving through doorways with both canes in one hand is the same as when using one cane. In the illustrations for this section the patient is demonstrating the use of two canes.

Door Opens Toward the Patient

The patient approaches the latch edge of the door, standing outside the arc through which the opening door will move. The patient shifts her weight onto the cane on the side away from the hand that will be placed on the door handle. Holding the cane, the unweighted hand grasps the door handle. Preferably, weight is shifted to the side closest to the door handle, and the hand toward the hinge edge is used to pull open the door.

Using a pulling motion, the door is opened wider than the width of the patient. Opening the door wider than the patient is necessary because the door will start to close automatically before the patient can progress through the doorway. To block the automatic closing of the door, the patient turns into the doorway and places the tip of the cane closest to the door on the floor in the path of the door. This acts as a door stop, permitting the patient to move into the doorway without being struck by the closing door.

Continuing to use the tip of the cane as a door stop, the patient ambulates through the doorway using an appropriate gait pattern. As the patient moves through the doorway, the tip of the cane is used as a door stop by placing it progressively closer to the hinge edge of the door. The therapist and patient must be aware that as the tip of the cane gets closer to the hinge edge of the door, it becomes more difficult to hold open the door.

Once the patient has moved completely through the doorway, the door closes behind the patient.

Door Opens Away from the Patient

LO-15

The patient faces the door and shifts her weight onto the cane away from the hand that is closest to the door handle. Holding the cane, the unweighted hand grasps the door handle.

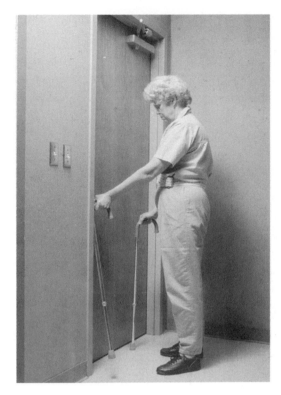

Figure 9.14–44. Grasping door handle and cane in one hand.

Using a pushing motion, the door is opened part way, and the automatic closing of the door is blocked by the tip of the cane closest to the door.

As the patient moves through the doorway, the door is pushed open in increments. Continuing to use the tip of the cane as a door stop, the patient ambulates through the doorway using the chosen gait pattern.

Once the patient has moved completely through the doorway, the door closes behind the patient.

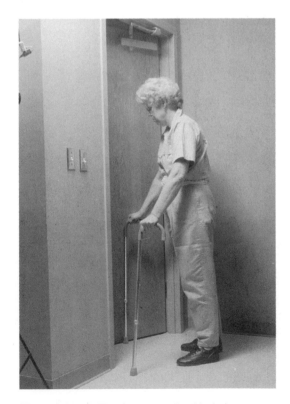

Figure 9.14–45. Tip of cane used to block door closing.

9.15 REVIEW QUESTIONS

1. What are the general guidelines for instructing a patient in the use of assistive devices and gait patterns?

2. Which components of assistive devices should be checked for safety?

3. What activities should be taught to a patient learning to use an assistive device?

4. List assistive devices in the order a) providing the most stability to the least stability, b) requiring the most patient coordination to the least patient coordination.

5. What are the indications for the selection of specific assistive devices?

6. Describe the five major gait patterns used with assistive devices.

7. Which gait patterns can be used with each assistive device?

8. What are the criteria for selection of gait patterns when using assistive devices?

9. What is the purpose of using the tilt table in gait training?

10. Describe how to fit each assistive device.

11. How does a therapist guard a patient ambulating using an assistive device on level surface, stairs, and through doorways?

12. How is the wheelchair properly prepared for a patient to move in or out of the wheelchair when using assistive devices?

9.16   SUGGESTED ACTIVITIES

1. Demonstrate the procedures presented in this chapter to students.

2. Students practice the procedures working in pairs. Students should rotate partners during the practice sessions.

3. Students practice fitting each assistive device to at least three different people.

4. Students practice demonstrating gait patterns with each assistive device.

5. Students practice guarding partners using each assistive device with various appropriate gait patterns on level surfaces, stairs and curbs, the assumption of sitting from standing and standing from sitting, moving through doorways, falling without injury, and resumption of ambulation after falling.

6. Students practice teaching partners how to use assistive devices on level surfaces, stairs and curbs, the assumption of sitting from standing and standing from sitting, moving through doorways, falling without injury, and resumption of ambulation after falling, as partners role-play various diagnoses. Students role-playing a patient can add "character" to the role-play by being cooperative, noncooperative, in pain, hard of hearing, or faint to enhance the activity. The patient must role-play the diagnosis and character consistently (see Case Studies for suggested patient roles).

7. Students monitor vital signs and check for signs of circulatory problems of the lower extremities as appropriate.

8. Students document treatment using the SOAP note format.

CASE STUDIES

1. The patient is a 16-year-old male high school soccer player who sustained a left knee injury in a game the night before. He is to ambulate using axillary crutches, with a non-weight-bearing gait pattern until a diagnosis is determined following a MRI in 2 days.

2. The patient is a 63-year-old female with a left CVA, presenting with right hemiplegia. She has sufficient motor control and balance to ambulate with a small base quad cane.

3. The patient is a 78-year-old male who had a left total hip replacement 1 day ago. He is to ambulate using a walker, with weight bearing as tolerated.

4. The patient is a 49-year-old female with severe rheumatoid arthritis who received a right total knee joint replacement 2 days ago. She is to ambulate using a platform walker, with weight bearing as tolerated.

5. The patient is a 21-year-old male with a complete L3-4 spinal cord injury. He is ready to begin gait training using Lofstrand crutches and knee-ankle-foot orthoses (KAFOs). His upper extremity strength is adequate for ambulating with these assistive devices.

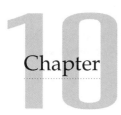

Chapter

Americans With Disabilities Act

 Learner Objectives

The student will be able to:

1 State the purpose of the Americans With Disabilities Act (ADA).
2 List the government agencies responsible for developing rules and regulations, and enforcing the ADA law.
3 List sources of updated information on ADA.
4 Be able to locate specific requirements for an accessible environment: accessible routes, alarms, assembly and auditorium areas, business and mercantile areas, clear space areas, control mechanisms, curb ramps, doors and doorways, drinking fountains, elevators, grab bars, ground and floor surfaces, handrails, hotels, libraries, parking spaces, platform lifts, ramps, reach heights, restaurant and food service areas, restrooms and bathrooms, signage, stairs, telephones, and transportation facilities.

INTRODUCTION

In 1990, Congress passes the **Americans With Disabilities Act (ADA)** (Public Law 101-336). Composed of five titles,

Title I—Employment
Title II—Public Services and Transportation
Title III—Public Accommodations
Title IV—Telecommunications
Title V—Other Provisions

LO-1

CLINICAL NOTE

Eliminate
discrimination

the purpose of the ADA is to provide "a clear and comprehensive national mandate for the elimination of discrimination against individuals with disabilities." Title II provides for accessible transportation which permits individuals with disabilities "to gain employment," and which "allows individuals with disabilities to enjoy cultural, recreational, commercial and other benefits that society has to offer." Title III provides individuals with disabilities the "full and equal enjoyment of the goods, services, facilities, privileges, advantages, or accommodations of any place of public accommodation."[1]

The purpose of this chapter is to provide basic information concerning how requirements of the ADA affect accessibility. This chapter will examine the basic requirements of accessibility as they apply to Title II (Public Services and Transportation) and Title III (Public Accommodations) because it is primarily in these areas that accessibility guidelines are addressed. This chapter contains specifics of space and configuration as required by the ADA. The philosophy or interpretation of ADA guidelines is *not* discussed.

10.1   BACKGROUND

LO-2

**AGENCIES
RESPONSIBLE**

EEOC
DOJ

The ADA was passed on 26 July, 1990. Phased implementation of Titles II and III was mandated to follow the schedule in Table 10–1.

It is not appropriate, nor is it possible, for the language of a law to contain provisions for every potential situation intended to be covered by the law. Therefore, **rules, regulations,** and **guidelines** for implementation of laws are promulgated following passage of a new law. In the case of the ADA, the government agencies primarily responsible for developing rules and regulations, and enforcing the law, are the **Equal Employment Oppor-**

TABLE 10–1 Implementation Schedule ADA Titles II and III

Title	Effective Date
II—Public Services, Public Transportation	26 January, 1992
	New vehicles—26 August, 1990
	Paratransit—26 January, 1992
III—Public Accommodations	26 January, 1992
	New construction—26 January, 1993 (ready for first occupancy after 26 January, 1993)
	Alterations—26 January, 1992 (initial work on alterations begun after 26 January, 1992)
Private Transportation	New vehicles—26 August, 1990
Over-the-Road Buses	Large providers—26 July, 1996
	Small providers—26 July, 1997

tunity Commission (EEOC) and the **Department of Justice (DOJ).** More specific interpretation of the law, and its rules, regulations, and guidelines will occur as the result of administrative rulings and legal opinions in response to complaints and lawsuits filed by those who believe they have been subjected to discrimination as defined by the ADA. In many cases, the most definitive interpretation of specific requirements of the ADA will only become known as the result of such administrative rulings or legal opinions.

10.2   RESOURCES

Because public laws, and their rules and regulations, are subject to constant change and interpretation, information that is updated on a regular basis is very important. Access to resources that are continually updated becomes a vital part of being informed. The resources listed below are not meant to be all-inclusive, and listing of a resource is not meant to be an endorsement. The resources listed are those that have been available over a period of years, and have been found to be useful.

LO-3

CLINICAL NOTE

Update information regularly

1. Building Officials & Code Administrators International, Inc. The BOCA National Building Code/1993, 1993.
   Building Officials & Code Administrators International, Inc.
   4051 W. Flossmoor Road
   Country Club Hills, IL 60478-5795
   (708) 799-2300

   This resource covers all design factors and requirements for the construction and occupancy of buildings. Requirements listed are not only related to issues of accessibility, but include such items as natural light requirements, fireproof ratings of walls, etc.
   This resource is the foundation of local building codes in the vast majority of jurisdictions that enforce building codes. The code is updated annually, and is reprinted in its entirety every 3 years.

2. Council of American Building Officials American National Standard—Accessible and Usable Buildings and Facilities (CABO/ANSI Standard A117.1-1992), 1992.
   Council of American Building Officials
   5203 Leesburg Pike, #708
   Falls Church, VA 22041
   (703) 931-4533

   This resource covers all design factors for accessibility in the construction of buildings, not just standards that apply to accessibility for individuals with disabilities. The previous version was ANSI Standard A117.1, a 1986 publication.
   The organization that developed and approved these standards, the Council of American Building Officials (CABO), then requested approval of their process from the American National Standards Institute (ANSI). ANSI approval permits the CABO standards to become an American National Standard. ANSI standards are the primary standards in many industries and for many products.

3. Thompson Publishing Group
  Americans With Disabilities Act—ADA Compliance Guide
    Thompson Publishing Group, Inc.
    1725 K Street N.W., Suite 200
    Washington, D.C. 20006
    (800) 424-2959

This resource is published by a private publishing group, which updates the material monthly. Information includes, but is not limited to, monthly bulletins, commentary on implementation and interpretation, changes in rules and regulations, charts and tables of specific requirements, and abstracts of relevant administrative rulings and legal opinions. Specific information and requirements of the Uniform Federal Accessibility Standards (UFAS) and of the Americans With Disabilities Accessibilities Guidelines (AADAAG) are included and updated as necessary.

The publication is produced by a proprietary group, which is one of many groups that research and provide such information on a variety of topics. The cost of a service such as this is higher than government or quasi-government publications. The benefits of such services are more timely and in-depth research and information.

10.3   GENERAL CONSIDERATIONS

RULES AND REGULATIONS

Pertain to needs of many
Written for greatest need

Requirements for accessibility must take into account a variety of people with different abilities. In many cases, such as ground and floor surfaces, many people may consider the effect of ground and floor surfaces on wheelchair use as the defining factor. Many people, however, are affected by the condition of ground and floor surfaces. Transitions greater than 1/4 inch may provide an unexpected bump or impediment for wheelchair users, and they can also provide an obstacle to trip over for the visually impaired. The same thinking process may be true for the consideration of clear space areas. Many people who have mobility impairments use assistive devices other than wheelchairs. While the clear space area requirements for maneuvering are greatest in a wheelchair, all users of assistive devices require increased clear space areas. Therefore, it is important to consider all aspects of accessibility for the general population, rather than identifying each barrier to accessibility with a single impairment.

LO-4

10.4   SPECIFIC REQUIREMENTS

Within each area of a public accommodation, such as a public office or a restroom, there are specific components that must be examined, and criteria that must be met. If a public accommodation encompasses a collection of areas, such as both an office and a restroom, then all components and criteria for each must be applied to the appropriate area. For example, the criteria for doorways must be applied to both areas, but the criteria for toilets need only be applied to the restroom.

When evaluating an area for accessibility, all appropriate components and criteria must be considered for the specified area. Many items, such as doorway widths, will need to be evaluated multiple times. The clear open width of a door must be no less than 32 inches. This requirement is true of doors, whether they are for an entry into an office or a restroom.

Listed on the following pages are the requirements for the majority of specific areas of accessibility that may be encountered in public accommodations. Each area is listed as a heading. Specific components and criteria for a given area are listed under the area heading. The list of area headings is alphabetical. Under each area heading, specific components, and criteria for each component, are also listed alphabetically.

While certain components or criteria are applied in a large variety of circumstances, there are some components or criteria that are not applied very often. For this reason, and because of space considerations, the following list does not include every individual requirement for accessibility. It does cover the vast majority of accessibility requirements. For a list of every requirement, and increased details concerning each requirement, reference to one of the resources is recommended.

In the following list, reference may be made to areas previously listed, or to areas that follow later in the list. These are areas that appear in a number of environments, and have common criteria, regardless of the area in which they are required. This method is used to reduce redundancy, but is limited to avoid the need for constant cross-reference searching.

COMMON CRITERION FOR REPEATED OCCURRENCES

Standard width for all doors
Ramp grades

Accessible Route

A minimum of one route within the path from public access via public transportation, accessible parking spaces, and public streets must be available. Such a route must also be available to connect additional accessible buildings at the same site. Stairs, steps, or escalators are not included in an accessible route.

LO-4

Grade:	Not greater than 1:20 (5%) unless requirements for a ramp are met.
Height:	Not less than 80 inches vertical clearance.
	If vertical clearance along an accessible route is less than 80 inches, a warning barrier must be provided.
Protrusions:	Not greater than 4 inches in the horizontal dimension; in the vertical area between 27 inches and 80 inches above the floor.
	Protrusions in the vertical area less than 27 inches above the floor may protrude any amount.
	Not greater than 12 inches in the horizontal dimension; in the vertical area between 27 inches and 80 inches above the floor when the object is mounted on a free standing post or pylon.
	May not reduce required amount of clear space required on an accessible route.
Width:	Not less than 36 inches.

Alarms

LO-4

Audible: Not less than 15 dbA greater than prevailing sound level or not less than 5 dbA greater than any maximum sound level that persists for greater than 60 seconds.

Visual: Must be integrated into building alarm system.
Must be within 50 feet of all sites required to have a visual signal unit.
Not less than 75 candela intensity.
Between 1 Hz and 3 Hz flash rate.
At 80 inches above floor level, or 6 inches below ceiling level, whichever is lower.

Assembly and Auditorium Areas

LO-4

Clear Area: *In series/Front or Rear access*
Not less than 66 inches in width by 48 inches in length for two spaces in series.
In series/Side access
Not less than 66 inches in width by 60 inches in length for two spaces in series.

Location: Must provide a variety of lines of sight and admission prices comparable to those available to the general public.
In assembly areas with capacity greater than 300, accessible wheelchair areas must be located in more than one location.
Readily movable seating may be used in wheelchair accessible spaces if they are not required for wheelchair use. Seating must be removed if seating by users of wheelchairs is requested, and is not available in other locations.
Must be configured in conjunction with assistive listening systems.
Must be on an accessible route with access to accessible emergency exits.
Must have access to accessible restrooms.

Business and Mercantile Areas

LO-4

Check-out Aisles: Number of accessible aisles required is

Total Aisles	Accessible Aisles
1 to 4	1
5 to 8	2
9 to 15	4
More than 15	3, plus 20% of aisles over 15

Counters: Must be on accessible routes.
Not greater than 36 inches above floor level.
Areas with fixed counters greater than 36 inches in

Security Barriers: height must have a portion of the counter not less than 36 inches in length with a height not greater than 36 inches above floor level. Accessible counters must be located throughout the building.
Devices used to prevent shopping carts from being removed from store may not prevent access for users of wheelchairs.

Clear Space Areas

Accessible Route: Not less than 32 inches in width at a single point.
Not less than 36 inches in width along a continuous pathway.
Landing: Not less than 60 inches by 60 inches.
Passing: Not less than 60 inches in width.
If width of 60 inches is not available, then areas 60 inches by 60 inches must be available for passing at distances not to exceed 200 feet.
Stationary: Not less than 30 inches by 48 inches.

LO-4

Control Mechanisms

Force: Not greater than 5 pounds force to operate.
Grasp: Easy to grasp with one hand.
Must not require tight grasping, tight pinching, or twisting of wrist to operate.
Reach: Not less than 15 inches above floor level.

LO-4

Curb Ramps

Grade: Not greater than 1:12 (8.3%) for new construction, with a vertical rise of not greater than 30 inches.
Not greater than 1:10 (10%) for existing sites, with a vertical rise of not greater than 6 inches if space does not permit construction of a grade of 1:12 or less.
Not greater than 1:8 (12.5%) for existing sites, with a vertical rise of not greater than 3 inches if space does not permit construction of a grade of 1:12 or less.
Width: Not less than 36 inches, exclusive of the flared sides.

LO-4

Doors and Doorways

Access to each area requires that entrances be accessible. Revolving doors and turnstiles may not be the only method of entrance. Gates must meet requirements if on an accessible route. For double-leaf doorways, at least one leaf by itself must meet the requirements, and this leaf must be the active leaf.

LO-4

Automatic Doors: Time to open not greater than 3 seconds.
Not greater than 15 pounds force to stop movement.

Closers:	Time to close not greater than 3 seconds for closing from 70 degrees open to a point where the leading edge of the door is 3 inches from the latch. Fire door opening force must be the minimum required by the local administrative entity (ie, Fire Department, Department of Public Safety, etc.). Not greater than 5 pounds force for interior hinged doors. Not greater than 5 pounds force for sliding or folding doors. Latches or other hardware do not come under these force requirements.
Depth:	The depth of the opening in which a door is placed not greater than 24 inches. If the depth is greater than 24 inches, this area must be considered part of an accessible route.

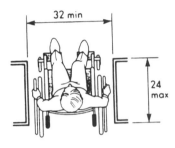

Figure 10.4–1. Maximum doorway depth and minimum doorway width.

Handles:	Easy to grasp with one hand. Must not require tight grasping, tight pinching, or twisting of wrist to operate. Mounted not higher than 48 inches above the floor.
Maneuvering Area: (clear space)	*Hinged door approached from the front/Door pulls open toward the person* (Figure 10.4–2A) Not less than 60 inches from doorway wall. Not less than 18 inches (24 inches preferred) on both left and right sides of the door opening. *Hinged door approached from the front/Door pushes open away from the person* (Figure 10.4–2B) Not less than 48 inches from doorway wall. Not less than 12 inches on the latch edge of the door opening if the door has a closer.

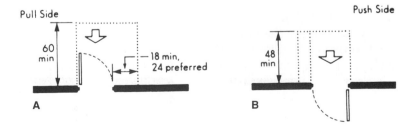

Figure 10.4–2. Maneuvering area at doorways for front approach. A. Door opens toward patient. B. Door opens away from patient.

Hinged door approached from the hinge edge (the opening door prohibits direct movement through the doorway)/Door pulls open into the area of approach (Figure 10.4–3)

Two space configurations are possible.

1. Not less than 60 inches from doorway wall with not less than 36 inches on the latch edge of the door opening.
2. Not less than 54 inches from doorway wall with not less than 42 inches on the latch edge of the door opening. In no case may the clear space from the doorway wall be less than 54 inches.

Hinged door approached from the hinge edge/Door pushes open away from the area of approach (Figure 10.4–3B)

Not less than 42 inches from doorway wall. Not less than 48 inches from doorway wall if door has a closer.

Not less than 22 inches on hinge edge of doorway opening.

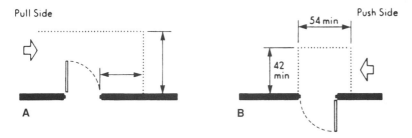

Figure 10.4–3. Maneuvering area at doorways for side approach at hinge edge. A. Door opens toward patient. B. Door opens away from patient.

Hinged door approached from the latch edge (the opening door does not prohibit direct movement through the doorway)/Door pulls open into area of approach (Figure 10.4–4A)

Not less than 48 inches from doorway wall. Not less than 54 inches from doorway wall if the door has a closer.

Not less than 24 inches on the latch edge of the door opening.

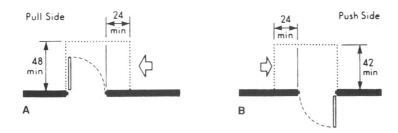

Figure 10.4–4. Maneuvering area at doorways for side approach at latch edge. A. Door opens into hall. B. Door opens away from patient.

Hinged door approached from latch edge/Door pushes open away from the area of approach (Figure 10.4–4B)
>   Not less than 42 inches from doorway wall.
>   Not less than 48 inches from doorway wall if door has a closer.
>   Not less than 24 inches on the latch edge of the doorway opening.

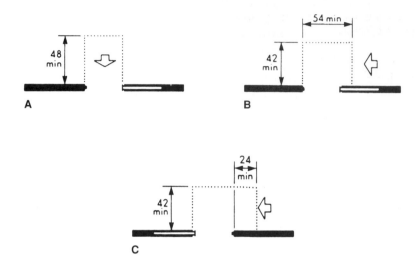

Figure 10.4–5. Maneuvering area at sliding doors. A. Front approach. B. Slide side approach. C. Latch side approach.

Sliding & Folding doors/Front approach
>   Not less than 48 inches from doorway wall.

Sliding & Folding doors/Slide side approach
>   Not less than 42 inches from doorway wall.
>   Not less than 22 inches on slide side of doorway opening.

Sliding & Folding doors/Latch edge approach
>   Not less than 42 inches from doorway wall.
>   Not less than 24 inches on latch edge of doorway opening.

Two hinged doors in series
>   Must not open in opposite directions *into* the intervening vestibule between the doorways.

Two hinged doors in series/Both doors open in same direction (first door opens away from intervening vestibule and second door opens into intervening vestibule)
>   Not less than 48 inches measured between the doorway wall of the first door and the latch edge of the second door when it is open at a 90-degree angle into the intervening vestibule.

Two hinged doors in series/Both doors open away from intervening vestibule (doors open opposite directions)
>   Not less than 48 inches between doorway walls.

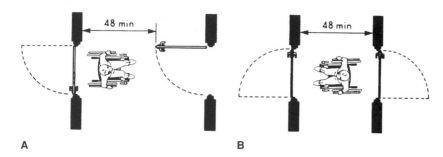

Figure 10.4–6. Maneuvering area at doorways in series. A. Doors open same direction. B. Doors open opposite directions.

Thresholds:	Not greater than 3/4 inch for sliding doors.
	Not greater than 1/2 inch for all other doors.
	Bevel not greater than 1:2 (50%).
Width:	Not less than 32 inches, measured between the face of the door and the opposite stop with the door open to 90 degrees.
	When the depth of the opening in which a door is placed is greater than 24 inches, the path to the door must be considered part of an accessible route, and the width must be no less than 36 inches except at the doorway.

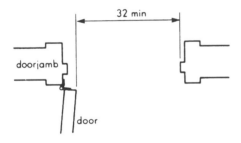

Figure 10.4–7. Minimum clear doorway width.

Drinking Fountains

Clearance:	Knee space between floor level and underside of the unit of not less than 27 inches in height, 30 inches in width, and 17 to 19 inches in depth.
	Not less than 30 inches by 48 inches for approach area.
Controls:	Must be mounted on the front of the unit, or on the side of the unit near the front.
	Must meet the requirements listed under "Control Mechanisms."
	Must not require tight grasping, tight pinching, or twisting of wrist to operate.
	Not greater than 5 pounds force to operate.

LO-4

Height: Spout height must be no greater than 36 inches from
                 the floor.
Spout: Must be near the front edge of the unit.
Water flow: No greater than 3 inches from the front of the unit.
                 No less than 4 inches in height.

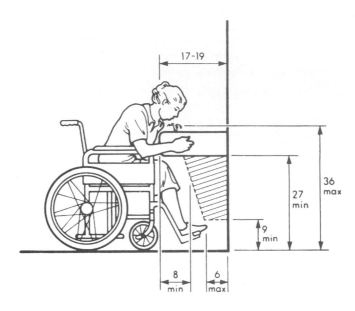

Figure 10.4–8. Drinking fountain clearance dimensions.

Elevators

LO-4

To be considered accessible, an elevator must be on an accessible route. Unless freight elevators are used for the general public as combination passenger and freight elevators, freight elevators may not be used to meet the requirement of an accessible elevator. Requirements of an accessible elevator are:

Car Controls: Must be located on a front wall for elevators with the
                 door opening in the center of the front wall.
                 Must be located on the side wall nearest the door, or
                 on the front wall, for elevators with the door opening
                 set to one side of the front wall.
                 Not greater than 48 inches above floor level for a
                 front-only approach.
                 Not greater than 54 inches above floor level for a side
                 approach.
                 Not less than 3/4 inch for smallest dimension.
                 Must be mounted raised or flush.
                 Must provide a visual indication by becoming lit
                 when floor is called and become dark when the floor
                 call is answered.
                 Must have both raised and Braille signage placed to
                 the left of the applicable button.
                 Must have a raised star placed to the left of the call

button for the floor that contains the main building entry.

Must have emergency controls grouped at the bottom of the control panel, with the center line for the emergency controls no less than 35 inches above the floor level.

Any emergency two-way communication system that is provided must be mounted with the uppermost control not greater than 48 inches above the floor.

Dimensions: Door width not less than 36 inches.

Elevators with the door opening in the center of the front wall may not be less than 80 inches in width and 51 inches in depth.

Elevators with the door opening set to one side of the front wall may not be less than 68 inches in width and 54 inches in depth.

Hall Call Buttons: Centered at 42 inches.

Not less than 3/4 inch for smallest dimension.

Must be mounted raised or flush.

Must not have projections greater than 4 inches in horizontal dimension mounted below them.

The up button must be on top.

Must have both raised and Braille signage.

Hall Signals: Must contain a visual and audible signal at each hoistway.

Centered not less than 72 inches above floor level.

Not less that $2 \frac{1}{2}$ inches for smallest dimension.

Audible signal must sound once for up and twice for down, or must have verbal annunciators capable of saying "up" or "down."

Leveling: Self-leveling mechanisms must bring the elevator car to within 1/2 inch of floor under the full rated load range.

Operation: Must be automatic.

Position Indicator: Must be placed over the control panel or above the door.

Must have numerals with a minimum dimension of 1/2 inch in height.

Must provide a sound not less than 20 dbA, with a frequency not higher than 1500 Hz, or have a verbal annunciator that provides an automatic announcement of the floor number for each floor at which the elevator stops.

Must provide both a visual and audible signal for each floor passed.

Grab Bars

The general size of grab bars is between $1 \frac{1}{4}$ and $1 \frac{1}{2}$ inches in diameter, or a shape that provides an equivalent gripping surface. When mounted adjacent to a wall, the space between the wall and grab bar should be $1 \frac{1}{2}$ inches.

LO-4

Ground and Floor Surfaces

LO-4

Ground and floor surfaces must be stable, firm, and slip-resistant.

Carpet: Must be securely attached.
                   Have a pile thickness no greater than 1/2 inch.
                   Exposed edges must be fastened to the floor and have trim along the full length of the exposed edge.

Gratings: Spaces must be no greater than 1/2 inch.
                   If elongated openings are used, the long dimension of the opening must be oriented perpendicular to the dominant direction of travel.

Transitions: Up to 1/4 inch may be left untreated.
                   Between 1/4 inch and 1/2 inch must have a beveled edge with a slope no greater than 1:2 (50%).
                   Greater than 1/2 inch must be achieved by use of a ramp.

Handrails

LO-4

The general size of handrails is between 1 1/4 and 1 1/2 inches in diameter, or a shape that provides an equivalent gripping surface. When mounted adjacent to a wall, the space between the wall and handrail should be 1 1/2 inches. Handrails may be placed in a recess in a wall if the recess is not greater than 3 inches, and there is not less than 18 inches of clear space in the recess above the upper edge of the handrail.

Continuous: Handrails must be continuous along a flight of stairs or the run of a ramp.
                   Inside rails on changes of direction for stairs and ramps must always be continuous.
                   If not continuous, the rail must extend not less than 12 inches beyond the top riser or top end of the ramp run.
                   At the top of a flight of stairs or a ramp run, the rail extension must be parallel to the floor or ground.
                   If not continuous, the rail must extend not less than 12 inches plus the depth of one tread beyond the bottom riser.
                   At the bottom of a flight of stairs, the rail extension must continue to slope past the bottom riser for a distance equal to the depth of one tread, and the remaining length of the extension must be horizontal.
                   If not continuous, the rail must extend not less than 12 inches beyond the bottom end of a ramp run.
                   At the bottom of a ramp run, the rail extension must be parallel to the floor or ground.

Distance
  from Wall: Clear space between a handrail and wall must be 1 1/2 inches.

Ends: Rail ends must be rounded or returned smoothly to the floor, a wall, or a post.

Height:	Top of gripping surface of the rail must be between 34 inches and 38 inches above the floor or ground surface for a ramp, or above the stair nosing for a stairway.
Rotation:	Rails must not rotate within fittings.

Hotels (Transient Lodging)

LO-4

Accessible Elements:	Auxiliary visual alarms.
	Visual notification devices for telephone.
	Visual notification devices for doors.
	Notification devices must not be connected to auxiliary visual alarms.
	Volume controls on telephone.
	Not greater than 48 inches between telephone connection and electrical outlet.
Individuals Units:	Must be on an accessible route.
	Include living area, dining area, at least one sleeping area, and patios/terraces/balconies.
	Available units must be dispersed among the entire range of units available to the general public in terms of facilities and size, cost, and number of beds provided.
	Not less than 36 inches clear space on each side of a bed. In rooms with two beds, a common clear space between them may be shared.
	Doors and doorways must meet the requirements listed under "Doors and Doorways."
	Storage areas must meet the requirements listed under "Reach."
	Bathrooms must meet the requirements listed under "Restrooms and Bathrooms."
Number:	Number of rooms required to be accessible, required to have roll-in showers, and to have accessible elements such as visual alarms, notification devices, and telephones is shown below.

Number of Rooms	Accessible Rooms	Rooms with Roll-in	Accessible Elements
1 to 25	1	0	1
26 to 50	2	0	2
51 to 75	3	1	3
76 to 100	4	1	4
101 to 150	5	2	5
151 to 200	6	2	6
201 to 300	7	3	7
301 to 400	8	4	8
401 to 500	9	4, plus one for each 100 over 400	9
501 to 1000	2% of total		2% of total
Over 1000	20 plus one for each 100 over 1000		20 plus one for each 100 over 1000

Public/
Common Areas: Must be on an accessible route.

Must meet accessibility requirements for the facilities provided.

Libraries

LO-4

Card Catalogs: Not less than 36 inches in width.

Not less than 18 inches above floor level for bottom of catalog.

Not greater than 54 inches above floor level (48 inches preferred) for top of catalog.

Check-out Area: Must be on an accessible route.

Counter height not greater than 36 inches above floor level over a distance not less than 36 inches in length.

Seating
Clear Area: Not less than 30 inches by 48 inches.

Clear area may not overlap knee space by more than 19 inches.

Knee Area: Not less than 27 inches in height, 30 inches in width, and 19 inches in depth.

Security Devices: Security devices or gates may not prohibit access to facilities by users of wheelchairs.

Stacks: Not less that 36 inches (42 inches preferred) in width. Stack height is not restricted.

Study Areas: Must be on an accessible route.

Not less than 5%, or a minimum of 1, of each type of area (fixed seating, carrel, table), must be available.

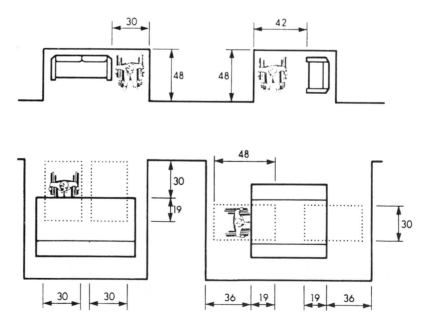

Figure 10.4–9. Clear and knee area dimensions for seating.

Medical Facilities

In general, each specific area of a medical facility must comply with the appropriate requirements for the designated type of area. There are some specific differences, however.

Bathroom:	Each accessible room must have a bathroom that complies with the requirements for an accessible toilet and sink.
Bedside Clear Area:	Not less than a 60-inch diameter maneuvering area (preferably between the two beds in a double room). Not less than 36 inches along each side of a bed, with an accessible path to each side of a bed.
Doors:	The requirements listed under "Doors" apply to medical facilities. For in-patient facilities, an exception is made for maneuvering space on the latch edge of the door if the doorway opening is not less than 44 inches in width.

Parking Spaces

Accessible parking spaces must be designated to be on the shortest possible path from the parking area to an accessible entrance via an accessible route. Access to parking spaces may not be behind other parked cars. Such spaces must be designated with a posted sign that cannot be obscured by a vehicle parked in the space. A sign or symbol painted on the ground is not acceptable.

Area:	Not less than 96 inches wide. Not less than 240 inches long.
Aisle:	Adjacent aisle not less than 60 inches wide by 240 inches long. Adjacent accessible spaces may share the same aisle. One of every 8 accessible spaces must have an adjacent 96-inch-wide aisle.
Grade:	Not greater than 1:50 (2%).
Height:	Vehicle access routes to accessible spaces must have a minimum vertical clearance of 114 inches. Accessible spaces must have a minimum vertical clearance of 98 inches.
Ramp:	An accessible curb ramp that is not obstructed by a parking space must be available when necessary.

Space:

Total Parking Lot Size	Required Minimum Number Accessible Spaces
1 to 25	1
26 to 50	2
51 to 75	3
76 to 100	4
101 to 150	5
151 to 200	6
201 to 300	7
301 to 400	8
401 to 500	9
501 to 1000	2% of total
1000 and over	20, plus 1 for each 100 over 1000

Platform Lifts

LO-4

Platform lifts are used for building entrances, in building interiors, and with transportation vehicles. In any of these settings, the requirements for platform lifts must be followed.

Clear Space:	Not less than 30 inches by 48 inches for the surface of the lift platform.
	Approach areas must meet requirements for clear space.
	Not less than 60 inches by 60 inches is required for a landing.
Controls:	Not greater than 49 inches in vertical height for forward reach only.
	Not greater than 54 inches in vertical height for side reach.
	Not less than 15 inches above the floor.
	Must meet the requirements listed under "Control Mechanisms."

Ramps

LO-4

Any portion of an accessible route with a grade greater than 1:20 (5%) must be considered a ramp.

Grade:	The least possible slope must be used.
	Not greater than 1:12 (8.3%) for new construction, with a vertical rise of not greater than 30 inches.
	Not greater than 1:10 (10%) for existing sites, with a vertical rise of not greater than 6 inches if space does not permit construction of a grade of 1:12 or less.
	Not greater than 1:8 (12.5%) for existing sites, with a vertical rise of not greater than 3 inches if space does not permit construction of a grade of 1:12 or less.

	Cross slope must be no greater than 1:50 (2%).
Handrails:	Required for a rise of 6 inches or more, or for a horizontal run of 72 inches or more.
	Must be provided along both sides of the ramp.
	Must meet the general requirements listed above under "Handrails."
Landing Length:	Not less than 60 inches.
Landing Placement:	At top and bottom of each run.
Landing Width:	At least as wide as the ramp run leading up to the landing.
	Not less than 60 inches if the landing is at a place where the ramp changes direction, or at a doorway.
Rise:	Not greater than 30 inches for any one run, except as noted above for existing construction.
Transitions:	Not greater than 1/4 inch.
Width:	Not less than 36 inches.

Reach Heights

High Forward:	Not greater than 48 inches when only a forward approach is possible.
	Not greater than 44 inches when a high forward reach must be made over an obstruction.
High Side:	Not greater than 54 inches when a parallel approach is possible.
	Not greater than 46 inches when a high side reach must be made over an obstruction.
Low Forward:	Not less than 15 inches above the floor when only a forward approach is possible.
Low Side:	Not less than 9 inches above the floor when a parallel approach is possible.

LO-4

Restaurants and Food Services

Counter Height:	Between 28 inches and 34 inches above floor level. Areas with fixed counters greater than 34 inches in height must have a portion of the counter not less than 60 inches in length with a height between 28 inches and 34 inches above floor level.
Seating	
Clear Area:	Not less than 30 inches by 48 inches.
	Clear area may not overlap knee space by more than 19 inches.
Knee Area:	Not less than 27 inches in height, 30 inches in width, and 19 inches in depth.
Service Lines:	Not less than 36 inches in width: 42 inches in width preferred.
	Condiment and tableware areas must be accessible, and comply with the requirements listed under "Reach."
Vending Areas:	Must be on an accessible route.
	Must comply with the requirements listed under "Reach."

LO-4

The figure in the section on "Libraries" presents the clear and knee area dimensions required for seating in a restaurant or food service area.

Restrooms and Bathrooms

LO-4

Aproach:	Must be on an accessible route.
	Doors are not permitted to swing into the clear area required for any fixture.
Bathtub	*Definitions of walls for bathtubs:*
	Foot wall refers to the wall at the end of the bathtub at which the controls are placed, which is the end of the bathtub where the feet are placed when sitting within the bathtub.
	Back wall refers to the wall opposite the side from which a person enters the bathtub.
	Head wall refers to the wall at the head of the bathtub, which is the end of the bathtub where the head is when sitting within a bathtub.
Area:	*Parallel approach*
	Not less than 30 inches from side of bathtub.
	Not less than the length of the bathtub (60 inches) or the length of the bathtub plus seat (75 inches) if a seat is provided at the head of the bathtub.
	Perpendicular approach
	Not less than 48 inches from side of bathtub.
	Not less than the length of the bathtub (60 inches) or the length of the bathtub plus seat (75 inches) if a seat is provided at the head of the bathtub.
	Enclosures that require tracks to be mounted on the bathtub rim, that obstruct transfers, or that obstruct controls are not permitted.
Controls:	Located towards the edge of bathtub used for entry.
	A shower spray unit that can be used as both a fixed shower head and a hand-held spray unit with a hose not less than 60 inches in length.
Grab Bars:	Between 33 inches and 36 inches from floor level.
	Must not rotate within fittings.
	Bathtub only/Back wall
	Not less than 24 inches in length.
	Mounted starting not more than 12 inches from wall at foot (control end) of bathtub.
	Mounted starting not more than 24 inches from wall at head of bathtub.
	Bathtub only/Head wall
	Not less than 12 inches in length.
	Mounted starting at the edge of bathtub used for entry.
	Bathtub only/Foot wall
	Not less than 24 inches in length.
	Mounted starting at the edge of bathtub used for entry.
	Bathtub with seat at head/Back wall
	Not less than 48 inches in length.

Mounted starting not more than 12 inches from wall at foot (control end) of bathtub.

Mounted starting not more than 15 inches from wall at head of bathtub with seat.

Bathtub with seat at head/Head wall

No grab bar is required in this configuration.

Bathtub with seat at head/Foot wall

Not less than 24 inches in length.

Mounted starting at the edge of bathtub used for entry.

Seats: Must be provided either at the head of the bathtub or within the bathtub.

Must be mounted to prevent movement during use.

Lavatory Area: Not greater than 34 inches from floor level to top rim of lavatory.

Not less than 29 inches between floor level and lowest portion of counter apron.

Not less than 8 inches depth under front edge of counter apron before lavatory projections decrease clear height under counter to less than 27 inches.

Not less than 9 inches clearance between lowest pipe or lavatory projection and floor level.

Not greater than 6 inches between back wall and front edge of any pipes or lavatory projections under counter.

All exposed drain and hot water pipes must be insulated or isolated from user contact.

Not greater than 40 inches from floor level to bottom of any mirror or paper dispenser.

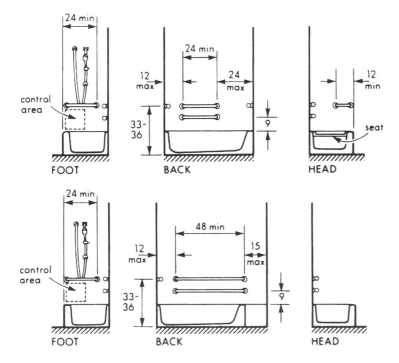

Figure 10.4–10. Dimensions for bathtub grab bars and seats.

Faucets:	Must meet the requirements listed under "Control Mechanisms."
	Self-closing valves must remain open for not less than 10 seconds.
Shower Stalls	
Area:	Not less than 36 inches by 36 inches.
	Enclosures that obstruct transfers, or that obstruct controls are not permitted.
	Curbs not greater than 1/2 inch in height in stalls 36 inches by 36 inches.
	Curbs are not permitted in stalls 30 inches by 60 inches or larger.
Controls:	Located towards the edge of stall used for entry.
	Not less than 38 inches between floor level and the bottom of controls.
	Not greater than 48 inches between floor level and the top of controls.
	A shower spray unit that can be used as both a fixed shower head and a hand-held spray unit with a hose not less than 60 inches in length.
Grab Bars:	Between 33 inches and 36 inches above floor level.
	18 inches in length along back wall, mounted starting at control wall of stall.
	Full depth of stall along control wall.
	No grab bar required along seat wall.
Seats:	Between 17 inches and 19 inches above floor level.
	Mounted on wall opposite controls.
	"L" shaped, with long leg of "L" along side wall and shorter foot of "L" along back wall.
	Runs full depth of stall.

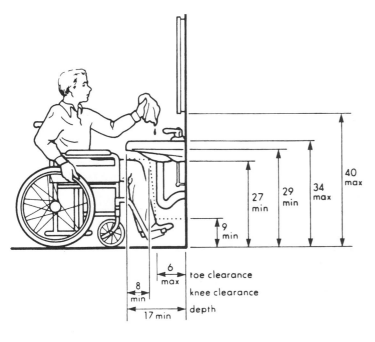

Figure 10.4–11. Lavatory clearance dimensions.

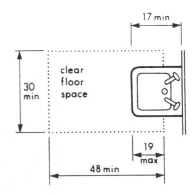

Figure 10.4–12. Maneuvering area at lavatories.

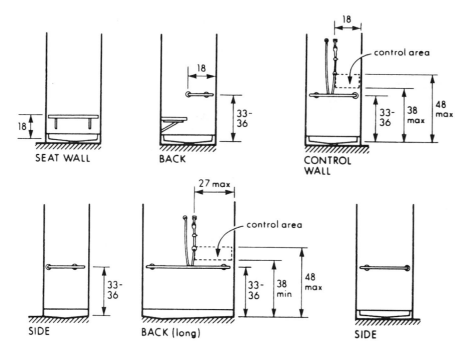

Figure 10.4–13. Dimensions for shower stall grab bars.

Not greater than 23 inches width along back wall.
Width dimension along back wall (short foot of "L")
may not be carried further forward to front edge of
stall for a distance greater than 15 inches.
Width dimension along front edge of stall may not be
greater than 16 inches.
Space between edges of seat and stall walls may not
be greater than 1 $^1/_2$ inches.

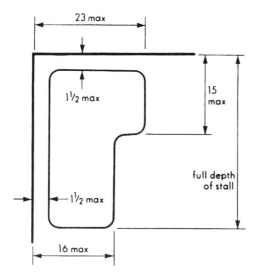

Figure 10.4–14. Dimensions for shower seats.

Urinal Area:	Not greater than 17 inches above floor level to top of rim.
	Not less than 30 inches by 48 inches clear space in front of each urinal.
Controls:	Controls must meet the requirements listed for "Control Mechanisms."
Water Closet Area:	Not less than 42 inches of approach width if approach is made to latch edge of door.
	Not less than 48 inches of approach width if approach is made to hinge edge of door.
	Door openings not less than 32 inches in width.
	Not less than 18 inches from center of water closet to wall on both sides of water closet (36 inch total minimum width).

NOT IN TOILET STALLS

    Front approach

       Not less than 48 inches in width.

       Not less than 66 inches in depth.

    Side approach

       Not less than 48 inches in width.

       Not less than 56 inches in depth.

    Front or Side approach

       Not less than 60 inches in width.

       Not less than 56 inches in depth.

IN TOILET STALLS

    Front entry standard stall

       Not less than 60 inches in width.

       Not less than 56 inches in depth for a wall mounted water closet.

       Not less than 59 inches in depth for a floor

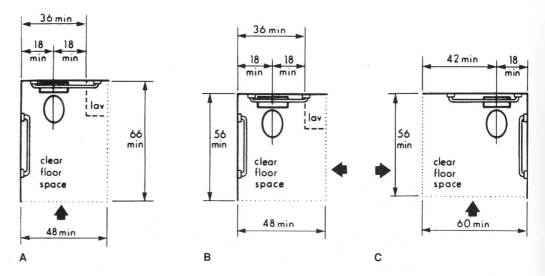

Figure 10.4–15. Maneuvering area at water closets not in toilet stalls. A. Front approach. B. Side approach. C. Front or side approach.

        mounted water closet.
       Side entry end of row stall
         Not less than 60 inches in width.
         Not less than 92 inches in depth for a wall
         mounted water closet.
         Not less than 95 inches in depth for a floor
         mounted water closet.

Controls: Not greater than 44 inches above floor level.
        Mounted on wide side of water closet area.
        Must meet the requirements listed under "Control
        Mechanisms."

Grab Bars: Between 33 inches and 36 inches above floor level.
        Not less than 36 inches in length.
        Must not rotate within fittings.
         Behind water closet
          Must extend not less than 12 inches beyond one
          side of water closet (or water tank).
         Along side water closet
          Must be mounted no closer than 12 inches from
          rear wall behind water closet.

Seats: Between 17 inches and 19 inches in height from floor
        level to top of toilet seat.
        Seats with a spring return to the up position are not
        permitted.

Toilet Paper: Not less than 19 inches from floor level.

Signage

The purpose of signs is to provide

LO-4

1. Information concerning room numbers
2. Names of occupants or activities in specific areas or offices
3. Instructions for specific locations
4. Instructions for the location and path of accessible routes

 In general, signage must be in upper case, sans serif, or simple serif type. Type must be accompanied by Grade 2 Braille. Pictograms must be accompanied with appropriate type and braille signage.

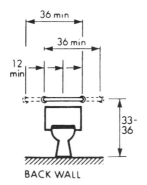

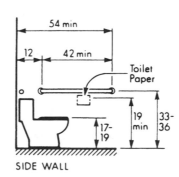

Figure 10.4–16. Dimensions for water closet grab bars, toilet paper, and seats.

This is an example of sans serif type.
    UPPER CASE
    lower case
This is an example of simply serif type.
    UPPER CASE
    lower case

Contrast:	Not less than 1/32 inch raised contrast for both type and braille.
	Nonglare finishes must be used for background and characters.
Location Walls:	At 60 inches above floor level.
	On wall adjacent to latch edge of door for identification of rooms.
	Access to within 3 inches of signate without obstruction or protruding objects.
Suspended:	Not less than 80 inches above floor level.
Size:	Ratio measurements are taken using an upper case "X."
	Between 3:5 and 1:1 width to height ratio.
	Between 1:5 and 1:10 stroke width to height ratio.
	Character heights sized with respect to viewing distance. Lower case letters must meet the requirement for character height chosen.
	Not less than 3 inches in height (lower case letters) for a suspended sign.
	Not less than 6 inches in height for a pictogram.

Stairs

LO-4

Handrails:	Must be provided along both sides of the stairway.
	Must meet the general requirements listed under "Handrails."
Moisture:	Outdoor stairs and paths must be designed to avoid accumulation of moisture.
Nosing:	Must project not more than 1 1/2 inches.
	Not greater than 1/2 inch radius of curvature for the front edge.
	Must not have an abrupt or sharp underside.
	An underside must be angled not less than 60 degrees from the horizontal unless risers are sloped forward.
Riser Height:	Must be uniform on any given set of stairs.
	Open risers are not permitted.
Tread Depth:	Not less than 11 inches, measured from riser to riser.
	Must be uniform on any given set of stairs.

Telephones

LO-4

Clear Area:	Not less than 30 inches by 48 inches for a forward or parallel approach.
	Wall mounted telephones or pole mounted telephones must comply with the requirements listed under "Accessible Route—Protrusions."

Cord: Not less than 29 inches in length.
Longer length required if handset must reach an acoustic coupler or other required text equipment.

Electrical: An electrical outlet and a fixed shelf must be available for telephones designed to accommodate portable text equipment.

Height: Not greater than 48 inches for forward reach only to top of controls.
Not greater than 54 inches for side reach to top of controls.
Not less than 15 inches above floor level to bottom of controls.

Transportation Facilities

Many areas and components within transportation facilities appear elsewhere on this list, such as "Restrooms, Telephones," etc., and must meet all individually listed criteria. Criteria specific to transportation facilities are listed below.

LO-4

Clear Area: Must be on an accessible route.
Not less than 96 inches in length parallel to path of bus travel.
Not less than 60 inches in width from curb.
May be limited by site constraints.

Fare Gates: Must be on an accessible route.
Automatic fare gates may not prohibit accessible entry to a transit system.
Not less than one accessible fare gate must be available.
Not less than 32 inches in width clear opening at fare collection devices.
Smooth and continuous surfaces between 2 inches and 27 inches above floor level.

Fare Vending: Reach limits must meet the requirements listed under "Reach."

Grade: Parallel to roadway must be as close to grade of roadway as possible.
Not greater than 1:50 (2%) perpendicular to roadway.

Loading Gaps: No less than one door per vehicle or car must meet these requirements.
Gap is measured from edge of platform surface to edge of transportation vehicle or car floor.
Existing Stations
    No greater than $1\,^1/_2$ inches vertical gap.
    No greater than 3 inches horizontal gap.
New Stations
    No greater than 5/8 inch vertical gap.
    No greater than 3 inches horizontal gap.
    No greater than 1 inch horizontal gap for low speed automated "people mover" systems.

Location: To greatest extent possible, routes should follow path comparable to path used by the general public.

	Distances along accessible route must be minimized to the greatest extent possible.
Platform Edges:	Must be protected by screens or guard rails.
	When not protected by screens or guard rails, detectable warnings must be in place.
Shelters:	Must be on an accessible route.
	Not less than 30 inches by 48 inches clear area entirely within shelter.
Signage:	Must comply with requirements listed under "Signage."
	Signs that are the maximum size permitted by local ordinance are deemed to have met signage requirements.
	Not less than one sign per stop must meet the requirements of "Signage," and list the station.
	Lists of stations, route, and destinations served by the route must meet the requirements of "Signage."
	Schedules, time tables, or maps posted at bus stops need not meet signage requirements.

10.5 REVIEW QUESTIONS

1. What is the purpose of the Americans With Disabilities Act (ADA)?

2. What are the effective dates of the ADA?

3. List general considerations and specific requirements of the ADA.

4. How does the ADA improve accessibility of facilities for people with physical impairments?

10.6 SUGGESTED ACTIVITIES

1. Assign students specific areas to be assessed for accessibility. Suggested areas are classrooms, restrooms, library, building entry, cafeteria, dormatory rooms, and access to floors other than the ground floor.

2. Students evaluate assigned areas playing the role of the therapist or patient. Suggested modes of ambulation when role-playing as patient include using crutches, wheelchair, or a walker.

3. Students spend at least 2 hours in a public area while using an assistive device for ambulation. Students are to consistently and appropriately role-play the need for the assistive device. Students are to observe, and write a report about, the public reaction to their presence, their own reaction to using assistive devices in a public place, and any architectural barriers encountered.

10.7 References

1. United States Congress (101st), Americans With Disabilities Act (PL 101-336), 1990.

Index

AAROM (active assisted range-of-motion), 134
Abduction, 138, 139t
  D1, 153–155
  D2, 156–159
  defined, 136
  fingers, 175
  hip, 143, 153–159
  shoulder, 160, 162
  thumb, 177
Accessibility
  ADA requirements, 468–492. *See also specific item, e.g.* Handrails; Hotels
  general considerations, 468
Accessible route, ADA requirements, 469
Active assisted range-of-motion, 134
Active range-of-motion, 134
ADA. *See* Americans with Disabilities Act
Adduction, 138, 139t
  D1, 153–155
  D2, 156–159
  defined, 136–137
  fingers, 175
  hip, 143–144, 153–159
  shoulder, 160, 163
  thumb, 177
Afebrile, 46
Airborne transmission, of infection, 95
Alarms, 470
Ambulation with assistive devices. *See* Assistive devices; *specific device*
Americans with Disabilities Act, 466–492
  accessibility requirements, 468–492. *See also specific item*
  general considerations, 468
  implementation schedule, 466t
  passage and purpose, 466–467
  resources for, 467–468
Amputee frame wheelchairs, 216

Anatomical planes of motion. *See also* Passive range-of-motion exercises
  defined, 136–137
  head, neck, and trunk, 187–189
  lower extremity, 140–152
  upper extremity, 160–178
Ankle exercises, 139t, 148–150, 153–159
Antimicrobial-containing products, 58
Antitipping devices, wheelchair, 206
Apparel, aseptic techniques for, 55–56
Armrests, wheelchair, 200
  fitting, for patient, 219
  and sitting
    with quad cane, 408–409
    with standard cane, 414–415, 418–419
    with two canes, 438–439, 443
    with walker, 318–319, 322–323
  and standing
    with quad cane, 406–407
    with standard cane, 412–413, 416–417
    with two canes, 437
    with walker, 320–322
AROM (active range-of-motion), 134
Aseptic techniques, 50–112. *See also specific technique*
  for apparel, 55–56
  for cleansing and sterilizing, 84–89, 86t–87t
  definitions, 50–52
  for gloving, 66–75
  for gowning, 65
  for handwashing, 56–58
  for housekeeping, 92–93
  isolation, 93–112
  for laundry, 91–92
  for rinsing, 63–64
  for scrubbing, 59–64
  sterile field guidelines, 52–55
  universal precautions, 52
  for waste disposal, 89–90
  for wound dressings, 76–83

Assembly areas, 470
Assessment, SOAP notation, 5–6
Assistance, levels and types of, 226
Assisted standing pivot transfer, 257–258
  guarding in, 258–261
  from treatment table to wheelchair, 264–266
  from wheelchair to treatment table, 262–263
Assisted transfers, 226
  sliding board, 248–249
  standing pivot, 257–266
  two-person lift, 242–245
Assistive devices, 288–464
  ambulation techniques with. *See also specific device*
    cane(s), 297, 404–461
    choosing gait patterns for, 298–300
    crutches. *See* Axillary crutches; Forearm crutches
    curbs and, 20–23, 309
    doorways and. *See* Doorways
    fatigue and, 288
    parallel bars, 288
    patient concentration and, 288–289
    on stairs. *See specific assistive device*
    tilt table and, 310–312
    walkers, 292–295, 313–343
    weight bearing and, 289
  selection, 290–297
  sitting with. *See* Sitting position, assuming
  standing with. *See* Standing position, assuming
  wheelchairs, 194–222
Audit, of medical records, 8
Auditorium areas, ADA requirements, 470
Axillary crutches, 296, 344–373
  ambulation techniques with
    ascending stairs, 364–365, 366–367
    descending stairs, 368–369

Axillary crutches (*cont.*)
  ambulation techniques withdoorways
      and (*cont.*)
    four-point gait, 358–359
    three-point gait, 354–357
    two-point gait, 360
  assuming sitting position with, 348–349,
      352–353
  assuming standing position with,
      345–347, 350–351
  falling with, 361–363
  fitting patient for, 345
Axillary temperature, 45, 46

Backward lift independent transfer,
    272–275
Backward method of stair ambulation,
    400–403
Bacterial barrier, 50
Band-Aid, 78
Barriers
  bacterial, 50
  protective, 52
Bathrooms, ADA requirements, 484–489
Biceps femoris, exercise for, 141
Blood and Body Fluid Precautions, 52,
    107–108
Blood pressure
  age and, 42t
  defined, 39
  hypertension/hypotension levels, 42, 42t
  measurement, 39–41
  norms, 41–42
Bodies, postmortem handling, 101
Body fluid precautions, 52, 107–108
Body mechanics, 13–14
Brachial pulse, 37
Bradycardia, 39
Brakes, wheelchair, 195–197
Bridging the gap, 117
Building Officials & Code Administrators
    International, Inc., 467
Burn patients, isolation precautions, 111–112
Business areas, ADA requirements, 470–471

Cafeterias, 483
Cane(s), 297, 404–461
  assuming sitting position with
    quad cane, 408–409, 411
    standard cane, 414–415, 418–419
    two canes, 438–439, 442–443
  assuming standing position with
    quad cane, 406–407, 410
    standard cane, 412–413, 416–417
    two canes, 437, 440–441
  doorways, ambulation through, 432–436
    460–461
  fitting patient for, 404–405
  moving in and out of wheelchair with
    standard cane, 412–419
    two canes, 437–443

  single cane ambulation, 432–436
  stair ambulation with, 422–423
    ascending, 424–425, 428–429, 450–451,
        454–455, 458
    descending, 426–427, 430–431, 451–453,
        456–457, 459
    four-point-gait pattern, 454–457
    standard cane, 422–431
    three-point-gait pattern, 450–453
    two canes, 449–459
    two-point-gait pattern, 458–459
  standard cane ambulation, 420–421
  two cane ambulation, 437–461
    doorways and, 460–461
    four-point gait pattern, 446–447
    three-point gait pattern, 444–445
    two-point gait pattern, 448
Carotid pulse, 36
Cart
  transfer to/from
    sliding method, 228–229
    three-person carry, 230–232
  transportation via, 18–19
Case manager, 4
Caster wheels, 198
"Category-Specific" isolation precautions,
    101–108
  for blood and body fluids, 107–108
  contact isolation, 103–104
  for drainage and secretion, 106–107
  for enteric diseases, 105–106
  respiratory isolation, 104–105
  strict isolation, 102–103
  tuberculosis isolation, 105
CDC (Center for Disease Control and
    Prevention)
  address for, 50
  recommendations
    for cleansing and sterilization, 88–89
    for handwashing, 57–58
    for housekeeping, 92–93
    for laundry, 91–92
    ranking scheme, 51
    for waste disposal, 90
Center for Infectious Diseases
  address for, 50
  recommendations ranking scheme, 51
Chemicals, sterilization with, 84–89, 86t–
    87t
CID. *See* Center for Infectious Diseases
Cleaning, isolation precautions, 100–101
Cleanliness, levels of, 51
Cleansing
  CDC recommendations, 86–89, 86t–87t,
      88–89
  general considerations for, 84–86
Clear space areas, ADA requirements, 471
Clothing, isolation precautions, 98
Compression wraps, 83
Contact isolation, 103–104
Contact transmission, of infection, 94–95
Contaminated, defined, 51
Contaminated gloves, removal, 74–75
Control mechanisms, ADA requirements,
    471

Coronal plane, 136
Council of American Building Officials, 467
Crutches
  axillary. *See* Axillary crutches
  forearm (Lofstrand). *See* Forearm
      crutches
Curb ramps, ADA requirements, 471
Curbs, 309
  ascending via wheelchair
    backward method, 22
    forward method, 23
  descending via wheelchair
    backward method, 20
    forward method, 21
  ramps, ADA requirements, 471

Database, 3
Department of Health and Human
    Services, 50
Department of Justice, 466–467
Dependent transfers, 226
  one-person, 267–270
  standing pivot, 246–247
Depression, of scapula, 139t, 160
Deviation, of wrist, 170
Diagonal patterns of motion, PNF. *See also*
    Passive range-of-motion exercises
  defined, 138–139, 138f, 139t
  lower extremity, 153–159
  upper extremity, 179–186
Diastolic pressure, 40
Discharge note, 3
Diseases
  requiring isolation precautions, 103–107.
      See also Isolation precautions
    in burn patients, 111–112
    in infants and newborns, 109–111
    in intensive care, 109
    in severely compromised patients, 111
  transmission, prevention of, 50
Dishes, isolation precautions, 98
Disinfection
  gloves and, 85
  for microorganisms, 86, 86t–87t
Disposal
  of needles, 98
  of personal articles, 97, 99
  of waste, 89–90
Documentation. *See* Medical Records
Doors, ADA requirements, 471–475
Doorways
  accessibility requirements, 471–475
  ambulation through, 309
    with axillary crutches, 370–373
    with cane(s), 432–436, 460–461
    with walker, 340–343
    with wheelchair, 24–27
Dorsal pedal pulse, 38
Dorsiflexion, 139t
  ankle, 149–150, 153–159
    D1, 153–155
    D2, 156–159
  gastrocnemius, 150

Downward rotation, of scapula, 139t, 182, 186
Drainage precautions, 106–107
Draping, 15–16
Dressings. *See* Wound dressings
Drinking fountains, ADA requirements, 475–476
Drinking water, isolation precautions, 99
Drive wheels, 199
Dry heat sterilization, 84
Dry-to-dry dressing, 77

EEOC (Equal Employment Opportunity Commission), 466–467
Elbow exercises, 139t, 166–167, 179–181, 183–185
Elevating legrests, wheelchair, 204–205
Elevation, of shoulder, 160
Elevators
    accessibility requirements, 476–477
    wheelchair entry and exit, 30
End feel, 134
Enteric precautions, 105–106
Environment, management of, 12–13
Equal Employment Opportunity Commission, 466–467
Ethylene oxide gas sterilization, 84
Eversion, 139t
    ankle, 153, 155–159
    D1, 153, 155
    D2, 156–159
    defined, 137
    foot, 151
Exercises, ROM. *See* Range-of-motion exercises
Expiration date, 52
Extension, 138, 139t
    ankle, 153–159
    biceps femoris, 141
    D1, 153–155
    D2, 156–159
    defined, 136
    elbow, 167
    extensor digiti minimi, 172
    extensor digitorum, 172
    extensor indicis, 172
    fingers, 171, 174
    flexor digitorum profundus, 172
    flexor digitorum superficialis, 172
    head, 187
    hip, 140–142, 144, 153–159
    knee, 153–159
    neck, 187
    palmaris longus, 172
    PNF diagonals, 139t
    semimembranosus, 141
    semitendinosus, 141
    shoulder, 161
    thumb, 178
    toes, 152
    wrist, 169
Extensor digiti minimi, 172
Extensor digitorum, 172

Extensor indicis, 172
External rotation, 138, 139t
    D1, 153–155
    D2, 156–159
    defined, 137
    hip, 145, 153–159
    shoulder, 165
Eye protection, 55–56

Falling
    with axillary crutches, 361–363
    with forearm crutches, 390–395
Fatigue, during gait training, 288
Febrile, 46
Feces, isolation precautions, 99
Femoral pulse, 37
Figure-of-eight wrap, 80
Fingers. *See also* Thumb exercises
    nail cleaning, 60–61
    PROM exercises, 139t, 171–175, 179–181, 183–185
Flexion, 138, 139t
    ankle, 148–150, 153–159
    biceps femoris, 141
    D1, 153–155
    D2, 156–159
    defined, 136
    elbow, 166, 167
    extensor digiti minimi, 172
    extensor digitorum, 172
    extensor indicis, 172
    fingers, 171, 174
    flexor digitorum profundus, 172
    flexor digitorum superficialis, 172
    head, 187
    hip, 140–141, 153–159
    knee, 146–147, 154–155, 158
    neck, 187
    palmaris longus, 172
    PNF diagonals, 139t
    semimembranosus, 141
    semitendinosus, 141
    shoulder, 161, 166
    thumb, 178
    toes, 152
    wrist, 169
Flexor digitorum profundus, 172
Flexor digitorum superficialis, 172
Floor mat, turning patient on, 126
Floor surfaces
    accessibility requirements for, 478
    falling and getting up from, with forearm crutches, 390–395
    transfer to/from via wheelchair
        dependent one-person transfer, 267–270
        independent transfer, 270–283
        two-person lift from wheelchair, 242–245
Folding, of wheelchairs, 207, 210–211
Food services, ADA requirements, 483–484
Foot exercises, 151

Footplates, wheelchair, 201–202, 221
Footrests, wheelchair, 202–203
Forearm
    PROM exercises, 139t, 168, 179–181, 183–185
    scrubbing procedures, 62–64
Forearm crutches, 296, 374–403
    ambulation techniques with, 396
        ascending stairs, 396–397, 400–401
        backward method (stairs), 400–403
        descending stairs, 398–399, 402–403
        forward method (stairs), 396–399
        swing-through gait, 388–389
        swing-to gait, 386–387
    assuming sitting position with
        power method, 384–385
        turn around method, 378–381
    assuming standing position with
        power method, 382–383
        turn around method, 375–377
    falling and getting up with, 390–395
    fitting patient for, 374
Forward independent transfers, 270–271, 280–283
Forward method of stair ambulation, 396–399
Fountains (drinking), ADA requirements, 475–476
Four-point gait pattern, 299
    with axillary crutches, 358–359
    with canes
        on level surface, 446–447
        on stairs, 454–457
Frame wheelchair, amputee, 216
Front rigging, wheelchair, 201–205
Frontal plane, 136

Gait patterns
    choosing. *See also specific gait pattern*
        four-point, 299
        swing-through, 300
        swing-to, 299–300
        three-point, 299
        two-point, 298
    weight bearing in, 298
Gait training, with assistive devices. *See also* Assistive devices
    considerations in, 288–290
    gait belt for, 301
    guarding in, 14, 301–305
Gas sterilization, 84
Gastrocnemius, exercise for, 150
Gauze dressing and wrap, 78–79
Gloves
    contaminated, removal, 74–75
    donning. *See* Gloving
    infection/disinfection and, 85
    purpose, 56
Gloving, aseptic techniques, 66–75
    with clean gown, 70–73
    with sterile gown, 66–69
Goals of treatment, 5–6
Gowning, 65

Gowns
  clean, gloving with, 70–73
  donning, aseptic technique, 65
  purpose and use, 56
  sterile, gloving with, 66–69
Grab bars, ADA requirements, 477
Ground surfaces, ADA requirements, 478
Guarding
  in gait training, 14, 301–305
  in transfers, 258–261

Hand(s)
  gloving. See Gloving
  placement, in PROM exercises. See
    also Passive range-of-motion
    exercises
    for head, neck, and trunk, 187–189
    for lower extremities, 140–159
    for upper extremities, 160–186
  scrubbing, 59–64
  washing, 56–75
Hand scrubbing, 59–64
Handrails
  accessibility requirements, 478–479
  use
    with axillary crutches, 364–369
    with single cane, 422, 424–431
Handwashing, 56–58
Head, exercises for, 187
Health and Human Services, 50
Heart rate, 34–39
  bradycardia, 39
  maximal, 39
  measurement. See Pulse
  norms, 39
  tachycardia, 39
  target, 39
Hip exercises, 139t, 140–145, 147, 153–159,
  189
Horizontal adduction, of shoulder, 163
Hotels, ADA requirements, 479–480
Housekeeping, 92–93
Hydraulic lift
  components and function, 233–235
  transfer via, 236–241
Hydrotherapy equipment, sterilization,
  85–86
Hypertension, 42, 42t
Hyperthermia, 46
Hypotension, 42, 42t
Hypothermia, 46

Immersion pools/tanks, sterilization, 85–
  86
Independent transfers, 270–283
  backward lift, 272–275
  forward lowering, 270–271
  forward to floor, 280–283
  with step stool, 274–275
  turn around methods, 276–279
Infants, isolation precautions, 109–111

Infection
  isolation precautions, 93–95. See also
    Isolation precautions
  nosocomial, 51, 56
  transmission, 50, 94–96
Initial note, 3
Instructions, giving to patient, 14–15
Intensive care, isolation precautions, 109
Interim note, 2
Internal rotation, 138, 139t
  D1, 153–155
  D2, 156–159
  defined, 137
  hip, 145, 153–159
  shoulder, 164
Inversion, 139t
  ankle, 153–159
  D1, 153, 155
  D2, 156–159
  defined, 137
  foot, 151
Involuntary muscle contractions, 134–135
Isolation precautions, 93–112
  blood and body fluids, 52
  for blood and body fluids, 107–108
  for burn patients, 111–112
  "Category-Specific," 101–108
  cleaning and, 100–101
  contact isolation, 103–104
  "Disease-Specific," 101, 108–112
  disposal procedures, 97
  drainage and secretion, 106–107
  enteric, 105–106
  for equipment, materials, and substances,
    97–99
  general considerations, 93–95
  for infants and newborns, 109–111
  in intensive care, 109
  methods, 95–96
  in patient transport, 100
  for postmortem handling of bodies,
    101
  private room and, 96
  respiratory isolation, 104–105
  roommates and, 96–97
  for severely compromised patients,
    111
  strict isolation, 102–103
  tuberculosis isolation, 105
  visitors and, 99–100

Joint range-of-motion. See also specific
    joint
  defined, 134
  methods and purpose, 134–135

Knee
  in forward independent transfers,
    280–283
  PROM exercises for, 139t, 140–141,
    146–147, 153–159

Laboratory specimens, isolation
    precautions, 99
Lateral rotation. See External rotation
Laundry, 91–92
Levels of assistance, 226
Libraries, ADA requirements, 480
Lift, hydraulic. See Hydraulic lift
Linen, isolation precautions, 98
Liquid chemicals, sterilization with, 84–89,
    86t–87t
Lofstrand crutches. See Forearm crutches
Long sitting position, 129
Long-term goals, 5–6
Lower extremity PROM exercises, 140–
  159
LTG (long-term goals), 5–6

Masks, 55
Maximal heart rate, 39
Medial rotation. See Internal rotation
Medical equipment, sterilization, 84–89,
    86t–87t
Medical facilities, ADA requirements, 481
Medical records, 2–8
  audit of, 8
  formats, 2–3
  narrative notes, 4
  patient's chart, isolation precautions, 99
  POMR, 2–3
  problem list, 3
  procedure for, 3–4
  purpose, 2
  requirements, 7
  SOAP notes, 4–7
  source oriented method, 2
Mercantile areas, ADA requirements,
    470–471
Microorganisms, pathogenic
  disinfection levels for, 86, 86t–87t
  resistance to, 95. See also Isolation
    precautions
  transmission, 94–96
Midsagittal plane, 136
Motion
  anatomical planes of. See Anatomical
    planes of motion
  diagonal patterns of. See Diagonal
    patterns of motion, PNF
  PROM exercises. See Passive range-of-
    motion exercises
  ROM exercises, 134–135
Muscle range-of-motion, 134–135
Muscles
  biceps femoris, 141
  flexor digitorum profundus, 172
  flexor digitorum superficialis, 172
  gastrocnemius, 150
  involuntary contractions, 134–135
  palmaris longus, 172
  range-of-motion, 134–135
  rectus femoris, 147
  semimembranosus, 141
  semitendinosus, 141

tensor fascia latae, 144
triceps brachii, 166

Nail cleaning, 60–61
Narrative format, of medical records, 4
Neck exercises, 187–188
Needles, disposal and isolation, 89, 98
Newborns, isolation precautions, 109–111
Non-weight bearing gait
  with axillary crutches, 356–357
  with walkers, 298
Nonsterile, 52
Nosocomial infection
  defined, 51
  handwashing and, 56
Note formats
  narrative, 4
  SOAP, 4–7

Objective data, SOAP notation, 5
Occlusive dressing, 77
One-arm drive wheelchairs, 212–215
Opposition, of thumb, 137, 139t, 176
Oral temperature, 45

Palmaris longus, 172
Parallel bars, 288
Parking spaces, ADA requirements,
  481–482
Passive range-of-motion exercises, 140–189
  anatomical planes of motion, 136–137
  ankle, 148–150, 153–159, 155–159
  biceps femoris, 141
  diagonal patterns of motion, 138–139,
    139t
    D1, 153–155, 179–182
    D2, 156–159, 183–186
  elbow, 167
  fingers, 171, 172–173, 174, 175
  foot, 151, 153, 155–159
  forearm, 168
  gastrocnemius, 150
  head, 187
  hip, 140–142, 143–144, 144, 145, 153–159,
    189
  knee, 146, 153–159
  neck, 187–188
  rectus femoris, 147
  semimembranosus, 141
  semitendinosus, 141
  shoulder, 161–166
  tensor fascia latae, 144
  thumb, 176, 177, 178
  toes, 152
  trunk, 189
  wrist, 169, 170
Patency, 34
Pathogenic microorganisms. See
  Microorganisms, pathogenic

Patient care equipment categories, 51
Patient care skills. See also specific skill
  ambulation with assistive devices,
    288–461
  aseptic techniques, 50–112
  body mechanics, use of, 13–14
  communication, 14–15
  documentation, 2–8
  environment, management of, 12–13
  patient preparation, 15–16
  range-of-motion exercise, 134–189
  transfers, 226–283
  transporting, 16–30
  turning and positioning, 116–131
  vital signs, measurement, 34–46
  wheelchairs, knowledge about, 194–222.
    See also Wheelchair(s)
Patient concentration, 288–289
Patient's chart, 99
Pedal pulse, 38
Pelvic slide, 254
Personal articles, disposal, 97, 99
Plan, SOAP notation, 4
Plantar flexion, 139t
  ankle, 148, 153–159
  D1, 153–155
  D2, 156–159
Platform lifts, ADA requirements, 482
PNF (proprioceptive neuromuscular
  facilitation approach), 135. See also
  Diagonal patterns of motion, PNF;
  Passive range-of-motion exercises
POMR (problem oriented medical record
  method), 2–3
Popliteal pulse, 38
Positioning, 116–131. See also Turning and
  positioning
Postmortem handling of bodies, 101
Precautions
  isolation, 93–112. See also Isolation
    precautions
  for PROM exercises
    ankle, 148–150, 153–159
    biceps femoris, 141
    D2, 157, 183
    elbow, 167
    fingers, 173, 183
    foot, 151, 153, 155–159
    forearm, 168, 183
    gastrocnemius, 150
    head, 187
    hip, 140–145, 153–159, 189
    knee, 153–159
    neck, 187–188
    rectus femoris, 147
    semimembranosus, 141
    semitendinosus, 141
    shoulder, 161–162, 164–165, 183–185
    tensor fascia latae, 144
    thumb, 183
    toes, 152
    trunk, 189
    wrist, 170, 183
Private room, isolation precautions and,
  96

Problem list, 3
Problem oriented medical record method,
  2–3
Progress note, 2
PROM exercises. See Passive range-of-
  motion exercises
Pronation, 139t
  defined, 137
  of forearm, 168
Prone position
  defined, 122
  PROM exercises from
    hip, 142, 147
    knee, 147
  turning from supine position to, 118–121
  turning to supine position from, 123–125
Proprioceptive neuromuscular facilitation
  approach, 135. See also Diagonal
  patterns of motion, PNF; Passive
  range-of-motion exercises
Protective barrier, 52
Protraction
  defined, 137
  of shoulder, 160
Pulse
  defined, 34
  measurement, 34–38
  norms, 39
Push-up transfer techniques, 250–251, 255
Push wheels, 199

Quad cane
  fitting patient for, 405
  getting in and out of wheelchairs with,
    406–411

Radial deviation, of wrist, 170
Radial pulse, 36
Ramps, ADA requirements
  curb ramps, 471
  in general, 482–483
Range-of-motion exercises
  anatomical planes of motion, 136–137
  diagonal patterns of motion, 138–139,
    139t
  passive. See Passive range-of-motion
    exercises
  types and methods, 134–135
Reach heights, ADA requirements, 482–483
Reciprocal walker, 295
Reclining-back wheelchairs, 209–211
Recommendations ranking scheme, 51
Rectal temperature, 45, 46
Rectus femoris, exercise for, 147
Respiration
  measurement, 42–44
  norms, 44
Respiratory cycle, 42
Respiratory isolation, 104–105
Restaurants, ADA requirements, 483
Restrooms, ADA requirements, 484–489

Retraction
    defined, 137
    of shoulder, 160
Reusable equipment, isolation and, 97
Reverse walker, 295
Rigid dressings, 77
Rigidity, muscular, 135
Ring walker, 295
Rinsing, following scrubbing, 63–64
ROM exercises. See Range-of-motion
        exercises
    passive. See Passive range-of-motion
        exercises
Roommates, isolation precautions, 96–97
Rotation, 138, 139t
    D1, 153–155, 179–182
    D2, 156–159, 183–186
    hip, 145, 153–159, 189
    neck, 188
    scapula, 182, 186
    shoulder, 164, 165
    trunk, 189
    types of, 137

Sagittal plane, 136
Scapula, exercises for, 139t, 182, 186
Scrub suits, 55
Scrubbing, 59–64
Seat belts, wheelchair, 198
Secretion precautions, 106–107
Semimembranosus, exercise for, 141
Semitendinosus, exercise for, 141
Severely compromised patients, isolation
        precautions, 111
Shelf life, sterile products, 51, 52–53
Short-term goals, 5–6
Shoulder exercises, 139t, 160–166, 179–181,
        183–185
Shower stalls, ADA requirements, 486–487
Side-to-side weight shifting, 252–253
Sidelying position
    assuming, from supine position, 127
    assuming sitting position from, 130
    defined, 128
    PROM exercises from
        D1, 182
        D2, 186
        hip, 142, 144
        shoulder, 160, 161
Signage, ADA requirements for, 489–490
Sitting position, assuming, 129
    with cane(s)
        quad cane, 408–409, 411
        standard cane, 414–415, 418–419
        two canes, 437, 440–441
    with crutches
        axillary, 348–349, 352–353
        forearm, 378–381, 384–385
    power method, 384–385
    on side of treatment table, 130–131
    from supine position, 129
    turn around method, 378–381
    with walker, 307–308, 317–319, 322–323

Sitting push-up, 255
Sliding board transfer, 248–249
Sliding transfer, 228–229
SOAP note format, 4–7
Source oriented method, 2
Spasticity, 135
Sphygmomanometer, 40, 98
Spiral wrap, 79
Stair climbing walker, 330–335
Stairs. See also specific gait or assistive device
    accessibility requirements, 490
    ascending and descending, 308
        with axillary crutches, 364–369
        with cane(s), 422–431, 449–459
        with forearm crutches, 396–403
        with four-point gait pattern, 454–457
        with three-point gait pattern, 450–453
        with two-point gait pattern, 458–459
        with walker, 330–339
Standard measurements, wheelchair, 222t
Standing pivot transfer
    assisted, 257–266
    dependent, 246–247
Standing position, assuming
    with cane(s)
        quad cane, 406–407, 410
        standard cane, 412–413, 416–417
        two canes, 437, 440–441
    with crutches
        axillary, 345–347, 350–351
        forearm, 375–377, 382–383
    power method, 382–383
    transfer techniques, 246–247, 257–266
    turn around method, 375–377
    unassisted, 306
    with walker, 314–316, 320–321
Steam sterilization, 84
Step stool, use in transfers, 262–263,
        274–275
Sterile, 51
Sterile drapes, 53
Sterile field
    defined, 51
    guidelines for, 52–55
Sterilization
    CDC recommendations, 86–89, 86t–87t,
        88–89
    general considerations for, 84–86
    types of, 84–85
Stethoscope, 98
STG (short-term goals), 5–6
Straight let raise, 141
Strict isolation, 102–103
Subjective data, SOAP notation, 4–5
Supination
    defined, 137
    of forearm, 168
Supine position, 140, 141
    assuming sitting position from
        long sitting, 129
        to side of treatment table, 131
    defined, 118
    PROM exercises from
        ankle, 148–150
        D1, 153–155, 179–181

D2, 156–159, 183–185
    elbow, 166, 167
    fingers, 171–175
    foot, 151
    forearm, 168
    head, 187
    hip, 140–141, 143, 145
    knee, 146
    lower trunk, 189
    neck, 187–188
    shoulder, 161–166
    thumb, 176–178
    toes, 152
    wrist, 169, 170
    turning
        to prone position from, 118–121
        from prone position to, 123–125
        to sidelying position from, 127
Swing-through gait pattern, 300, 388–389
Swing-to gait pattern, 299–300
    with forearm crutches, 386–387
    with walker, 329
Syringes, disposal and isolation, 89, 98
Systolic pressure, 39–40

Tachycardia, 39
Target heart rate, 39
Telephones, ADA requirements, 490–491
Telfa pads, 78
Temperature
    measurement, 44–46
    norms, 46, 46t
Thermometers
    isolation precautions, 98
    measuring temperature with, 45–46
    types, 44–45
Thompson Publishing Group, ADA
        Compliance Guide, 468
Three-person carry, 230–232
Three-point gait pattern, 299
    with axillary crutches, 354–357
    with two canes
        on level surface, 444–445
        on stairs, 449–453
    with walker, 326–328
Thumb exercises, 139t, 176–181, 183–185
Tilt-in-space wheelchairs, 212
Tilt table, 310–312
Toes
    PROM exercises, 139t, 152
    toe touch weight bearing, 298
Toilet stalls, ADA requirements, 488–489
Transfer belts, 227
Transfers, 226–283
    assisted standing pivot, 257–266
    dependent, 226
        one-person, 267–270
        standing pivot, 246–247
    to/from floor. See Floor surfaces
    to front edge of chair, 252–255
    guarding in, 258–261
    hydraulic lift, 236–241
    independent. See Independent transfers

levels of, 226
pelvic slide, 254
push-up, 250–251
sitting push-up, 255
sliding, 228–229
sliding board, 248–249
three-person carry, 230–232
transfer belts, 227
to treatment table, 256
from treatment table to wheelchair, 262–263
two-person lift, 242–245
types of, 226
using a step stool, 262–263
Transient lodging, ADA requirements, 479–480
Transportation facilities, ADA requirements, 491–492
Transportation of patient, 16–30
via cart, 18–19
isolation precautions, 100
patient preparation for, 15–16
via wheelchair, 20–30
ascending curbs, 22–23
descending curbs, 20–21
doorway navigation, 24–27
elevator usage, 30
wheelies, 28–29
Transverse plane, 136
Treatment, patient preparation for, 15–16
Treatment table
assuming sitting position on, 130–131, 256
transfer to/from, 262–263
assisted standing pivot transfer, 257–266
via hydraulic lift, 236–241
push-up transfer, 250–251
sliding board transfer, 248–249
sliding transfer, 228–229
via three-person carry, 230–232
using a step stool, 262–263
Triceps brachii, 166
Trunk exercise, 189
Tuberculosis (AFB) isolation, 105
Turn around method
with forearm crutches, 375–381
independent transfers, 276–279
Turning and positioning, 116–131
assuming sitting position, 129–131
floor mat turning, 126
general procedures, 117
positioning goals, 116
positions, defined
prone, 122
sidelying, 128
supine, 118
prone to supine turning, 123–125
supine to prone turning, 118–121
supine to sidelying turning, 127
Two-person lift, 242–245
Two-point gait pattern, 298
with axillary crutches, 360

with two canes
on level surface, 448
on stairs, 458–459
Types of assistance, 226

Ulnar deviation, of wrist, 139t, 170
United States
CDC. See CDC (Center for Disease Control and Prevention)
CID. See Center for Infectious Diseases
Department of Health and Human Services, 50
Department of Justice, 466–467
Universal precautions, 52
Unsterile, 52
Upper extremity PROM exercises, 160–186
Urinals, ADA requirements, 488–489
Urine, isolation precautions, 99

Vectorborne transmission, of infection, 95
Vehicle route of transmission, of infection, 95
Verbal commands, 14–15
Visitors, isolation precautions and, 99–100
Vital signs, 34–46. See also Pulse; specific sign
blood pressure, 39–42
heart rate, 34–39
respiration, 42–44
temperature, 44–46

Walkers, 292–295, 313–343
ambulation techniques, 324–325
ascending stairs, 330–333, 336–337
descending stairs, 334–335, 338–339
swing-to gait, 329
three-point gait, 326–328
through doorways, 340–343
weight bearing and, 298, 326–327
assuming sitting position with, 307–308, 317–319, 322–324
assuming standing position with, 314–316, 320–321
fitting patient for, 313
specialized, 294–295
Waste disposal, 89–90
Water for drinking, isolation precautions, 99
Weight bearing
axillary crutches and, 354–357
defined, 298
degrees of, 298
instructional techniques, 289
walkers and, 298, 326–327
Weight shifting, as transfer technique, 252–253

Wet-to-dry dressing, 77
Wet-to-wet dressing, 77
Wheelchair(s), 194–222
assist to front edge of, 252–255
components
antitipping devices, 206
armrests, 200
brakes, 195–197
footplates, 201–202, 221
footrests, 202–203
front rigging, 201–205
legrests, 204–205
seat belts, 198
wheels, 198–199
folding of, 207, 210–211
getting into and/or out of. See also Transfers; specific assistive device
with cane(s), 406–419, 437–443
with crutches, 345–353, 375–385
power method, 382–385
sitting, 306, 307–308
standing, 306
turn around method, 375–381
with walker, 307–308, 314–323
measurement, for patient, 217–221
armrest height, 219
back height, 218
seat depth, 217, 222t
seat height, 222t
seat-to-footplate length, 219–220
seat width, 218, 222t
propulsion
on and off elevators, 30
one-arm, 212–215
over curbs, 20–23
through doorways, 24–27
via wheelies, 28–29
specialized types of, 208–216
amputee frame, 216
one-arm drive, 212–215
reclining-back, 197, 209–211
tilt-in-space, 212
standard measurements for, 222t
Wheelchair wheelies, 28–29
Wheeled walker, 294
Wheels, wheelchair
caster, 198
drive (push), 199
Work area, management of, 12–13
Wound dressings, 76–83
application
compression wraps, 83
figure-of-eight wrap, 80–83
gauze wrap, 79
materials, 78
methods, 77–78
spiral wrap, 79
isolation precautions, 99–100
preparation for, 77
purpose, 76
wound evaluation and, 76–77
Wrist exercises, 139t, 169–170, 179–181, 183–185